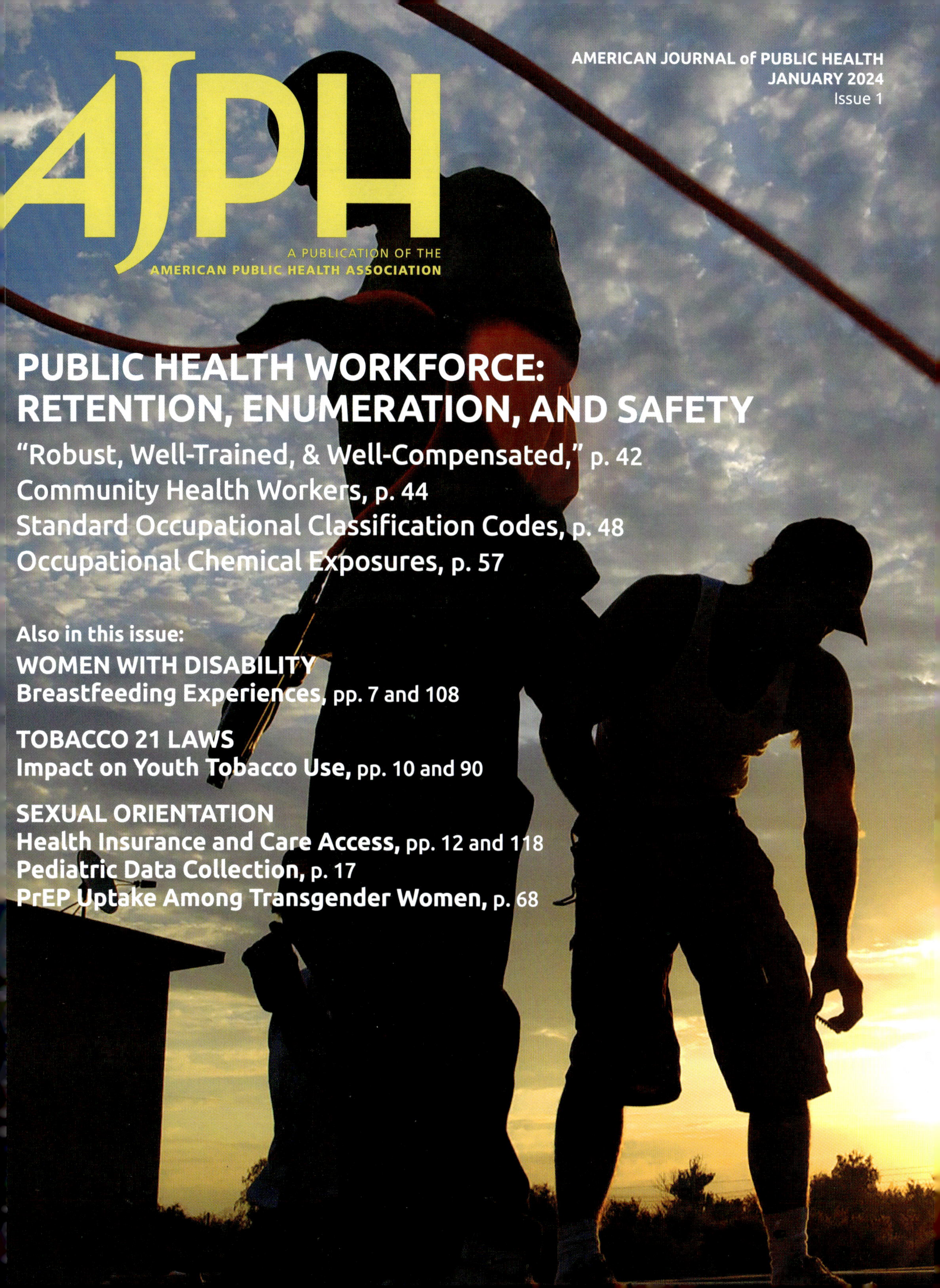

AJPH

A PUBLICATION OF THE
AMERICAN PUBLIC HEALTH ASSOCIATION

AMERICAN JOURNAL of PUBLIC HEALTH
JANUARY 2024
Issue 1

PUBLIC HEALTH WORKFORCE: RETENTION, ENUMERATION, AND SAFETY

"Robust, Well-Trained, & Well-Compensated," p. 42
Community Health Workers, p. 44
Standard Occupational Classification Codes, p. 48
Occupational Chemical Exposures, p. 57

Also in this issue:

WOMEN WITH DISABILITY
Breastfeeding Experiences, pp. 7 and 108

TOBACCO 21 LAWS
Impact on Youth Tobacco Use, pp. 10 and 90

SEXUAL ORIENTATION
Health Insurance and Care Access, pp. 12 and 118
Pediatric Data Collection, p. 17
PrEP Uptake Among Transgender Women, p. 68

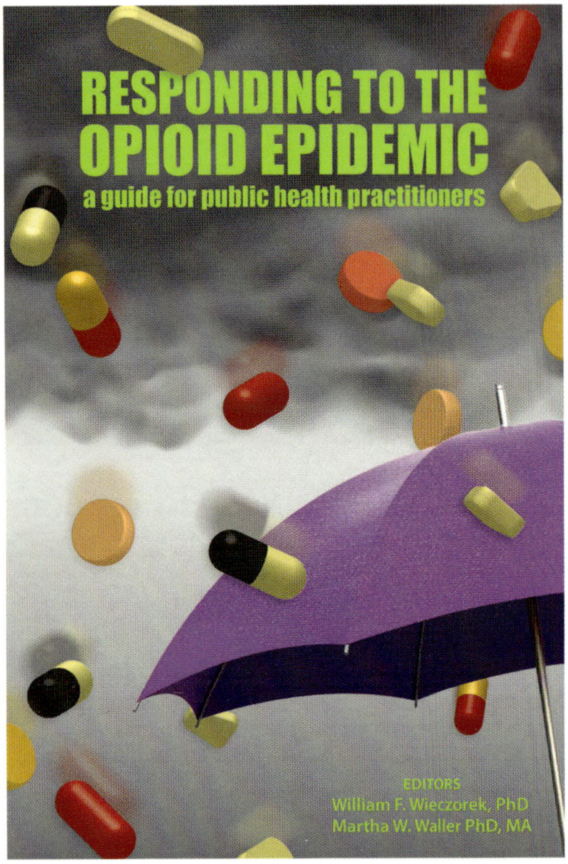

ISBN 978-0-87553-344-5, 400 PP., 2024,
SOFTBOUND/PRINT-ON-DEMAND

Responding to the Opioid Epidemic: A Guide for Public Health Practitioners

Edited by: William F. Wieczorek, PhD and Martha W. Waller PhD, MA

It's impossible to completely prevent the substance misuse defining the opioid epidemic, and it's impossible to treat the problem away. This reality requires a continuum of care (COC) approach, which includes promotion, prevention, case-finding, treatment, and recovery. This book presents research-informed interventions aligned with the COC approach to guide how communities, first responders, lay persons, medical providers, policymakers, treatment providers, and others can respond to the opioid epidemic at an individual, community, state, and national level.

APHABOOKSTORE.ORG

APHA PRESS

AN IMPRINT OF AMERICAN PUBLIC HEALTH ASSOCIATION

APHA
AMERICAN PUBLIC HEALTH ASSOCIATION
For science. For action. For health.

AJPH®, published monthly, is the official Journal of the American Public Health Association®, 800 I St NW, Washington, DC 20001-3710; (202) 777- APHA; TDD (202) 777-2500. APHA is a nongovernmental professional society founded in 1872, representing all disciplines and specialties in public health.

APHA OFFICERS

Ella Greene-Moton
President

Chris Chanyasulkit, PhD, MPH
Immediate Past-President

Deanna Wathington, MD, MMPH, FAAFP
President-Elect

Robert K. Ross, MD
Vice President (USA)

Vamini Selvanandan, MD, MPH
Vice President (Canada)

Jarbas Barbosa, MD, PhD
Vice President
(Latin America and the Caribbean)

Benjamin H. Hernandez, MBA
Treasurer

M. Aaron Guest, PhD, MPH
Speaker, Governing Council

Georges C. Benjamin, MD
Executive Director/Secretary

APHA EXECUTIVE BOARD

E. Oscar Alleyne, DrPH, MPH (2024)
Moose Alperin, EdD, MPH (2025)
Georges C. Benjamin, MD
Executive Director/Secretary
Jessica Boyer, MSW, MPH (2027)
Monique Brown, PhD, MPH, FGSA (2027)
Bryan O. Buckley, DrPH, MPH (2025)
Chris Chanyasulkit, PhD, MPH (2024)
Immediate Past-President
Shontelle Dixon, MPH, CHES (2026)
Ella Greene-Moton (2025)
President
M. Aaron Guest, PhD, MPH, MSW (2026)
Speaker, Governing Council
Benjamin H. Hernández, MBA (2025)
Treasurer
Claude A. Jacob, MPH (2026)
Amy Lee, MD, MPH, MBA (2025)
Nandi A. Marshall, DrPH, MPH (2024)
Stephen Modell MD, MS (2026)
Chair, Education Board
Padmini Murthy, MD, MPH, MS (2024)
Chair, Intersectional Council
Shirley Orr, MSH, APRNA (2027)
David Reyes, DNP, MN/MPH, RN (2024)
Gopal Sankaran, MD, DrPH (2026)
Anthony Santella, DrPH, MCHES (2024)
Chair, Action Board
Denise Strehlow, MPH, MSW (2024)
Chair, Council of Affiliates
Kevin Sykes, PhD, MPH (2024)
Chair, Science Board
Veena Thamilselvan (2024)
Chair, Student Assembly
Deanna Wathington, MD, MMPH (2026)
President-Elect

The *American Journal of Public Health*® (*AJPH*) (print ISSN: 0090-0036; electronic ISSN: 1541-0048), first published in 1911, is the official journal of the American Public Health Association® (APHA). The oldest and largest organization of public health professionals in the world, APHA represents approximately 30 000 members from more than 50 occupations of public health.

Submissions: Visit www.editorialmanager.com/ajph or ajph.edmgr.com for online manuscript preparation and submission guidelines. Contributions of original unpublished research, social science analyses, scholarly essays, critical commentaries, departments, and letters to the editor are welcome. Questions? Write ajph.submissions@apha.org or call APHA at (202) 777-2469.

Print plus online subscriptions: Institutional price (print copy with online access for a single institution and all authorized users, regardless of geographic location) varies by size of organization and ranges from $993–$1445 for US organizations, and $1073–$1526 for international organizations (air delivery); multiple campuses not permitted without special arrangement. Details of the tiered pricing system at https://subscriptionoffice.com/pages/apha-landing-page. To order, write apha.subscriptions@apha.org.

Online-only subscriptions: Institutional price for one institution and its authorized users (regardless of geographic location) is $878–$1307. To order, write apha.subscriptions@apha.org. For academic consortia or multisite corporate subscriptions, contact apha.subscriptions@apha.org.

Print-only subscriptions: Institutional price is US $701, $782 international.

Back print issues: A limited number of print issues are for sale. Single copies are US $49, $55 international (air delivery). Shipping included; prepay only. To order, write apha.subscriptions@apha.org.

Reprints: For prices and ordering information on 50 or more reprints, check the Reprints section at www.ajph.org. To order smaller quantities of reprints (rush delivery), use the "Purchase Article" link on the article site itself.

Electronic access: Online articles more than 10 years old are available free for personal use at www.ajph.org. Recent articles are available through pay-per-view: single PDF article for $24, single issue access for 24 hours for $33, or entire site access for 24 hours for $38.

Postal information: Periodicals postage paid at Washington, DC, and additional mailing offices. Postmaster: Send address changes to American Journal of Public Health, 800 I St NW, Washington, DC 20001-3710.

Address changes: Send to AJPH, Membership Department (members) or AJPH Subscriptions (subscribers), APHA, 800 I St NW, Washington, DC 20001-3710. Or write to membership.mail@apha. org (members) or apha.subscriptions@apha.org (subscribers).

Advertising: For pricing and other information, see www.ajph.org. Please write to ashell.alston@apha.org or call (202) 777-2470 for other advertising opportunities. Ask about special exhibit packages and sponsorships. Acceptance of advertising by the *Journal* does not imply endorsement of products.

Copyright: Copyright © 2024 by the American Public Health Association. Opinions expressed by authors of articles summarized, quoted, or published in full in this *Journal* represent only the opinions of the authors and do not necessarily reflect the official policy of the American Public Health Association or the institution with which the author(s) is (are) affiliated, unless so specified.

Any report, article, or paper prepared by employees of the US government as part of their official duties is, under the Copyright Act, a "work of the United States Government" for which copyright protection under Title 17 of the US Code is not available. However, the *Journal* format is copyrighted and pages may not be photocopied, except in limited quantities, or posted online, without permission of APHA. Copying done for other than personal or internal reference use—such as copying for general distribution, for advertising or promotional purposes, for creating new collective works, or for resale—without the expressed permission of APHA is prohibited. Requests for special permission should be sent to permissions@apha.org.

Indexes: Publications that index or abstract articles from AJPH include the following: Ageline, Assia (Applied Social Science Index and Abstracts), Biological Abstracts, Chemical Abstracts, CINAHL, Criminal Justice Abstracts, EMBASE, EMCare, Environmental Abstracts, e-psyche, ERIC, ETOH (Alcohol and Alcohol Problems Science Database), Excerpta Medica, Food Science and Technology, General Science Index, Grateful Med, Hospital Literature Index, Human Resources Abstracts, International Pharmaceutical Abstracts (IPA), Medline, Physical Education Index, Pollution Abstracts, Psychological Abstracts, PsychINFO, Safety Science Abstracts, Sage Family Studies Abstracts, Sage Human Resources Abstracts, Science Citation Index, SCOPUS, SIIC Data Bases, Social Work Research and Abstracts, and Statistical Reference Index (SRI)/LexisNexis.

Medscape Publishers' Circle

AJPH
A PUBLICATION OF THE
AMERICAN PUBLIC HEALTH ASSOCIATION

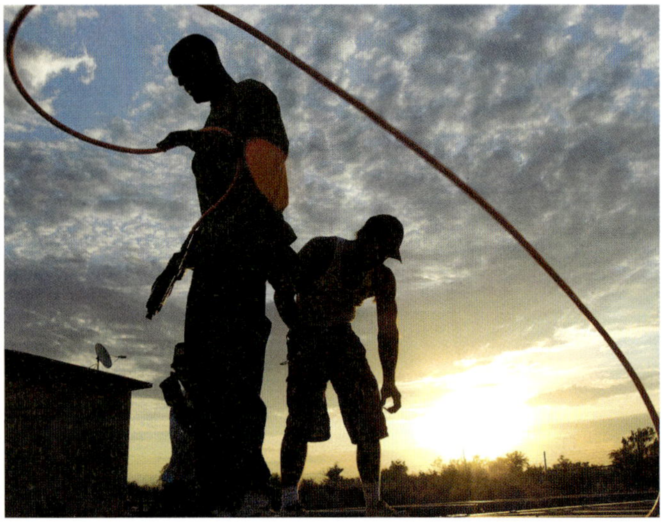

COVER: Construction workers in extreme heat. Roofing construction workers arrive at work before sunrise at 4:30 am to beat the extreme heat by mid-morning, August 8, 2003 in Needles, California.

Cover concept and selection by Aleisha Kropf. Photo by Bob Riha Jr/Getty Images. Printed with permission.

APHA
AMERICAN PUBLIC HEALTH ASSOCIATION
For science. For action. For health.

Promoting public health research, policy, practice, and education is the *AJPH* mission. As we widen our scope to embrace global issues, we also sharpen our focus to support the needs of public health practitioners. We invite contributions of original unpublished research, opinion and commentary, and letters to the editor.

The *Journal* is printed on acid-free recycled paper.

AJPH January 2024, Vol. 114, No. 1

EDITOR-IN-CHIEF
Alfredo Morabia, MD, PhD

SENIOR DEPUTY EDITOR
Michael C. Costanza, PhD

DEPUTY EDITOR
Farzana Kapadia, PhD

DEPUTY STATISTICAL EDITOR
Hua He, PhD

DEPUTY EDITOR FOR OPEN ACCESS SUPPLEMENTS
Steven C. Fiala, MPH

IMAGE EDITOR
Aleisha Kropf

ASSISTANT EDITOR
Keira McCarthy, MA

STUDENT EDITOR
Katherine M. Anderson, MPH

EDITORS
Luisa Borrell, DDS, PhD
Lisa Bowleg, PhD, MA
Theodore M. Brown, PhD
B. Ethan Coston, PhD
Nabarun Dasgupta, PhD, MPH
Paul C. Erwin, MD, DrPH
Laura Ferguson, PhD, MSc, MA
Daniel M. Fox, PhD
Robert J. Kim-Farley, MD, MPH
Stewart J. Landers, JD, MCP
Tanya Telfair LeBlanc, PhD
Jonathan I. Levy, ScD
Jihong Liu, ScD
Evan Mayo-Wilson, DPhil
Vickie Mays, PhD
Marian Moser Jones, PhD, MPH
Bisola Ojikutu, MD, MPH
Wendy Parmet, JD
Kenneth Rochel de Camargo Jr, MD, PhD
Cassia Roth, PhD
Julian Santaella-Tenorio, DVM, DrPH, MSc
Lorna Thorpe, PhD
Roger Vaughan, DrPH, MS
Eric R. Walsh-Buhi, PhD, MPH

EDITORIAL BOARD
Moya L. Alfonso, PhD, MSPH (2024)
Amy Hagopian, PhD, MHA (2024), Chair
Michael T. Halpern, MD, PhD, MPH (2024)
Kenneth Hoekstra, PhD (2024)
Shawn M. Kneipp, PhD, RN, ANP (2024)
Laura A. Nabors, PhD, MA (2024)
Georgios Nikolopoulos, DDS, PhD, MSc (2026)
A.G. Palladino-Davis, MPH, MJ, MS (2026)
Laura Schwab Reese, PhD, MA (2026)
Martha Romney, RN, MS, JD, MPH (2025)
Janet Rosenbaum, PhD (2026)
Gulzar H. Shah, PhD, MStat, MS (2024)
Mark A. Strand, PhD, MS (2026)
Joseph Telfair, DrPH, MSW, MPH (2024)
Cynthia Williams, PhD, MHA, PT (2025), Vice Chair

FORMER EDITORS-IN-CHIEF
Mary E. Northridge, PhD, MPH (Editor Emerita)
Mervyn Susser
Michel Ibrahim
Alfred Yankauer
George Rosen
Abel Wolman
Charles-Edward A. Winslow
Harry S. Mustard
Mazÿck Ravenel

STAFF
Georges C. Benjamin, MD
Executive Director/Publisher
Ashell Alston
Director of Publications
Brian Selzer
Deputy Director of Publications
Michael Henry
Associate Production Editor (Sr)
Avery Ferguson, MA
Associate Production Editor
Shokhari Tate, MPH
Journal Project Liaison
Jane Shealy
Associate Production Editor – Special Publications
Kristin Crocker, MFA
Journal Production Coordinator
Emily Dalton
Digital Publications Specialist

FREELANCE
Kelly Burch
Greg Edmondson
Aisha Jamil
Gary Norton
Michelle Quirk
Sarah Cook
Copyeditor
Aisha Jamil
Sinéad Schenk
Proofreader
Vanessa Sifford
Graphic Designer
Michelle Sarah Livings, MPH
Data Presentation Specialist

OPEN ACCESS | ONLINE ONLY | PODCAST | DATA SUPPLEMENT AVAILABLE

EDITOR'S CHOICE

5 Public Health Should Lead the Charge on Improving Life Expectancy
A. Vasan

OPINIONS, IDEAS, & PRACTICE

EDITORIALS

7 Time to Count the Breastfeeding Experiences of Women With Disabilities in Health Surveillance Efforts
H. K. Brown and Y. Lunsky

10 Moving Beyond Policy Adoption—The Necessity of Understanding the Whys and Hows
A. C. Liber

12 To Reduce Sexual Minority Health Care Disparities, Advocate for Expanded Health Insurance Coverage and LGBTQ+ Rights
A. R. Wootton

15 The Value of Peace: A Public Health of Consequence, January 2024
F. Kapadia

PERSPECTIVES

17 Advancing Pediatric Sexual Orientation and Gender Identity Data Collection
M. Liu, C. Grasso, H.-H. Kim, K. H. Mayer, and A. S. Keuroghlian

21 Living Systematic Reviews and Living Guidelines to Maintain the Currency of Public Health Guidelines
R. K. Hodder, J. P. Vogel, L. Wolfenden, and T. Turner

27 Built Environment and Public Health: More Than 20 Years of Progress
K. A. Rollings, A. L. Dannenberg, H. Frumkin, and R. J. Jackson

NOTES FROM THE FIELD

34 Wastewater-Informed Digital Advertising as a COVID-19 Geotargeted Neighborhood Intervention: Jefferson County, Kentucky, 2021–2022
L. B. Anderson, H. D. Ness, R. H. Holm, and T. Smith

THE PUBLIC HEALTH WORKFORCE

38 Evaluation of the Ontario Mandatory Working-at-Heights Training Requirement in Construction, 2012–2019
L. S. Robson, V. Landsman, P. M. Smith, and C. A. Mustard

42 Public Health Workforce: Retention, Enumeration, and Safety
A. Morabia

RESEARCH & ANALYSIS

THE PUBLIC HEALTH WORKFORCE

44 Retention of Community Health Workers in the Public Health Workforce: Public Health Workforce Interests and Needs Survey, 2017 and 2021
C. Kirkland, J. S. Dill, and H. Karnik

48 Standard Occupational Classification Codes: Gaps in Federal Data on the Public Health Workforce
H. Krasna, M. Venkataraman, M. Robins, I. Patino, and J. P. Leider

57 Characterizing the Burden of Occupational Chemical Exposures by Sociodemographic Groups in the United States, 2021
S. C. Stephan-Recaido, T. K. Peckham, J. Lavoué, and M. G. Baker

PERSPECTIVES FROM THE SOCIAL SCIENCES

68 Preexposure Prophylaxis Uptake Among Spanish-Speaking Transgender Women: A Randomized Controlled Trial in North and South Carolina, 2019–2022
S. D. Rhodes, J. Alonzo, L. Mann-Jackson, L. R. Aviles, A. E. Tanner, C. A. Galindo, P. A. Bessler, C. Courtenay-Quirk, M. Garcia, A. D. Sucaldito, B. D. Smart, T. Goldenberg, and B. A. Reboussin

POLICY

79 Untangling Concepts of Financial Circumstances for Public Health Professionals and Scholars: A Glossary and Concept Map
C. I. J. Nykiforuk, A. P. Belon, and L. KA. Scott

SURVEILLANCE

90 Tobacco 21 Laws and Youth Tobacco Use: The Role of Policy Attributes
A. S. Friedman and M. F. Pesko

98 Cannabis Use Among Adults in Cigarette Smoking Cessation Treatment in Ontario, Canada: Prevalence and Association With Tobacco Cessation Outcome, 2015–2021
S. Voci, S. Veldhuizen, A. Ivanova, O. C. Melamed, P. Selby, and L. Zawertailo

OPEN-THEMED RESEARCH

108 Breastfeeding by Disability Status in the United States: Pregnancy Risk Assessment Monitoring System, 2018–2020
S. Ramer, A. T. Nguyen, J. Nelson, M. K. Whiteman, L. Warner, J. M. Thierry, S. Folger, B. S. von Essen, and K. Kortsmit

118 Health Insurance Coverage and Access to Care by Sexual Orientation During the COVID-19 Pandemic: United States, January 2021–February 2022
K. H. Nguyen, T. W. Levengood, H. L. Allen, and G. Gonzales

BACKMATTER

OTHER DEPARTMENTS

136 Subscription Form

APHA 2024
ANNUAL MEETING & EXPO
Minneapolis | Oct. 27-30

CALL FOR
ABSTRACTS

Rebuilding Trust in Public Health and Science

MAKE YOUR MARK
ON PUBLIC HEALTH!

APHA.org/AnnualMeeting

Opening Date:
Jan. 2, 2024

Submission Deadline:
Mar. 29, 2024

Submit your abstract to
Apha.confex.com/apha/2024/cfp.cgi

Public Health Should Lead the Charge on Improving Life Expectancy

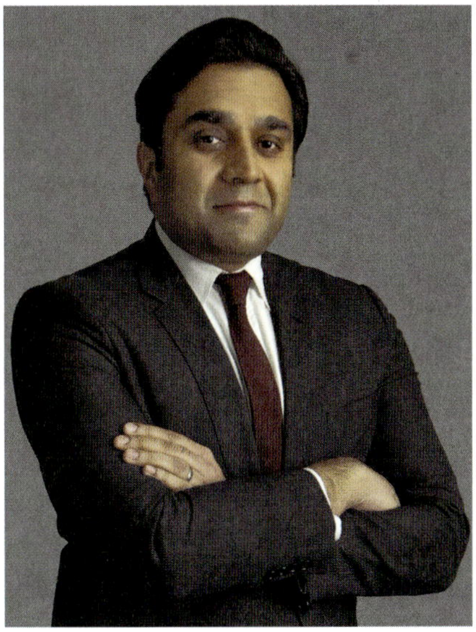

Ashwin Vasan, MD, PhD, Commissioner of the New York City Department of Health and Mental Hygiene

As the health commissioner for New York City, I lead one of the largest public health agencies in the world. Yet, when I talk to New Yorkers, I often find myself explaining the basic functions of public health. "So you're the City's doctor," people ask, "but you aren't seeing patients [I still do, but why argue?]? What exactly do you do?"

It is a fair question. Often, as public health professionals, we struggle to articulate our place in the health ecosystem. We are not providers, nor insurers, nor any of the other health care players that patients interact with on a day-to-day basis and that have come to shape their understanding of health. In New York City, people might associate our department's work with anything from restaurant health code violations, to school health, to subway and television ads that encourage vaccination against COVID-19.

At the same time, people intuitively understand that government should be in charge of and focused on improving the health of people in the place they live. In the same way they expect their tax dollars to pay for trash pickup and firefighters, they expect those dollars to go toward protecting and improving health.

They also intuitively understand we are not getting healthier as a society. They may experience this decline in their own lives and in those of their loved ones, and see it in the communities where they live, work, play, and raise children.

The cold reality is that Americans are suffering more and dying sooner. On average, as a nation, we have lost roughly three years of life span since 2020 (https://on.cfr.org/3QQMtLT). New York City observed a staggering 4.6-year drop in 2020—the steepest decline in the country (https://nyti.ms/467t9yf). COVID-19 is but a partial explanation, as gains in life expectancy began to stagnate well before the pandemic.

While other wealthy, industrialized nations had higher life expectancies to begin with and have recovered much of their losses from 2020 and 2021, the United States has not. As public health is a discipline focused on the health of entire populations across the life course from birth to death and that works across all of the sectors that shape and influence health, reversing this decline should be a defining focus of our profession. In the modern era, there has never been a greater need for the kind of population-wide strategies to extend and improve life, which public health is uniquely equipped to design, oversee, implement, and measure.

Increasing life expectancy will require a coordinated effort across levels of government, as well as the private and nonprofit sectors, and even individual New Yorkers, who are ultimately the key to better health. It will also require us to lead with prevention. In New York City, we have set a bold goal of boosting life expectancy to 83 years by 2030 from its recent nadir of 78.1 years in 2020, while

Continued on page 6...

HISTORY CORNER

96 YEARS AGO

Medico-Legal Aspects of Occupational Disease

[I]t is a common feeling that the industrial hazards to which workmen are exposed are a definite factor in the reduction of their life expectancy, but there are no data that definitely state what this reduction is. Such data as exist, the mortality statistics by occupation, are not necessarily conclusive. They are by industries rather than by occupations and lump together a large number of widely varying employments. Although no statistics are available, it would seem rational and equitable to all concerned to compensate sick and injured workers on the basis of the reduction of their life expectancy. . . . If sufficient data could be gathered and tabulated to form a basis of such an appraisal, they could be used and checked up later by actual experience. . . Dublin estimates the diminished life expectancy of industrial workers as 8 years compared to non-industrial workers.

From *AJPH*, March 1928, p. 278

65 YEARS AGO

Occupational Health and Local Health Department Activities

[E]very local health department should determine how employees could be kept healthy and productive on the job in the extreme adversities and conditions which would result from an enemy attack upon the community. This would be unlikely if not impossible unless an effective occupational health program had already been established. In this era every local health director should be able to say how he would undertake such an employee health program essential to restoring his community as a functional entity, and how he would return and keep workers on jobs essential to maintaining the community and doing community work essential to effective war production. One who has no reasonable assurance along this line should search his conscience now, for he may be a serious menace to his ensuring measurable gains across racial and ethnic groups. We are working toward this ambitious goal through an initiative called HealthyNYC (https://bit.ly/3uMx6M1), which is designed to tackle the leading drivers of this decline, and the leading causes of death, excess death, and premature death head-on. This includes action in areas such as diet-related chronic diseases, overdoses, suicide, violence, and widening inequity in Black maternal mortality.

Beneath each of these primary drivers of life expectancy loss, HealthyNYC defines bundles of strategies, skewing toward prevention, to help achieve our goals while ensuring that no one is left behind. These bundles are organized within three main pillars: (1) leveraging population-wide risk-factor-reduction strategies (e.g., reducing tobacco use and added salt and sugar, calorie labeling); (2) centering equity-focused, place-based approaches to reduce premature mortality, knowing that the majority of people who die before age 65 years in New York City are Black and Latino; and (3) to our understanding, including for the first time in an overall population health strategy, planning around vulnerable communities—defined by age, disability, underlying conditions, or congregate or unstable setting (e.g., unhoused or incarcerated populations)—who comprise significant excess deaths, especially because of COVID-19 and other preventable infections. HealthyNYC is explicit—there is no means to achieving our overall goals without centering equity and marginalized peoples.

HealthyNYC is also clear that there are indirect or cross-cutting drivers that impact mortality, trends like worsening mental health and social isolation; access to community-based, affordable health care; and climate change—to say nothing of social and economic drivers. Other recent New York City blueprints and plans address these other cross-cutting drivers, reinforcing interagency collaboration to ensure that New York City makes progress toward HealthyNYC's quantitative goals for life expectancy.

HealthyNYC is different in theory and in action from many past public health plans. First, it focuses on concrete steps that people can take immediately—like tobacco cessation, better nutrition, increased activity and social connection, and overdose prevention—in addition to policy and institutional strategy, ensuring that everyday people feel seen and a part of this citywide health agenda. It emphasizes individual buy-in, at scale, as a way to promote population-level progress and ensure sustainability of the agenda. Put more plainly, it recognizes the need for simple and clear communication and messaging that individuals can understand and act upon.

Second, HealthyNYC brings into the planning process a broad swath of city agencies that might not think of themselves as related to health. We know that decisions about transportation, housing, economic development, and education factor immensely into how well and how long people can expect to live. HealthyNYC's approach positions the Health Department as New York City's health strategist, with the support of the mayor and City Hall, which pulls together stakeholders to align initiatives, track progress, and work toward coordinated action and investment in health, including a focus on social determinants of health that fall mainly outside of the remit of conventional public health agency structure. We can debate whether life expectancy is the best measure of health, but make no mistake: it is an important measure, and one we can organize and plan around, not just talk or write about.

Finally, HealthyNYC embraces, not avoids, advocacy. Most of us did not get into this line of work to play politics, but the truth is that life expectancy figures are indelibly tied to health, social, and economic policies, which, in turn, are products of underlying political actions (or inactions). Rather than ignore this reality, public health must advocate the policies—including at the state and federal level—that we know will make us healthier, and that means understanding and becoming more adept at navigating the political contours of key health decisions. In addition, we are working with the New York City Council on legislation that would require us to track and update core features of HealthyNYC at regular intervals in local law, ensuring that the long-term work of improving health and healthy longevity, for all people, does not end with one mayor, one administration, or one health commissioner.

Faced with drastic declines in overall health and persistent inequities that concentrate the worst of the damage, we have a choice. And for those of us in public health leadership today, this decline is happening on our watch. So, we can refuse to evolve or battle amongst ourselves as to what is most important, leading to deserved irrelevance. Or we can expand the boundaries of public health and align behind a common agenda that engages all of us and gives the nation and the world an unequivocal answer to the question of what we do: help Americans live longer, healthier lives—perhaps the most important litmus test of progress of our civic project in America. AJPH

DOI: https://doi.org/10.2105/AJPH.2023.307460

HISTORY CORNER

community because their reliance upon him may be unjustified.

From *AJPH*, March 1959, p. 359

38 YEARS AGO

Asbestos Examinations for Construction Workers

[A] model program for construction workers, the Western States Asbestos Health Plan, was initiated in the late 1960s by Drs. Cooper and Tabershaw of the University of California and Asbestos Workers Local 16 in the San Francisco area. It was extended to almost all of the insulation workers' locals in the Western United States by 1970, predating both OSHA and any of OSHA's asbestos standards. . . . Each provider conducts the protocol of tests approved by the trustees of the plan, then sends all of the medical records plus the original chest x-rays to the Plan's medical consultant who evaluates the information, using a uniform set of criteria. The individual participants receive a letter explaining the results of their examination as well as a separate letter describing any work limitations, including the use of respirators, plus a card indicating when the examination occurred. . . . The Plan's medical consultant also provides a perpetual archive for the medical records and chest x-rays. . . . This type of plan could be established in other areas of the country to alleviate the administrative problems raised by some in the construction industry regarding the feasibility of conducting medical examinations for their workers.

From *AJPH*, December 1986, p. 1389

Time to Count the Breastfeeding Experiences of Women With Disabilities in Health Surveillance Efforts

Hilary K. Brown, PhD, and Yona Lunsky, PhD, CPsych

ABOUT THE AUTHORS

Hilary K. Brown is with the Department of Health and Society at the University of Toronto Scarborough, and the Dalla Lana School of Public Health, University of Toronto, Toronto, Ontario, Canada. Yona Lunsky is with the Azrieli Adult Neurodevelopmental Centre at the Centre for Addiction and Mental Health, and the Department of Psychiatry, University of Toronto.

See also Ramer et al., p. 108.

Breastfeeding has established benefits for child and maternal health outcomes.[1] Under the Baby Friendly Hospital Initiative, the World Health Organization and United Nations Children's Fund recommend breastfeeding initiation within 1 hour of birth and exclusive breastfeeding to 6 months postpartum.[2] However, despite global efforts to promote breastfeeding, rates in the United States and elsewhere remain suboptimal.[3] Known risk factors for breastfeeding noninitiation and early cessation include young maternal age, poverty, low social support, smoking, and chronic illness.[4] Yet, few studies have examined breastfeeding in women with disabilities, despite their high rates of many of these risk factors.

NEW DATA ON DISABILITY AND BREASTFEEDING

Ramer et al. (p. 108) used data from the Pregnancy Risk Assessment Monitoring System (PRAMS) to compare breastfeeding initiation and breastfeeding at 1, 2, and 3 months in US women with and without disabilities, as well as their sources of information on breastfeeding. A positive finding was that, after adjusting for sociodemographic and pregnancy-related factors, women with self-reported impairments suggesting the presence of a disability had similar rates of breastfeeding initiation (86.7% vs 86.6%) and breastfeeding at 1 month (74.2% vs 76.4%) as women without disabilities. However, women with disabilities were less likely to breastfeed at 2 (62.6% vs 66.6%) and 3 months (54.7% vs 59.6%), demonstrating the presence of small but important disparities in breastfeeding duration. The study could not identify the reasons for these disparities. However, breastfeeding intentions and experiences, breastfeeding supports, and the social determinants of health may play important roles, each with implications for future research and for the development of accessible breastfeeding care.

Breastfeeding intentions are a critical determinant of later breastfeeding outcomes.[5] While Ramer et al. could not measure breastfeeding intentions, other studies have shown that women with disabilities are less likely to intend to breastfeed and that disparities in rates of breastfeeding are smaller after accounting for their intentions.[6] Future studies should examine breastfeeding intentions in women with disabilities and the factors that influence them. For example, barriers to reproductive health care and education across the life course for disabled women may lead to lower breastfeeding intentions because of discomfort and poorer breastfeeding self-efficacy and knowledge.[6] Studies should also examine disabled women's breastfeeding experiences, including why some women stop early and what helps others continue. Such data would be valuable for understanding if breastfeeding difficulties relate to specific challenges with breastfeeding (e.g., latching), problems related to the person's disability (e.g., pain, fatigue), or barriers accessing the right type of health care, suggesting areas for intervention.

Indeed, one barrier Ramer et al. were able to examine was lack of breastfeeding support. They found women with disabilities were as likely as those without disabilities to receive support from breastfeeding or lactation consultants (78.1% vs 75.3%) but were slightly less likely to receive support from health care providers and support professionals (89.3% vs 92.3%). The authors also found receipt of breastfeeding support from health care providers was associated with higher rates of breastfeeding initiation and breastfeeding at 1 and 2 months in the overall sample, but not in women with disabilities. Together, these findings suggest not only that health care providers are less likely to offer breastfeeding support to women with disabilities but also that the supports they do offer may be less useful to women with disabilities.

These findings show a need to understand why health care providers are less likely to offer breastfeeding support to this population and develop provider training resources to address negative attitudes or erroneous assumptions about disability and breastfeeding, such as when medications are or are not contraindicated. The data also show the need to improve health care providers' competencies in delivering accessible breastfeeding care. Equity does not mean giving every woman the same information in the same way; disabled women may benefit from tailored communication strategies and adaptive breastfeeding techniques. Health care providers such as family physicians and pediatricians may be the first point of contact for early questions about breastfeeding; however, they may not be aware of these considerations,[7] showing the need for better resources and collaborative care with lactation consultants.

As acknowledged by Ramer et al., the broader social determinants of health may also play a role in the observed disparities. Adjustment for sociodemographic and pregnancy-related characteristics attenuated the magnitude of the disparities. This attenuation suggests efforts to improve disabled women's breastfeeding behaviors, and the supports available to them, will not be effective without attending to their broader social and medical needs. Disabled women face pervasive social inequities, including poverty, that have downstream effects on pregnancy outcomes.[8] Breastfeeding promotion in this population, therefore, needs to be done in tandem with initiatives to address the social determinants of health for women with disabilities.

The research by Ramer et al. clearly has implications for optimizing breastfeeding outcomes in women with disabilities. However, efforts to educate health care providers on disability and breastfeeding and to develop accessible breastfeeding supports for disabled women must be sensitive to the ways in which breastfeeding is wrapped up in other pressures experienced by many women with disabilities. Women with disabilities experience heightened scrutiny around infant care, driven by historical eugenic notions about disability and pregnancy, and ableist assumptions about their parenting abilities.[8] As such, the pressure to breastfeed may be particularly acute for women with disabilities,[7] which carries implications for postpartum mental health when difficulties are encountered or their decisions do not align with health care providers' advice. This is a critical point because women with disabilities are already at elevated risk for postpartum depression.[9] It is therefore important that breastfeeding promotion efforts for this population, and for all women, focus on informed decision-making and identify ways of supporting women whose circumstances or medical needs do not allow them to breastfeed—reflecting what women need and want and their comfort with their breastfeeding decisions.

DISABILITY IDENTIFIERS IN MATERNAL–NEWBORN HEALTH SURVEILLANCE

The study by Ramer et al. makes an important contribution to the literature. Past research using administrative data shows women with disabilities have lower breastfeeding initiation rates,[6] and qualitative studies show barriers to breastfeeding—but not on a population level.[7] The work by Ramer et al. provides new data on longer-term breastfeeding outcomes and generates clues about the structural barriers women may experience. This study was possible because of inclusion of disability identifiers in PRAMS, initiated in 2019 when the National Institutes of Health and Centers for Disease Control and Prevention responded to a need for population-based data to understand the perinatal experiences of disabled women.[10] PRAMS is notable because inclusion of disability items in maternity surveys is rare, driven by historical assumptions that pregnancy is uncommon in women with disabilities and is, therefore, not a public health priority. The research by Ramer et al. is an example of what can be gleaned when disability identifiers are included in maternal–newborn health surveillance efforts. It is also a reminder to be aware of who is counted in such surveys; Ramer et al. found 6.0% of their sample had a disability, but the prevalence of disability in pregnant women is higher, at approximately 13%.[11] Cognitive and communication barriers to survey participation remain, underscoring the need for continued efforts to improve disability inclusion and identification in health surveillance efforts to ensure everyone is counted.

As many as one in eight pregnancies are to women with a disability.[11] The work by Ramer et al. demonstrates the importance of counting maternal and child health outcomes in this population and of ensuring that the data structures exist to do so. AJPH

CORRESPONDENCE

Correspondence should be sent to Hilary K. Brown, PhD, Department of Health and Society, University of Toronto Scarborough, 1265 Military Trail, Toronto, Ontario, Canada, M1C 1A5 (e-mail: hk.brown@utoronto.ca). Reprints can be ordered at https://ajph.org by clicking the "Reprints" link.

PUBLICATION INFORMATION

Full Citation: Brown HK, Lunsky Y. Time to count the breastfeeding experiences of women with disabilities in health surveillance efforts. *Am J Public Health*. 2024;114(1):7–9.

Acceptance Date: October 23, 2023.

DOI: https://doi.org/10.2105/AJPH.2023.307514

CONTRIBUTORS

H. K. Brown undertook the conceptualization of the commentary and drafting of the article. Y. Lunsky contributed to the conceptualization of the commentary and critically revised the article for important intellectual content. Both authors approve the final version to be published and agree to be accountable for all aspects of the work.

ACKNOWLEDGMENTS

Hilary K. Brown is funded by the Canada Research Chairs Program.

CONFLICTS OF INTEREST

The authors have no conflicts of interest to disclose.

REFERENCES

1. Kramer MS, Kakuma R. The optimal duration of exclusive breastfeeding. *Cochrane Database Syst Rev*. 2012;2012(8):CD003517.
2. World Health Organization. Protecting, promoting and supporting breastfeeding in facilities providing maternity and newborn services: the revised Baby Friendly Hospital Initiative. Geneva, Switzerland: World Health Organization; 2018.
3. Vaz JS, Maia MFS, Neves PAR, Santos TM, Vidaletti LP, Victora C. Monitoring breastfeeding indicators in high-income countries: levels, trends and challenges. *Matern Child Nutr*. 2021;17(3):e13137. https://doi.org/10.1111/mcn.13137
4. Cohen SS, Alexander DD, Krebs NF, et al. Factors associated with breastfeeding initiation and continuation: a meta-analysis. *J Pediatr*. 2018;203:190–196.e21. https://doi.org/10.1016/j.jpeds.2018.08.008
5. Meedya S, Fahy K, Kable A. Factors that positively influence breastfeeding duration to 6 months: a literature review. *Women Birth*. 2010;23(4):135–145. https://doi.org/10.1016/j.wombi.2010.02.002
6. Brown HK, Taylor C, Vigod SN, et al. Disability and in-hospital breastfeeding practices and supports in Ontario, Canada: a population-based study. *Lancet Public Health*. 2023;8(1):e47–e56. https://doi.org/10.1016/S2468-2667(22)00310-3
7. Powell RM, Mitra M, Smeltzer SC, et al. Breastfeeding among women with physical disabilities in the United States. *J Hum Lact*. 2018;34(2):253–261. https://doi.org/10.1177/0890334417739836
8. Powell RM. Disability reproductive justice. *Univ Pa Law Rev*. 2022;170(7):1851–1904.
9. Mitra M, Iezzoni LI, Zhang J, Long-Bellil LM, Smeltzer SC, Barton BA. Prevalence and risk factors for postpartum depression symptoms among women with disabilities. *Matern Child Health J*. 2015;19(2):362–372. https://doi.org/10.1007/s10995-014-1518-8
10. D'Angelo DV, Cernich A, Harrison L, et al. Disability and pregnancy: a cross-federal agency collaboration to collect population-based data about experiences around the time of pregnancy. *J Womens Health (Larchmt)*. 2020;29(3):291–296. https://doi.org/10.1089/jwh.2020.8309
11. Brown HK, Chen S, Guttmann A, et al. Rates of recognized pregnancy in women with disabilities in Ontario, Canada. *Am J Obstet Gynecol*. 2020;222(2):189–192. https://doi.org/10.1016/j.ajog.2019.10.096

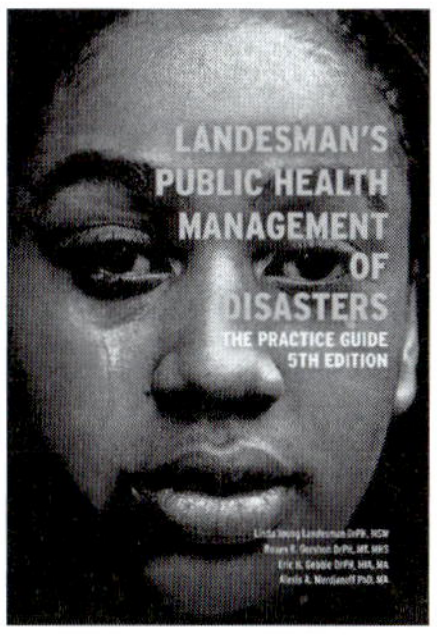

SOFTCOVER, 100 PAGES, 2021
ISBN 978-0-87553-312-6

Landesman's Public Health Management of Disasters: The Practice Guide, 5th Edition

By: Linda Young Landesman, DrPH, MSW; Robyn R. Gershon, DrPH, MT, MHS; Eric N. Gebbie, DrPH, MIA, MA; Alexis A. Merdjanoff, PhD, MA

This new edition is both a comprehensive textbook and an essential tool for those who have a role in disaster management. Every chapter now includes extensive sections on Covid-19 covering all of public health's responsibility as it relates to a pandemic.

APHABOOKSTORE.ORG

APHA PRESS
AN IMPRINT OF AMERICAN PUBLIC HEALTH ASSOCIATION

Moving Beyond Policy Adoption—The Necessity of Understanding the Whys and Hows

Alex C. Liber, PhD

ABOUT THE AUTHORS

Alex C. Liber is an assistant professor at the Lombardi Comprehensive Cancer Center, Georgetown University, Washington, DC.

See also Friedman and Pesko, p. 90.

As good research should, the newest article from Friedman and Pesko (published in this issue of *AJPH*; p. 90) raises more questions than it answers about policy to raise the minimum legal age for tobacco product sales to 21 years (Tobacco 21). In an age of polarized politics, Tobacco 21 grew from a local oddity in Needham, Massachusetts, to US federal policy in less than 7 years.[1] The policy, which at first represented a technocratic evidence-based incremental improvement over the status quo minimum age of 18 years, came to embody a commonsensical response to a growing epidemic of youth e-cigarette use.

By 2019, leading public health organizations and tobacco companies alike, although driven by different motives, supported Tobacco 21 laws.[2] A chapter of Karalyn Kiessling's recent University of Michigan doctoral dissertation contrasts the politics and policy process that drove the states of Colorado and Virginia to adopt Tobacco 21 laws.[3] Through thick description, she paints a vivid portrait of a policy process in Virginia in which lobbyists from Altria, the nation's largest tobacco company, which has headquarters in Richmond, Virginia, "[did] all the work" to pass Tobacco 21, including writing the bill, finding sponsors, finding medical professionals, and testifying in support of the legislation.[3(p136)]

By contrast, in Colorado, public health organizations Preventing Tobacco Addiction Foundation and Campaign for Tobacco-Free Kids served as policy entrepreneurs for the Tobacco 21 adoption effort. After an aborted statewide Tobacco 21 attempt in 2014 and several subsequent successful local adoption efforts, a statewide law pushed by public health organizations was finally adopted in 2020.

Based on its internally established best practices, the Preventing Tobacco Addiction Foundation assigns Virginia's Tobacco 21 law its lowest grade and Colorado's law its highest. Public health groups viewed the policy as a way to stem the rising tide of youth e-cigarette use, and tobacco companies likely viewed the policy as a way to forestall laws that would affect a wider slice of their customer base.[3]

Because the likely motives for, content of, and backers of policies that are both labeled "Tobacco 21" differ so much, it makes sense to explore whether the effects of different varieties of Tobacco 21 also vary. Although Kiessling's work documents that Tobacco 21 policies can arise through different policy pathways, it raises important questions about why we expect such policies to have similar outcomes.

Friedman and Pesko conducted quasiexperimental analyses that reinforce a growing base of evidence, finding that Tobacco 21 policies efficaciously reduce the use of tobacco products among young people in the United States. Importantly, they provide novel analyses that find that policies that continue to penalize young people for the purchase, use, or possession (PUP) of tobacco products yield higher youth tobacco use than policies without PUP provisions. Public health groups have advocated eliminating PUP rules alongside Tobacco 21 adoption. The Preventing Tobacco Addiction Foundation considers PUP elimination best practice because doing so shifts responsibility to the retailers that profit from underage sales.

However, other recommended best practices, including mandatory annual compliance checks and higher retailer penalties, were not found to affect tobacco use outcomes. Furthermore, Friedman and Pesko do not attempt to drill down on the PUP issue to determine which of these separate provisions drives their effect or to see whether states that removed some or all PUP provisions with Tobacco 21 adoption (e.g., California, Colorado, Illinois, Maryland, and Louisiana) saw different outcomes than those who did not have them in place before Tobacco 21 adoption (e.g., Massachusetts, New Jersey, New York, and Nevada).[4]

Some of these findings and analytic decisions can likely be attributed to inadequate statistical power available

AJPH January 2024, Vol. 114, No. 1

through these population surveys. Additionally, regression coefficients can tell us only a part of why Tobacco 21 policies worked better or worse in some places than others. In a sense, Friedman and Pesko's article has generated a series of new research questions that call for a mixed qualitative and quantitative methodological approach to be answered.

Well-constructed econometric studies can guess the mechanism behind why a law works. Still, an on-the-ground thick description is required to truly understand what is causing the behavior to change after policy shifts. As Friedman and Pesko point out in their discussion, work in the 2000s examining the effect of PUP provisions (including a randomized controlled trial of 24 Illinois communities[5]) found opposite results: PUP rules decreased youth smoking.[6(pp180–182)] However, previous work that looked into mechanisms often found that law enforcement officers did not place significant priority on enforcing PUP laws,[7,8] raising questions about whether changing PUP laws themselves changes youth behavior.

Mainline public health views about the efficacy of PUP laws appear to have changed during the Tobacco 21 diffusion period, too. The first statewide Tobacco 21 policy adopted in Hawaii was accompanied by an expansion of PUP laws, whereas every state that followed either removed or did not change PUP provisions.[4] Increasing visibility of problems surrounding the inequitable enforcement of policies, including PUP, among minoritized communities altered what was considered Tobacco 21 best practice to include eliminating these laws.

Although Friedman and Pesko's new research meets expectations of what practitioners expected Tobacco 21 policies to do, a great deal more work needs to delve into why this happened. Interest in adopting policies that are inspired by Tobacco 21 is growing around the world.[9] Policy entrepreneurs need to understand why the policy works, and a more detailed description of the on-the-ground mechanisms that lead to positive change is required. If Tobacco 21 diffusion outward from the US context is to replicate the success we have witnessed here, curious funders and public health organizations need to support this necessary work. AJPH

CORRESPONDENCE

Correspondence should be sent to Alex C. Liber, 2115 Wisconsin Ave NW, Washington, DC 20007 (e-mail: alex.liber@georgetown.edu). Reprints can be ordered at http://www.ajph.org by clicking the "Reprints" link.

PUBLICATION INFORMATION

Full Citation: Liber AC. Moving beyond policy adoption—the necessity of understanding the whys and hows. *Am J Public Health*. 2024;114(1):10–11.

Acceptance Date: October 26, 2023.

DOI: https://doi.org/10.2105/AJPH.2023.307521

ACKNOWLEDGMENTS

Thank you to Karalyn Kiessling for sharing an early version of her wonderful doctoral dissertation.

CONFLICTS OF INTEREST

A. C. Liber has received grants from the US Food and Drug Administration and the National Cancer Institute but otherwise has no conflicts of interest to report.

REFERENCES

1. Reynolds MJ, Crane R, Winickoff JP. The emergence of the Tobacco 21 movement from Needham, Massachusetts, to throughout the United States (2003–2019). *Am J Public Health*. 2019;109(11):1540–1547. https://doi.org/10.2105/AJPH.2019.305209
2. Whyte LE, Náñez DM. Why Big Tobacco and JUUL are lobbying to raise the smoking age. *USA TODAY*. May 23, 2019. Available at: https://www.usatoday.com/story/news/investigations/2019/05/23/why-big-tobacco-and-juul-lobbying-raise-smoking-age/3758443002. Accessed September 19, 2023.
3. Kiessling K. Tobacco Control in the 21st Century: Policies to Address Traditional and Emerging Tobacco Products [PhD dissertation]. Ann Arbor: University of Michigan; 2023. https://dx.doi.org/10.7302/8517
4. Centers for Disease Control and Prevention. State Tobacco Activities Tracking and Evaluation (STATE) System. October 20, 2023. Available at: https://www.cdc.gov/statesystem/index.html. Accessed September 14, 2023.
5. Jason LA, Pokorny SB, Adams M. A randomized trial evaluating tobacco possession–use–purchase laws in the USA. *Soc Sci Med*. 2008;67(11):1700–1707. https://doi.org/10.1016/j.socscimed.2008.09.028
6. Institute of Medicine; Bonnie RJ, Stratton K, Kwan LY, eds. *Public Health Implications of Raising the Minimum Age of Legal Access to Tobacco Products*. Washington, DC: National Academies Press; 2015. Available at: https://www.ncbi.nlm.nih.gov/books/NBK310405. Accessed October 10, 2023. https://doi.org/10.17226/18997
7. Hrywna M, Adler RK, Delnevo CD, Slade JD. Content analysis and key informant interviews to examine community response to the purchase, possession, and/or use of tobacco by minors. *J Community Health*. 2004;29(3):209–216. https://doi.org/10.1023/B:JOHE.0000022027.03119.38
8. Hahn EJ, Riker C, Butler KM, et al. Enforcement of tobacco purchase, use, and possession laws in four Kentucky communities. *Policy Polit Nurs Pract*. 2007;8(2):140–147. https://doi.org/10.1177/1527154407303500
9. Iacobucci G. England plans to raise legal age for buying tobacco each year to create "smoke-free" generation. *BMJ*. 2023;383:2297. https://doi.org/10.1136/bmj.p2297

To Reduce Sexual Minority Health Care Disparities, Advocate for Expanded Health Insurance Coverage and LGBTQ+ Rights

Angie R. Wootton, PhD, MSW

ABOUT THE AUTHOR

Angie R. Wootton is with the School of Social Welfare, University at Albany, State University of New York, Albany, NY.

See also Nguyen et al., p. 118.

AJPH January 2024, Vol. 114, No. 1

The *AJPH* article by Nguyen et al. (p. 118) begins answering key questions lesbian, gay, bisexual, transgender, queer, and other nonheterosexual and noncisgender (LGBTQ+) health equity scholars have been asking since the beginning of the COVID-19 pandemic: How will LGBTQ+ population health be affected by pandemic conditions? Will existing health care inequities compound in the presence of COVID-19–induced strains on economic and health care systems? These questions quickly arose at the pandemic's onset as there have been several decades of research documenting the disproportionate burden of economic hardships (e.g., poverty and homelessness) on LGBTQ+ people, alongside early indications of pandemic-related health care delays and interruptions.[1]

The early years of the COVID-19 pandemic spurred work and economic challenges for both LGBTQ+ and non-LGBTQ+ people alike that raised concerns about access to affordable health care. During the Fall 2020 COVID-19 surge, LGBTQ+ people faced more layoffs and furloughs than non-LGBTQ+ people, particularly in hard-hit industries that LGBTQ+ people were more likely to work in, such as hospitality.[2,3] Uncertainty about job security and employment income were notable stressors for many LGBTQ+ people during the pandemic, especially those already experiencing challenges in these areas, as shown by Nguyen et al. and others.[2] LGBTQ+ people of color were disproportionately affected by layoffs and furloughs relative to White LGBTQ+ people and non-LGBTQ+ people of color,[3] creating particularly difficult circumstances for sexual and gender minority women of color[4] and people experiencing multiple simultaneous forms of economic and social disadvantage. These layoffs led to income loss and often the loss of employer-sponsored health insurance, increasing the need for Medicaid or alternative forms of coverage for those affected.[3] Because of these economic impacts of the pandemic, LGBTQ+ individuals, particularly LGBTQ+ people of color, faced significant challenges in affording household essentials and housing compared with heterosexual and cisgender people,[3] financial concerns that could amplify financial barriers to accessing health care.

INSURANCE COVERAGE AND CARE ACCESS IN THE COVID-19 PANDEMIC

When comparing the health insurance status and access to care of more than 158 000 adults (aged 18–64 years) across 34 states in 2021–2022, Nguyen et al. found that sexual minority adults (e.g., lesbian, gay, and bisexual people) were more likely to lack health insurance coverage and experience health care as inaccessible during the COVID-19 pandemic, compared with heterosexuals. Sexual minority women were significantly more likely to lack health insurance coverage than heterosexual women, in part because of lower likelihood of having employer-sponsored health insurance, which was not the case for sexual minority men. Uninsurance widened sexual orientation–related disparities in access to health care for sexual minority women, including whether an individual had a personal doctor, received a check-up in the past 2 years, or reported an inability to afford needed care in the past year. For sexual minority men, underinsurance, or lack of access to care because of high costs despite having insurance, appeared to be of greater concern than uninsurance.

These findings highlight the importance of considering the specific health care experiences and needs of subgroups under the broader LGBTQ+ umbrella, such as sexual minority women, which can become obscured when researchers aggregate LGBQ+ respondents of all genders into a single sexual minority category for sample size reasons. Whenever possible, LGBTQ+ health research should conduct within-group analyses by both sexual orientation and gender, as Nguyen et al. did, to avoid the risk of making generalizations about a heterogeneous community. Unfortunately, the study does not discuss the experiences of transgender and gender-expansive people because of limitations with the questions asked of respondents. Further research on COVID-19 pandemic impacts on health insurance coverage and access to care for transgender and gender-expansive people is vital given that this community experiences many of the same economic stressors as sexual minority people along with additional stressors that may negatively impact health.

POLICY ADVOCACY TO PROMOTE LGBTQ+ HEALTH EQUITY

There are multiple avenues for policy advocacy to improve sexual minority people's access to health insurance and care during this wind down of the acute phase of the COVID-19 pandemic, many of which are recommended by Nguyen et al. Advocates can speak against threats to Medicaid (e.g., the 2023 wind down of continuous coverage protections for Medicaid enrollees) and advocate continued state-by-state Medicaid expansion as a means of decreasing health disparities for sexual minority adults, who have higher rates of Medicaid usage than heterosexuals. Given that uninsurance rates and access to care improved for sexual minority people after the implementation of the 2010 Affordable Care Act (ACA) and that the 2022 proposed ACA revision reinstates the prohibition of discrimination by insurers based on sexual orientation and gender, advocacy to protect the ACA and Medicaid is a critical way to promote LGBTQ+ health equity.

Antidiscrimination policies may also play a role in health insurance coverage and care access for sexual minority people, particularly within the current context of increasing anti-LGBTQ+ legislative efforts in some states, alongside gaps in existing antidiscrimination policies. In the study by Nguyen et al., states with more policies protecting LGBTQ+ equality had narrower disparities in health care unaffordability by sexual orientation. In other words, sexual minority people in states that protected their rights in the workplace and other societal domains appeared more able to afford health care than those who were vulnerable to workplace, economic, or other forms of discrimination. Although some LGBTQ+ affirmative policy changes in the past decade (e.g., the 2015 national legalization of same-sex marriage) have increased sexual minority people's sense of safety in being "out" and visible in the workplace, job security concerns persist for sexual minority people living in states without comprehensive antidiscrimination policies.[5]

To ensure that LGBTQ+ people who are insured through employers are not at risk for losing coverage because of discrimination (or simply not being hired in the first place), there is a need to advocate comprehensive federal antidiscrimination policies protecting LGBTQ+ people. Comprehensive antidiscrimination policies protecting sexual and gender minority people are currently in place in less than two thirds of states, and about 26% of the US LGBTQ+ population lives in states with a negative, anti-LGBTQ+ policy climate.[6] The Equality Act, which was reintroduced to Congress in June 2023, would provide all sexual and gender minority Americans with consistent antidiscrimination protections across the workplace, health care settings, and other social institutions implicated in these disparities in health insurance and access to care.[7,8] An alliance of public health, social work, nursing, and other medical and allied professionals could have a powerful voice in the national conversations on these issues given what our fields' research has shown about the negative health effects of discrimination on minority groups. AJPH

CORRESPONDENCE

Correspondence should be sent to Angie Wootton, 135 Western Ave, Richardson Hall #281, Albany, NY 12203 (e-mail: awootton@albany.edu). Reprints can be ordered at https://ajph.org by clicking the "Reprints" link.

PUBLICATION INFORMATION

Full Citation: Wootton AR. To reduce sexual minority health care disparities, advocate for expanded health insurance coverage and LGBTQ+ rights. *Am J Public Health*. 2024;114(1):12–14.

Acceptance Date: October 22, 2023.

DOI: https://doi.org/10.2105/AJPH.2023.307513

CONFLICTS OF INTEREST

The author has no conflicts of interest to declare.

REFERENCES

1. Papautsky EL, Rice DR, Ghoneima H, et al. Characterizing health dare delays and interruptions in the United States during the COVID-19 pandemic: Internet-based, cross-sectional survey study. *J Med Internet Res*. 2021;23(5):e25446. https://doi.org/10.2196/25446
2. Banerjee D, Nair VS. "The untold side of COVID-19": struggle and perspectives of the sexual minorities. *J Psychosexual Health*. 2020;2(2):113–120. https://doi.org/10.1177/2631831820939017
3. Sears B, Conron KJ, Flores AR. The impact of the Fall 2020 COVID-19 surge on LGBT adults in the US. UCLA School of Law, Williams Institute. February 2021. Available at: https://williamsinstitute.law.ucla.edu/wp-content/uploads/COVID-LGBT-Fall-Surge-Feb-2021.pdf. Accessed October 6, 2023.
4. Riggle EDB, Drabble LA, Bochicchio LA, et al. Experiences of the COVID-19 pandemic among African American, Latinx, and White sexual minority women: a descriptive phenomenological study.

Psychol Sex Orientat Gend Divers. 2021;8(2): 145–158. https://doi.org/10.1037/sgd0000510

5. Wootton AR, Drabble LA, Riggle EDB, et al. Impacts of marriage legalization on the experiences of sexual minority women in work and community contexts. *J GLBT Fam Stud.* 2019;15(3):211–234. https://doi.org/10.1080/1550428X.2018.1474829
6. Movement Advancement Project. Equality maps snapshot: LGBTQ equality by state. Available at: https://www.mapresearch.org/equality-maps. Accessed October 6, 2023.
7. Equality Act. S. 5, 118th Congress (2023-2024). June 21, 2023. Available at: https://www.congress.gov/bill/118th-congress/senate-bill/5/text. Accessed October 6, 2023.
8. Equality Act. H.R. 15, 118th Congress (2023-2025). June 21, 2023. Available at: https://www.govtrack.us/congress/bills/118/hr15. Accessed October 6, 2023.

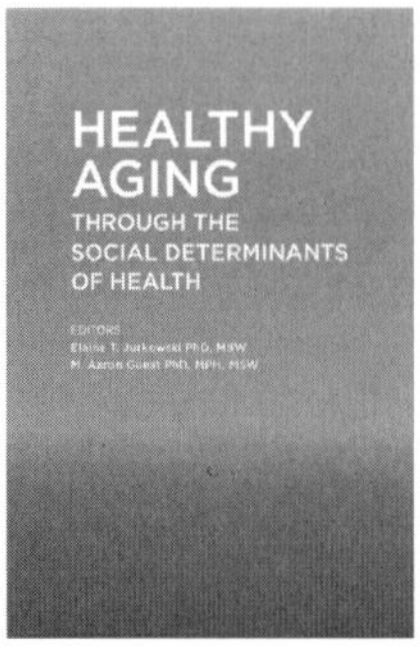

2021, SOFTCOVER,
350 PP, 978-087553-3155

APHABOOKSTORE.ORG

Healthy Aging Through The Social Determinants of Health

Edited by Elaine T. Jurkowski, PhD, MSW and M. Aaron Guest, PhD, MPH, MSW

This new book examines the link between social determinants of health and the process of healthy aging. It provides public health practitioners and others interacting with the older population with best practices to encourage healthy aging and enhance the lives of people growing older.

Healthy Aging: Through The Social Determinants of Health gives insight into the role each of these plays in the healthy aging process: health and health care; neighborhood and built environment; social support; education; and economics and policy.

APHA PRESS
AN IMPRINT OF AMERICAN PUBLIC HEALTH ASSOCIATION

The Value of Peace: A Public Health of Consequence, January 2024

Farzana Kapadia, PhD, MPH

ABOUT THE AUTHOR

Farzana Kapadia is the deputy editor of AJPH *and a professor in the Department of Epidemiology, New York University School of Global Public Health, New York.*

The latest trend data from the Uppsala Conflict Data Program, a leading resource on global conflicts, indicate that 56 active state-based armed conflicts and 45 one-sided conflicts involving government forces—defined as either those between nation-states or civil wars and internal conflicts—were being waged in 2023 (https://ucdp.uu.se/encyclopedia). Even more alarming is that these numbers manifest a steady increase in armed state-sponsored violence and conflict over the past 20 years. Although the wars in Ukraine and Palestine rightfully draw our attention currently, there are scores of other conflicts—across Sudan, Ethiopia, Mali, Myanmar, Syria, Afghanistan, and Yemen, to name just a few that persist. Although these ongoing wars and conflicts may not draw our attention, their persistence is a strong indicator that our world is becoming less peaceful and more violent.

In this Public Health of Consequence editorial, we review previous work published in *AJPH* that provides evidence of the both overt and insidious impacts of war on the health and humanity of our global community. We highlight how both the immediate and long-term impacts of war devastate already vulnerable societies and groups of people, which make recovery even more arduous. Finally, we summarize, providing evidence of initiatives that promote peace. In doing so, we call on public health practitioners and advocates to call for an end to violence and armed conflict—in all forms and in all places—to protect our global health and humanity.

WAR *AND* PUBLIC HEALTH

Since 2022, the absolute number of deaths caused by war and armed conflicts has increased dramatically. These increases in warfare-related mortality are driven largely by wars in Africa, Europe, and the Middle East (https://ourworldindata.org/war-and-peace). However, as we have witnessed throughout history, the number of direct warfare-related deaths are dwarfed by indirect warfare-related deaths and disease in civilian populations.

Specifically, mortality and morbidity among civilian adults and children increase during and after conflict because of an increase in infectious disease, homicide, suicide, sexual- and gender-based violence,[1] depression, and anxiety that occur in the weeks, months, and years following conflict.[2] Reporting on the war in Nicaragua in the 1980s, Garfield et al. noted, "Population movements, the establishment of new settlements, and war-related destruction of the primary health infrastructure are associated with recent epidemics of malaria, dengue, measles, and leishmaniasis."[4(p615)] Peterman et al., using population-based surveys and recent census data, estimated that the "number of women who have been the victims of rape and IPSV [intimate partner sexual violence] in the DRC [Democratic Republic of Congo] is several orders of magnitude higher than what has been cited in previous studies."[1(p1064)] Moreover, their results showed that women in regions experiencing the greatest burden of conflict—the DRC provinces of North Kivu and South Kivu—reported even higher rates of rape and intimate partner violence. And finally, in the decade following the US invasion of Iraq, outbreaks of vaccine-preventable disease among children, specifically measles, mumps, and rubella, ravaged the nation, whose health care infrastructure was already weakened by US sanctions.[3]

Beyond the toll of mortality and morbidity from war and armed conflict in a home country, for those who are displaced or forced to seek asylum, the long-term mental and physical health burdens can be devastating. Layered on the trauma of experiencing war are xenophobia and lack of support in a new host country, which can be further traumatizing. As has been well documented, refugees forced to flee to camps suffer from a lack of basic services, access to safe food and water, and adequate sanitation, which contribute to high rates of communicable disease in refugee camps. In reaction to the refugee crisis spawned by the war in Syria, Morabia and Benjamin have called for host countries to stem the rising tide of xenophobia against asylum seekers and to provide basic preventive health services to mitigate the mental and physical health harms resulting from mass displacement.[3]

WAR *ON* PUBLIC HEALTH

Alarming increases in attacks on medical facilities and medical personnel auger a new level of disregard of the First Geneva Convention articles that explicitly ban attacks on civilian hospitals and health care workers (https://bit.ly/46Et5Hy). A 2022 Safeguarding Health in Conflict Coalition report identified a 45% increase from 2021 to 2022 in the global incidence of attacks against health care facilities and health care workers across 32 countries and territories (https://bit.ly/3Fr3gOX). Even in conflicts that are not classified as wars, the international protections mandated in the Geneva Conventions are disregarded.[4] Not only does the destruction of health care facilities prevent care provision to anyone wounded, but it also prevents care delivery to the most vulnerable in a population: infants, children, the elderly, and the sick.

Finally, the years required to rebuild health care infrastructure and, more importantly, a health care delivery workforce in conflict settings can undermine population stability and safety during postconflict periods. For all of these reasons, the public health community must stand in solidarity against any and all military action against health care facilities and health care workers. Such attacks are war crimes, and all those responsible for such attacks should be held accountable.

THE VALUE OF PEACE FOR GLOBAL PUBLIC HEALTH

As peace is a requirement for global health, likewise global health and well-being are requirements for peace. To this point, the 1986 Ottawa Charter for Health Promotion lists peace as the first "fundamental condition and resource" for achieving and sustaining population health and well-being (https://bit.ly/46SlgxK). Furthermore, the World Health Organization (WHO) constitution clearly states, "The health of all peoples is fundamental to the attainment of peace and security and is dependent on the fullest cooperation of individuals and States" (https://bit.ly/491i7gP). Governments and public institutions that are able to provide safe, secure, and consistent access to basic public goods and services, especially health care–related services, are viewed as more legitimate and much less susceptible to political and military opposition. However, when these services are not provided or cease to be provided—as we have seen across the Middle East, Africa, Latin America, and Asia—governments and their institutions are more prey to destabilizing forces that can lead to armed hostility and conflict.

Although spending on public health infrastructure and public health and medical health care personnel is often a small fraction of government spending, the short- and long-term return on investment vis-à-vis safety, security, and peace are incalculable. One such example is the WHO Global Health and Peace Initiative, a model that focuses on "local level peace outcomes" and "building collaboration between different sides in a conflict on common topics like health governance and the delivery of health care" (https://bit.ly/3s1bASE). Critical to the success of such programs are efforts to design and implement health programs that "seek to contribute to improving the prospects for peace such as social cohesion, equity, inclusivity, dialogue, or community resilience to violence."

Such programs provide evidence that there is power and value in promoting peace as a means to ensuring a global public health of consequence. Consequently, we call on all public health professionals to advocate efforts to end all forms or violence and to support investments in health, social, and economic policies and practices that promote peace and recognize the human rights of all people. AJPH

CORRESPONDENCE

Correspondence should be sent to Farzana Kapadia, PhD, MPH, New York University, School of Global Public Health, 708 Broadway, Room 729, New York, NY 10003 (e-mail: farzana.kapadia@nyu.edu). Reprints can be ordered at http://www.ajph.org by clicking the "Reprints" link.

PUBLICATION INFORMATION

Full Citation: Kapadia F. The value of peace: a Public Health of Consequence, January 2024. *Am J Public Health*. 2024;114(1):15–16.

Acceptance Date: October 23, 2023.

DOI: https://doi.org/10.2105/AJPH.2023.307522

CONFLICTS OF INTEREST

The author has no conflicts of interest to disclose.

REFERENCES

1. Peterman A, Palermo T, Bredenkamp C. Estimates and determinants of sexual violence against women in the Democratic Republic of Congo. *Am J Public Health*. 2011;101(6):1060–1067. https://doi.org/10.2105/AJPH.2010.300070
2. Bruno W, Parmar P. US war with Iran: a narrowly avoided public health crisis and a continuing risk. *Am J Public Health*. 2020;110(7):986–987. https://doi.org/10.2105/AJPH.2020.305700
3. Garfield RM, Frieden T, Vermund SH. Health-related outcomes of war in Nicaragua. *Am J Public Health*. 1987;77(5):615–618. https://doi.org/10.2105/AJPH.77.5.615
4. Morabia A, Benjamin GC. The refugee crisis in the Middle East and public health. *Am J Public Health*. 2015;105(12):2405–2406. https://doi.org/10.2105/AJPH.2015.302929

Advancing Pediatric Sexual Orientation and Gender Identity Data Collection

Michael Liu, MPhil, Chris Grasso, MPH, Hyun-Hee Kim, MD, Kenneth H. Mayer, MD, and Alex S. Keuroghlian, MD, MPH

ABOUT THE AUTHORS

Michael Liu is with Harvard Medical School, Boston, MA. Chris Grasso, Kenneth H. Mayer, and Alex S. Keuroghlian are with the Fenway Institute at Fenway Health, Boston. Hyun-Hee Kim is with the Division of Child and Adolescent Psychiatry, Massachusetts General Hospital, Boston.

The population of youths reporting sexual and gender minority (SGM) identities is growing in the United States. The percentage of high school students identifying as nonheterosexual increased from 8.3% to 11.7% between 2015 and 2019.[1] Nearly 1.4% of youths aged 13 to 17 years identified as transgender between 2017 and 2019, whereas 0.5% of adults identified as transgender during a similar time period.[2]

SGM youths experience substantial physical, mental, and sexual health inequities relative to their heterosexual and cisgender counterparts. For example, they are significantly more likely than non-SGM youths to report school bullying, poor mental health, and suicidality.[3] The prevalence of risky behaviors such as engaging in condomless sexual intercourse, smoking, and using recreational drugs is also much higher among SGM youths.[3] These disparities are driven in part by minority stress associated with belonging to a marginalized group. Such stressors erode the health of SGM youths through a range of structural and interpersonal forces, including family rejection, economic marginalization, peer discrimination, and internalized stigma.[4]

The recent onslaught of anti-SGM legislation sweeping across the United States is poised to exacerbate minority stress and worsen health inequities among SGM youths. According to the Human Rights Campaign, 77 anti-SGM bills had been signed into law as of June 8, 2023, more than any previous year and double the number passed in the entire preceding year. These laws encompass those that censor discussion of SGM topics in classrooms, restrict gender minority people from using bathrooms and other facilities according to their gender identities, and criminalize the delivery of gender-affirming medical care for gender minority youths.

Such legislation directly hinders access to lifesaving services and contributes to a hostile climate that excludes, erases, and endangers SGM youths. For example, receipt of gender-affirming hormone therapy has been associated with improved psychosocial functioning, and exposure to bathroom discrimination has been associated with suicidality among transgender and gender diverse youths.[5,6] Actions that exacerbate stigma, obscure visibility, and signal rejection of SGM identities have been linked to poor mental health and suicidality among SGM youths.[7]

IMPORTANCE OF DATA COLLECTION

The health care sector has a responsibility to protect and promote the health of SGM youths, and this is dependent on knowledge of patient sexual orientation and gender identity (SOGI). Guidelines from the American Academy of Pediatrics have directed all pediatricians to create safe and inclusive environments for SGM patients.[8] Fundamentally, collecting pediatric SOGI data ensures continued visibility of SGM youths and stands in opposition to ongoing legislative efforts to erase this population. Moreover, a wealth of evidence has demonstrated that collection of SOGI data is critical for delivering responsive, affirming, and patient-centered care for SGM people.[3] Knowledge of pediatric SOGI facilitates delivery of appropriate anticipatory counseling and referral to gender-affirming care and mental health supports.

SOGI data collection is also important for quality improvement and the conduct of population health research to monitor and identify opportunities to improve SGM health inequities. A secondary analysis of a pragmatic trial conducted across the United States revealed that only one in three adolescent men who have ever engaged in condomless anal sex with other men have been tested for HIV, despite clinical recommendations for annual, if not more frequent, screening in this population.[9] SOGI data can be combined with other routinely collected sociodemographic data to understand the experiences and unique health needs of youths with multiple marginalized identities. For example, a pooled analysis of the 2005 and 2007 Youth Risk Behavior Survey found that sexual minority Hispanic youths were more likely to report suicide attempts in the preceding year than both non–sexual minority Hispanic youths and sexual minority White youths.[10]

BEST PRACTICES FOR DATA COLLECTION

Guidelines have recently been developed for the collection and documentation of SOGI data with pediatric patients.[11] Examples of recommended questions to elicit information about SOGI by health professionals are provided in these guidelines. Questions regarding sexual orientation might be relevant starting at the ages of 10 to 13 years depending on the developmental readiness of the patient. Informed by cognitive interviews and field tests, an expert panel recommended using the term "crush" to indicate attraction among children 10 to 13 years of age and the phrase "sexual attraction" among adolescents 14 to 17 years of age.[12] Questions regarding gender identity may be asked starting at the age of 3 years, the point in time when most children are able to self-label their gender identities.[11]

Asking about and documenting sex assigned at birth subsequently allow for health professionals to identify transgender and gender diverse patients whose gender identity and sex assigned at birth do not align with societal expectations. Providers should also periodically inquire—annually at the minimum—about patient pronouns and patient-affirmed names to create safe spaces for SOGI and broader health discussions. Such information should appear in highly visible locations in electronic health records (EHRs) that are accessible to all staff members of pediatric care settings.

Unfortunately, progress on SOGI data collection with pediatric patients has lagged considerably behind that with their adult counterparts.[8] There have been concerted efforts in recent years to promote SOGI data completeness for adult patients at federally qualified health centers (FQHCs). In 2016, the US Health Resources and Services Administration (HRSA) mandated reporting of SOGI data for all adult patients receiving care at FQHCs. Over six years of mandated data reporting, the percentage of missingness decreased from 77.1% to 29.1% for sexual orientation data and from 62.8% to 24.0% for gender identity data.[13]

Increases in SOGI data completeness are likely attributable to a number of factors, including HRSA reporting mandates, more inclusive social environments, and widespread training and technical assistance spearheaded by the National LGBTQIA+ Health Education Center at the Fenway Institute. Other key facilitators of SOGI data completeness include the requirement for all EHRs certified under the Office of the National Coordinator for Health Information Technology's Certification Program to have the capacity to collect SOGI data and the recent addition of SOGI to the United States Core Data for Interoperability.[4,8]

Many of the facilitators of increased SOGI data collection with adult patients can be transferred and adapted to promote pediatric SOGI data collection. First, the Department of Health and Human Services (DHHS) should consider expanding SOGI data collection mandates at FQHCs to eligible pediatric patients.[13] Similar requirements from other payers such as commercial insurers and Medicaid state agencies could increase data collection efforts across the health system and promote alignment.

Second, all EHRs used in pediatric care settings should have the capacity to collect SOGI data with standardized categories and terminology from current guidelines.[11] This should also be paired with updating and integrating international code sets to capture patient SOGI data, such as the Systematized Nomenclature of Medicine and Logical Observation Identifiers Names and Codes.[14] Standardization across EHRs should continue to align with DHHS interoperability standards and allow for performance benchmarking related to data collection efforts. EHRs should also incorporate free text fields for documentation of SOGI outside of standard categories; a recent analysis of a national sample of 17 112 SGM adolescents reported 26 distinct SOGI categories, including pansexual and nonbinary.[15]

Third, there is evidence suggesting that adult SGM patients in emergency department settings prefer SOGI data entry into registration forms as compared with verbal communication with staff.[16] Pediatric care settings should similarly provide opportunities for patients and families to disclose SOGI information through electronic or paper forms that can be directly linked or entered into EHRs. More research is required to evaluate the most effective and patient-centered clinical workflows to enable routine and structured data collection among pediatric patients in different clinical settings.

AJPH January 2024, Vol. 114, No. 1

Finally, training programs related to SOGI data collection should be delivered to all members of the health care workforce in pediatric care settings. Most clinicians from 18 health care organizations surveyed in a large-scale needs assessment reported rarely or never talking to patients about sexual orientation (55.4%) or gender identity (71.9%).[17] Commonly cited reasons for not discussing SOGI included the belief that such information is not relevant to care, lack of provider experience, and not being familiar with the appropriate language to talk about SOGI.

A related challenge is inadequate provision of SGM-related education during undergraduate and graduate medical training. A study of residents from 120 US internal medicine residency programs revealed mean scores of 50% to 52% on a baseline assessment of SGM health knowledge throughout all three years of training.[18] Standardized curricula that prepare clinicians to care responsively for SGM patients should be required for all pediatric residency programs certified by the Accreditation Council for Graduate Medical Education, as well as all medical schools.

BARRIERS TO DATA COLLECTION

Several challenges related to pediatric SOGI data collection must be considered by providers, health system leaders, and policymakers. The first is privacy and confidentiality. Prior to documenting patient SOGI data in EHRs, it is critical that providers offer minors a clear explanation of who can access such information and obtain informed consent. Unwanted disclosure of SOGI information could compromise the patient–provider relationship and may even compromise the safety and well-being of pediatric SGM patients, who are often stigmatized and discriminated against.

One safeguard is the development of separate patient and proxy portals that allow pediatric patients to determine what information is visible to guardians, a recommendation endorsed by the Society for Adolescent Health and Medicine.[11] Maintaining patient privacy is especially challenging because the 21st Century Cures Act bans the blocking of guardian access to patient clinical information and the extent of confidentiality varies across states.[19] Pediatric care practices should seek legal counsel to understand whether their existing clinical workflows and information systems protect against unwanted disclosure of patient SOGI information in the context of applicable state and federal laws.

The second challenge is that both sexual orientation and gender identity are fluid and especially likely to change during early development. Providers should inquire about SOGI at least annually, and EHRs should have the flexibility to enable SOGI data updates and notifications to staff members of any changes. Finally, the recent wave of anti-SGM legislation likely discourages pediatric patients from sharing SOGI information. A recent analysis showed that city-level SOGI nondiscrimination laws were associated with more SOGI data completeness at FQHCs.[20] Thus, ongoing legal challenges to anti-SGM legislation and progress toward policies that explicitly protect the fundamental rights of SGM people are essential for fostering safe environments and sociocultural norms that enable youths to share their SGM identities freely and without fear.

CONCLUSIONS

Protecting and promoting the health of SGM youths is a priority for the health system, and collection of SOGI data is a necessary step toward achieving this goal. Concerted efforts from providers, public health leaders, and policymakers are critical for addressing existing barriers to collecting SOGI information among pediatric patients.

There is also an urgent need for researchers to monitor progress in improving pediatric SOGI data completeness and to evaluate different methods and workflows for enhancing the acceptability, experience, and overall uptake of SOGI data collection with this population. The resulting patient SOGI data will serve as an important foundation for providing comprehensive and affirming care to SGM youths, as well as identifying and reducing population-level health inequities. Even the simple act of asking for and collecting SOGI data serves to draw attention to and safeguard this substantial population under continued threat of erasure and persecution. As they experience increasingly hostile social and policy environments, it has never been more vital for SGM youths to know that they are seen and supported by the health system and beyond. AJPH

CORRESPONDENCE

Correspondence should be sent to Alex S. Keuroghlian, MD, MPH, Fenway Institute, Fenway Health, Boston, MA 02215 (e-mail: akeuroghlian@mgb.org). Reprints can be ordered at http://www.ajph.org by clicking the "Reprints" link.

PUBLICATION INFORMATION

Full Citation: Liu M, Grasso C, Kim Hyun-Hee, Mayer KH, Keuroghlian AS. Advancing pediatric sexual orientation and gender identity data collection. *Am J Public Health*. 2024;114(1):17–20.

Acceptance Date: September 1, 2023.

DOI: https://doi.org/10.2105/AJPH.2023.307448

CONTRIBUTORS

M. Liu conceptualized the editorial, wrote the first draft, and oversaw the editing and review process. A. S. Keuroghlian provided overall supervision. All of the authors critically reviewed the editorial for important intellectual content and provided overarching suggestions and revisions.

CONFLICTS OF INTEREST

Alex S. Keuroghlian reports receiving royalties as an editor of a McGraw-Hill textbook on transgender and gender diverse health care. The other authors have no conflicts of interest to declare.

REFERENCES

1. Rapoport E, Athanasian CE, Adesman A. Prevalence of nonheterosexual identity and same-sex sexual contact among high school students in the US from 2015 to 2019. *JAMA Pediatr.* 2021;175(9):970–972. https://doi.org/10.1001/jamapediatrics.2021.1109
2. Herman JL, Flores AR, O'Neill KK. *How Many Adults and Youth Identify as Transgender in the United States?* Los Angeles, CA: Williams Institute; 2022.
3. Patterson CJ, Sepúlveda MJ, White J, eds. *Understanding the Well-Being of LGBTQI+ Populations.* Washington, DC: National Academies Press; 2020.
4. Liu M, Sandhu S, Keuroghlian AS. Achieving the triple aim for sexual and gender minorities. *N Engl J Med.* 2022;387(4):294–297. https://doi.org/10.1056/NEJMp2204569
5. Chen D, Berona J, Chan YM, et al. Psychosocial functioning in transgender youth after 2 years of hormones. *N Engl J Med.* 2023;388(3):240–250. https://doi.org/10.1056/NEJMoa2206297
6. Price-Feeney M, Green AE, Dorison SH. Impact of bathroom discrimination on mental health among transgender and nonbinary youth. *J Adolesc Health.* 2021;68(6):1142–1147. https://doi.org/10.1016/j.jadohealth.2020.11.001
7. Gordon JH, Tran KT, Visoki E, et al. The role of individual discrimination and structural stigma in the mental health of sexual minority youth. *J Am Acad Child Adolesc Psychiatry.* 2023 Jul 6;S0890-8567(23)00375-1. https://doi.org/10.1016/j.jaac.2023.05.033
8. Stokes ST, Lecuyer M. Inclusive and affirming care strategies for sexual and gender minority patients. *Pediatrics.* 2023;151(4):e2022057699. https://doi.org/10.1542/peds.2022-057699
9. Mustanski B, Moskowitz DA, Moran KO, Rendina HJ, Newcomb ME, Macapagal K. Factors associated with HIV testing in teenage men who have sex with men. *Pediatrics.* 2020;145(3):e20192322. https://doi.org/10.1542/peds.2019-2322
10. Bostwick WB, Meyer I, Aranda F, et al. Mental health and suicidality among racially/ethnically diverse sexual minority youths. *Am J Public Health.* 2014;104(6):1129–1136. https://doi.org/10.2105/AJPH.2013.301749
11. Goldhammer H, Grasso C, Katz-Wise SL, Thomson K, Gordon AR, Keuroghlian AS. Pediatric sexual orientation and gender identity data collection in the electronic health record. *J Am Med Inform Assoc.* 2022;29(7):1303–1309. https://doi.org/10.1093/jamia/ocac048
12. Temkin D, Belford J, McDaniel T, Stratford B, Parris D. Improving measurement of sexual orientation and gender identity among middle and high school students. Available at: https://cms.childtrends.org/wp-content/uploads/2017/06/2017-23LGBTSurveyMeasuresExecSum.pdf. Accessed June 20, 2023.
13. Liu M, King D, Mayer KH, Grasso C, Keuroghlian AS. Sexual orientation and gender identity data completeness at US federally qualified health centers, 2020 and 2021. *Am J Public Health.* 2023;113(8):883–892. https://doi.org/10.2105/AJPH.2023.307323
14. McClure RC, Macumber CL, Kronk C, et al. Gender harmony: improved standards to support affirmative care of gender-marginalized people through inclusive gender and sex representation. *J Am Med Inform Assoc.* 2022;29(2):354–363. https://doi.org/10.1093/jamia/ocab196
15. Watson RJ, Wheldon CW, Puhl RM. Evidence of diverse identities in a large national sample of sexual and gender minority adolescents. *J Res Adolesc.* 2020;30(suppl 2):431–442. https://doi.org/10.1111/jora.12488
16. Haider A, Adler RR, Schneider E, et al. Assessment of patient-centered approaches to collect sexual orientation and gender identity information in the emergency department: the EQUALITY Study. *JAMA Netw Open.* 2018;1(8):e186506. https://doi.org/10.1001/jamanetworkopen.2018.6506
17. Goldhammer H, Maston ED, Kissock LA, Davis JA, Keuroghlian AS. National findings from an LGBT healthcare organizational needs assessment. *LGBT Health.* 2018;5(8):461–468. https://doi.org/10.1089/lgbt.2018.0118
18. Streed CG, Hedian HF, Bertram A, Sisson SD. Assessment of internal medicine resident preparedness to care for lesbian, gay, bisexual, transgender, and queer/questioning patients. *J Gen Intern Med.* 2019;34(6):893–898. https://doi.org/10.1007/s11606-019-04855-5
19. Pasternak RH, Alderman EM, English A. 21st Century Cures Act ONC rule: implications for adolescent care and confidentiality protections. *Pediatrics.* 2023;151(suppl 1):e2022057267K. https://doi.org/10.1542/peds.2022-057267K
20. Almazan AN, King D, Grasso C, et al. Sexual orientation and gender identity data collection at US health centers: impact of city-level structural stigma in 2018. *Am J Public Health.* 2021;111(11):2059–2063. https://doi.org/10.2105/AJPH.2021.306414

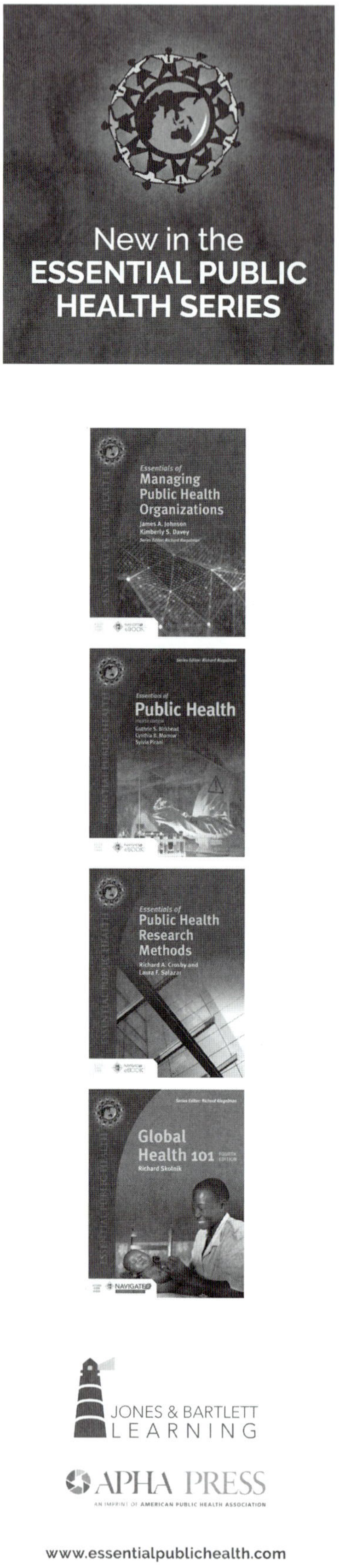

Living Systematic Reviews and Living Guidelines to Maintain the Currency of Public Health Guidelines

Rebecca K. Hodder, PhD, MAPPysc, Joshua P. Vogel, PhD, MBBS, Luke Wolfenden, PhD, and Tari Turner, PhD, MBus

ABOUT THE AUTHORS

Rebecca K. Hodder is with the College of Health Medicine and Wellbeing, The University of Newcastle, Callaghan, Australia and Hunter New England Population Health, Hunter New England Local Health District, Wallsend, Australia. Luke Wolfenden is with the College of Health Medicine and Wellbeing, The University of Newcastle, Callaghan, Australia and Cochrane Public Health, The University of Newcastle, Callaghan, Australia. Joshua P. Vogel is with the School of Public Health and Preventive Medicine, Monash University, Melbourne, Australia, and the Maternal, Child and Adolescent Health Program, Burnet Institute, Melbourne, Australia. Tari Turner is with the School of Public Health and Preventive Medicine, Monash University, Melbourne, Australia.

Globally, considerable resources and community trust are invested in the development of evidence-based guidelines for the prevention and treatment of a range of public health issues. Best practice guideline development processes draw on well-conducted systematic reviews of the contemporary evidence base to formulate recommendations. However, evidence underpinning many published public health guidelines may quickly become outdated.

Living systematic review methods, in which new research is continually identified and synthesized, can support the production of "living guidelines" that incorporate evidence into their recommendations as soon as it is available. Such processes have the potential to enhance the speed of translating the latest research evidence into public health practice and improve health outcomes. Living guidelines offer an opportunity to preserve the currency of guidelines and may be especially beneficial for priority public health issues in which the evidence base is uncertain and emerging. This opinion editorial aims to provide guidance and examples on how to apply living guidelines in public health to improve the quality of systematic reviews in public health.

PUBLIC HEALTH GUIDELINES

Guidelines are fundamental for public health to support evidence-based decision making by considering intervention options, scientific evidence to support their effects, and other important considerations (e.g., cost, equity). Ideally, they provide specific recommendations about the appropriate actions for stakeholders to take when addressing a health problem, enabling policymakers and health care providers to select the most effective interventions in the context of any feasibility or practical constraints.

Various international agencies, including the World Health Organization, the Centers for Disease Control and Prevention, and the National Health and Medical Research Council, provide standards for the process of developing public health guidelines.[1–4] Although there are subtle variations in these guideline development processes, the core expectations and processes for guideline development are consistent, including that they are informed by the best available and up-to-date evidence generated from high-quality systematic reviews.[1–5]

Traditional approaches to guideline development can be time consuming and sporadic. Guidelines can take years to produce, as they require the establishment of guideline development groups and the conduct of systematic reviews and deliberative processes that consider research evidence in the intended context. A years-long latency period between updates typically follows, often as a result of lack of funding. This means that the research evidence and the recommendations developed from that evidence can become quickly out of date, sometimes before the guideline is published. This slows translation of research evidence and delays health and health care improvements, often by many years.[6]

In the case of some topics, conclusions from research evidence remain stable over time because either little research is produced or the findings are consistent with or do not substantively challenge previous knowledge and understandings, and so no change to a recommendation is required. However, in active research areas, including priority public health research areas (e.g., COVID-19), evidence may be quickly generated with conclusions and recommendations rapidly changing. In such contexts, guideline recommendations are particularly susceptible to rapidly becoming out of date.[6] For such public health priorities, innovative solutions are required to reduce delays in the evidence to translation pathway.

LIVING SYSTEMATIC REVIEWS

Living systematic reviews (LSRs) offer an opportunity to preserve the currency of the systematic review evidence that underpins guideline recommendations. LSRs are defined as follows:

> a systematic review that is continually updated, incorporating relevant new evidence as it becomes available. . .this means continual surveillance for new research evidence through ongoing or frequent searches and the inclusion of relevant new information into the review in a timely manner so that the findings of the systematic review remain current.[7(p24)]

Proposed in 2014, the LSR approach to updating systematic review evidence adopts standard methods, albeit with a higher frequency of record searching, synthesis, and publication, specified a priori. Although the approach can be applied to any type of review, not all systematic review questions are appropriate for an LSR. Three key criteria are required to be met before an LSR is initiated: (1) the review question is a priority for decision making, (2) certainty in the existing evidence is low or very low, and (3) there is likely to be new research evidence.[7]

The feasibility of the LSR approach to updating evidence has been demonstrated in a number of case studies, including a mixed-methods evaluation that highlighted its potential for reducing time and resource requirements.[8] The feasibility of LSRs is also evidenced by their wide-scale adoption in a relatively short period of time. The first two LSRs were published in the Cochrane Library in 2017, and there are now more than 150 indexed in PubMed. Twenty LSRs have been published by Cochrane and 10 more are under way, three of which are related to public health. Published methods guidance is available to support the best practice conduct of LSRs.[9]

LIVING GUIDELINES

The application of LSR methods to guideline development is a recent innovation that addresses the issue of evidence currency and sporadic updating of guidelines. Living guidelines have been seminally defined as optimization of the guideline development process to allow updating of individual recommendations as soon as relevant new evidence becomes available.[10] Living recommendations are defined as recommendations that are updated as soon as relevant new evidence becomes available.

As with the LSR approach, a living guideline process can be applied to any health topic and applied to an entire guideline or individual recommendations. Similar to LSRs, criteria to consider whether a living guideline process is appropriate include the following: (1) the recommendation is a priority for decision making (e.g., areas of known variation in practice), (2) there is a reasonable chance that the existing recommendations will change with the emergence of new evidence, and (3) there is likely to be new research evidence emerging.[10]

Dozens of living guidelines are currently in production, with a number focused on public health priority areas, including COVID-19.[11–15] A framework for developing living practice guidelines in health care,[16] a handbook for developing living guidelines,[9] and a series of papers have recently been published to support best practice living guideline methods.[17–21]

GUIDELINE DEVELOPMENT PROCESS

Although living guideline steps are broadly similar to traditional approaches to guideline production, the more frequent generation of research evidence and subsequent guideline updates necessitates some modification to traditional approaches to enable rapid production. The following are the six key elements of traditional guideline development processes adapted for the production of living guidelines[10] (for more details, see Table A, available as a supplement to the online version of this article at http://www.ajph.org):

1. Identifying and synthesizing evidence via LSRs,
2. Generating a living evidence profile and evidence for a decision table,
3. Convening a living guideline panel and peer reviewers,
4. Engaging and supporting agencies that provide guideline approval,
5. Identifying appropriate living publication and dissemination pathways, and
6. Establishing a sufficient funding and production team.

Another important element is "living prioritization," which refers to ongoing review and consideration of which guideline recommendations meet the criteria for continual maintenance as a living approach.

CONSIDERATIONS FOR LIVING GUIDELINES IN PUBLIC HEALTH

Living guidelines have been successfully adopted across a broad range of health topics including stroke, diabetes, COVID-19, and maternal health.[14,15,22,23] Living review and guideline processes to date have been generically developed, and practical considerations for their operationalization (including methods for evidence surveillance and frequency) were discussed in a recent *Journal of Clinical Epidemiology* series.[17–21] However, there are a number of other aspects to consider when applying these methods to public health. A discussion of those we consider most important follows, including examples from existing living review and guideline development teams.

Study Designs and Outcomes

Although LSRs synthesizing research of any study design can underpin living guidelines, most to date have been applied to clinical care and treatment interventions, for which randomized controlled trials and outcomes amenable to synthesis via meta-analysis are standard. Many public health interventions and policies (e.g., COVID-19 mask mandates, infection control measures) are not as amenable to randomized designs. Therefore, evidence from nonrandomized studies, including opportunistic studies in which interventions may already have been implemented as part of standard care, may be required to form guideline recommendations. In such instances, existing public health surveillance data or existing clinical or other databases may be available for synthesis.

In addition, some important outcomes of public health interventions are not typically amenable to pooling via meta-analysis (e.g., acceptability) and are synthesized narratively. Synthesis without meta-analyses of findings from nonrandomized study designs and certain outcomes (e.g., qualitative outcomes) has the potential to increase the complexity and resource demand of LSRs and the development of living guidelines. Although these challenges require careful consideration, they are not insurmountable (see Table B, available as a supplement to the online version of this article at http://www.ajph.org).

Alignment of Research Questions and Living Guidelines

Identification of existing LSRs aligned with the focus of a living guideline can decrease resource requirements and increase feasibility. In such cases, surveillance for updated LSR results can be incorporated into the living guideline workflow. International databases of systematic reviews, such as PROSPERO[24] and Cochrane, provide a mechanism to identify prospectively registered LSRs and offer some information on progress.

The feasibility of using existing LSRs for living guidelines relies on the speed of their publication. For fast-moving public health topics (e.g., COVID-19), the possibility of existing or planned LSRs aligned with guidelines is more likely. In these cases, collaborations can be established between LSR author and guideline teams, including collaborations across guideline group jurisdictions to reduce duplication and improve efficiency. Sharing of review findings within these collaborations, including details on new studies or preprint review results, is important in enabling evidence to be incorporated into the guideline development process.

Existing LSRs may be less likely for other public health topics, and conversion of existing systematic reviews or establishment of new LSRs is required to enable a living guideline. Although there are obvious resource implications of initiating a new LSR, it allows an opportunity for direct alignment in research questions between the LSR and guideline, reducing complexity in the guideline development process.

Many challenges of using LSRs to underpin living guidelines are similar to those involved in using standard systematic reviews to inform standard guidelines. LSRs may not be updated rapidly enough, there may be multiple LSRs that cover the same trials, or LSRs might not cover the exact PICO of interest for the guideline. In these cases, existing LSRs can still be helpful in identifying studies or assessing analyses conducted by the guideline developers.

Editorial, Peer Review, and Publication Processes

Coordinated models of peer review, publication, and consideration by guideline approval agencies are necessary if LSRs and living guidelines are to provide timely and current evidence-based guideline recommendations. This can be challenging given that typical peer review to publication processes for systematic reviews can take up to 12 months, and guideline approval panels may meet less frequently than the frequency at which the living guideline is updated.

A growing number of journals and databases have modified their editorial, peer review, and publishing processes to support publication of LSRs (e.g., Cochrane, *BMJ*). The success of these editorial and publication models relies on the willingness to form close relationships and prompt communication between review author and editorial teams,[8] with time lines and expectations for submission, review, and publication mutually agreed on and adhered to. The adoption of living guidelines in public health topics will be partly influenced by how many journals recognize the potential impact of this approach and develop accommodating systems and processes.

In the case of living guidelines for which monthly or more frequent searching and synthesis of new evidence are conducted, a flexible approach to review and endorsement by guideline approval agencies outside of planned meetings may be required (see Table B). Online publication platforms are also vital for living guidelines. Platforms such as MAGICApp[25] and the Infectious Diseases Society of America's Practice Guideline App[26] can enable publication of multiple guideline versions, collaborative revision, and tracking of changes. Importantly, Web links for any derivative guidelines always take users to the most recent version of the guideline.

Resourcing and Sustainability

Similar to traditional guideline approaches, substantial resourcing (funding and people) is required to produce the initial iteration of a living guideline; however, significantly less resourcing is required to maintain the recommendations once the processes are established. In areas of public health priority that meet living guideline criteria, early experience suggests that although obtaining initial grant funding and engaging guideline development panel members are feasible,[27] sourcing ongoing funding (via grants or other mechanisms) and maintaining input over time may be challenging given that much funding operates on a project-based model. Living guidelines therefore may be most appropriate in cases in which stable funding is available (e.g., recurrent health agency funding).

Numerous technological enablers have been developed to reduce the resources required to conduct and maintain LSRs and living guidelines. This includes automation tools for database searching (e.g., machine learning) and identification of eligible research studies (e.g., crowd sourcing, Cochrane Crowd)[28] and online collaborative platforms for data extraction, analysis, and appraisal of study quality (e.g., Covidence, EPPIReviewer, Rayyan). Existing data sources (including big data) can also be leveraged for LSRs and living guidelines to reduce resource needs. Adoption of these tools can significantly reduce the resources required for evidence surveillance and generation and improve the sustainability of living guidelines (see Table B).

Living guidelines and LSRs are not intended to be maintained indefinitely. Similar to LSRs, guidance for living guidelines suggests that when any of the three criteria for considering a living guideline are not met, "living mode" should cease and instead standard guideline development methods should be adopted.[10] This can include the living guideline recommendations no longer being a priority for decision makers (e.g., reduced prevalence or mortality of a condition); high certainty of the evidence, in which case new evidence would be unlikely to change recommendations; or no active studies or new evidence of existing or new intervention approaches being imminent. This situation can apply to an entire guideline or recommendations within the guideline, and regular reviews against the criteria should be conducted to determine the ongoing appropriateness of a living approach (see Table B).

Knowledge Translation and Implementation

Knowledge translation is a key issue for living guidelines, and given the novelty of the approach there is still much to learn. The benefits of reliable, continually updated recommendations for public health and health care will be realized only if communication, dissemination and implementation strategies are in place that can respond on the time cycle of guideline updates.[29] Newsletters, social media, app-based notification systems, and other flexible, dynamic approaches are likely to be needed. It is vital that knowledge translation mechanisms are in place that clearly communicate the "what is new" in each updated version of the guideline so that health decision makers can remain up to date with recommendations as they are revised.

Concerns have been raised about potential knowledge translation challenges caused by "flip-flopping" recommendations; however, this has not occurred in our experience so far. Usually, knowledge translation efforts focus on "strong" guideline recommendations for which there is a high level of certainty in the underlying evidence. In their nature and with respect to both stroke and COVID-19 guidelines,[22] these types of recommendations established from a high level of certainty in the evidence have not substantively changed over time. In contrast, "conditional" or "weak" recommendations, in which the evidence is evolving and certainty in the evidence is low, are more likely to change over time and typically are not used to generate recommendations until the certainty of the evidence is higher.

There has been some limited investigation regarding the process of implementing updated living guideline recommendations[30] proportionate to their stage of innovation. The ongoing establishment of living guidelines and the creation of new guidelines will enable further investigation.

CONCLUSIONS

Living guidelines underpinned by LSRs offer an innovative, feasible, and effective solution to improving research on translation pathways by maintaining the currency of public health guidelines and ensuring that recommendations are based on the most up-to-date evidence. Although the feasibility of living guidelines for clinical care–focused public health topics has been demonstrated, adoption of living guidelines for other public health topics is evolving. Given the considerable potential for public health benefit, further application of living guidelines to other public health topics that meet living guideline criteria is warranted. AJPH

CORRESPONDENCE

Correspondence should be sent to Rebecca K Hodder, PhD, MAPPysc, Locked Bag 10, Wallsend, New South Wales 2287, Australia (e-mail: rebecca.hodder@health.nsw.gov.au). Reprints can be ordered at http://www.ajph.org by clicking the "Reprints" link.

PUBLICATION INFORMATION

Full Citation: Hodder RK, Vogel JP, Wolfenden L, Turner T. Living systematic reviews and living guidelines to maintain the currency of public health guidelines. *Am J Public Health*. 2024;114(1):21–26.

Acceptance Date: September 9, 2023.

DOI: https://doi.org/10.2105/AJPH.2023.307450

CONTRIBUTORS

All of the authors contributed to the drafting of the article and provided critical reviews.

ACKNOWLEDGMENTS

Rebecca K. Hodder is supported by an Australia National Health and Medical Research Council (NHMRC) early career fellowship (APP1160419). Luke Wolfenden is funded by an NHMRC investigator grant (APP1197022).

CONFLICTS OF INTEREST

The authors report no known conflicts of interest.

REFERENCES

1. Carande-Kulis V. CDC Guideline Development and Reporting Checklist. Available at: https://stacks.cdc.gov/view/cdc/81405. Accessed June 15, 2022.
2. National Health and Medical Research Council. 2016 NHMRC standards for guidelines. Available at: https://www.nhmrc.gov.au/guidelinesforguidelines/standards. Accessed June 15, 2022.
3. National Institute for Health and Care Excellence. How we develop NICE guidelines. Available at: https://www.nice.org.uk/about/what-we-do/our-programmes/nice-guidance/nice-guidelines/how-we-develop-nice-guidelines. Accessed June 15, 2022.
4. *WHO Handbook for Guideline Development*. 2nd ed. Geneva, Switzerland: World Health Organization; 2014.
5. Turner T, Misso M, Harris C, Green S. Development of evidence-based clinical practice guidelines (CPGs): comparing approaches. *Implement Sci*. 2008;3(1):45. https://doi.org/10.1186/1748-5908-3-45
6. Martínez García L, Sanabria AJ, García Alvarez E, et al. The validity of recommendations from clinical guidelines: a survival analysis. *CMAJ*. 2014;186(16):1211–1219. https://doi.org/10.1503/cmaj.140547
7. Elliott JH, Synnot A, Turner T, et al. Living systematic review: 1. Introduction—the why, what, when, and how. *J Clin Epidemiol*. 2017;91:23–30. https://doi.org/10.1016/j.jclinepi.2017.08.010
8. Millard T, Synnot A, Elliott J, Green S, McDonald S, Turner T. Feasibility and acceptability of living systematic reviews: results from a mixed-methods evaluation. *Syst Rev*. 2019;8(1):325. https://doi.org/10.1186/s13643-019-1248-5
9. Brooker J, Synnot A, McDonald S, et al. Guidance for the production and publication of Cochrane living systematic reviews: Cochrane Reviews in living mode. Available at: https://community.cochrane.org/sites/default/files/uploads/inline-files/Transform/201912_LSR_Revised_Guidance.pdf. Accessed June 15, 2022.
10. Akl EA, Meerpohl JJ, Elliott J, Kahale LA, Schünemann HJ. Living systematic reviews: 4. Living guideline recommendations. *J Clin Epidemiol*. 2017;91:47–53. https://doi.org/10.1016/j.jclinepi.2017.08.009
11. Lamontagne F, Agarwal A, Rochwerg B, et al. A living WHO guideline on drugs for covid-19. *BMJ*. 2020;370:m3379. https://doi.org/10.1136/bmj.m3379
12. English C, Bayley M, Hill K, et al. Bringing stroke clinical guidelines to life. *Int J Stroke*. 2019;14(4):337–339. https://doi.org/10.1177/1747493019833015
13. Tendal B, Vogel J, McDonald S, et al. Weekly updates of national living evidence-based guidelines: methods for the Australian Living Guidelines for Care of People with COVID-19. *J Clin Epidemiol*. 2021;131:11–21.
14. Vogel JP, Dowswell T, Lewin S, et al. Developing and applying a 'living guidelines' approach to WHO recommendations on maternal and perinatal health. *BMJ Glob Health*. 2019;4(4):e001683.
15. White H, Tendal B, Elliott J, Turner T, Andrikopoulos S, Zoungas S. Breathing life into Australian diabetes clinical guidelines. *Med J Aust*. 2020;212(6):250–251.e1. https://doi.org/10.5694/mja2.50509
16. El Mikati IK, Khabsa J, Harb T, et al. A framework for the development of living practice guidelines in health care. *Ann Intern Med*. 2022;175(8):1154–1160. https://doi.org/10.7326/M22-0514
17. Cheyne S, Fraile Navarro D, Buttery AK, et al. Methods for living guidelines: early guidance based on practical experience. Paper 3: selecting and prioritizing questions for living guidelines. *J Clin Epidemiol*. 2023;155:73–83. https://doi.org/10.1016/j.jclinepi.2022.12.021
18. Cheyne S, Fraile Navarro D, Hill K, et al. Methods for living guidelines: early guidance based on practical experience. Paper 1: introduction. *J Clin Epidemiol*. 2023;155:84–96. https://doi.org/10.1016/j.jclinepi.2022.12.024
19. Fraile Navarro D, Cheyne S, Hill K, et al. Methods for living guidelines: early guidance based on practical experience. Paper 5: decisions on methods for evidence synthesis and recommendation development for living guidelines. *J Clin Epidemiol*. 2023;155:118–128. https://doi.org/10.1016/j.jclinepi.2022.12.022
20. McDonald S, Sharp S, Morgan RL, Murad MH, Fraile Navarro D. Methods for living guidelines: early guidance based on practical experience. Paper 4: search methods and approaches for living guidelines. *J Clin Epidemiol*. 2023;155:108–117. https://doi.org/10.1016/j.jclinepi.2022.12.023
21. Synnot A, Hill K, Davey J, et al. Methods for living guidelines: early guidance based on practical experience. Paper 2: consumer engagement in living guidelines. *J Clin Epidemiol*. 2023;155:97–107. https://doi.org/10.1016/j.jclinepi.2022.12.020
22. Hill K, English C, Campbell BC, et al. Feasibility of national living guideline methods: the Australian Stroke Guidelines. *J Clin Epidemiol*. 2022;142:184–193. https://doi.org/10.1016/j.jclinepi.2021.11.020
23. White H, McDonald SJ, Barber B, et al. Care for adults with COVID-19: living guidelines from the National COVID-19 Clinical Evidence Taskforce.

Med J Aust. 2022;217(7):368–378. https://doi.org/10.5694/mja2.51718

24. National Institute for Health and Care Research. PROSPERO. Available at: https://www.crd.york.ac.uk/prospero. Accessed July 20, 2023.
25. MAGIC. Making Grade the Irresistible Choice (MAGIC). Available at: https://magicevidence.org. Accessed July 20, 2023.
26. Infectious Diseases Society of America. IDSA Practice Guidelines App. Available at: https://www.idsociety.org/practice-guideline/IDSA-practice-guidelines-app. Accessed July 20, 2023.
27. Turner T, Elliott J, Tendal B, et al. The Australian living guidelines for the clinical care of people with COVID-19: what worked, what didn't and why, a mixed methods process evaluation. *PLoS One*. 2022;17(1):e0261479. https://doi.org/10.1371/journal.pone.0261479
28. Thomas J, Noel-Storr A, Marshall I, et al. Living systematic reviews: 2. Combining human and machine effort. *J Clin Epidemiol*. 2017;91:31–37. https://doi.org/10.1016/j.jclinepi.2017.08.011
29. Wolfenden L, Mooney K, Gonzalez S, et al. Increased use of knowledge translation strategies is associated with greater research impact on public health policy and practice: an analysis of trials of nutrition, physical activity, sexual health, tobacco, alcohol and substance use interventions. *Health Res Policy Syst*. 2022;20(1):15. https://doi.org/10.1186/s12961-022-00817-2
30. Lynch EA, Lassig C, Turner T, Churilov L, Hill K, Shrubsole K. Prioritizing guideline recommendations for implementation: a systematic, consumer-inclusive process with a case study using the Australian Clinical Guidelines for Stroke Management. *Health Res Policy Syst*. 2021;19(1):85. https://doi.org/10.1186/s12961-021-00734-w

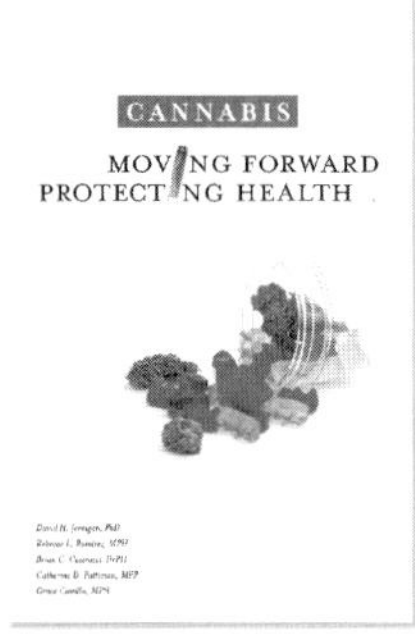

2021 | 300PP | SOFTCOVER
978-087553-3179

APHABOOKSTORE.ORG

Cannabis: Moving Forward, Protecting Health

Edited by: David H. Jernigan, PhD, Rebecca L. Ramirez MPH, Brian C. Castrucci, DrPH, Catherine D. Patterson, MPP, Grace Castillo, MPH

This new book addresses the ongoing debate on cannabis policy and provides guidance on how to regulate its sale and distribution. Instead of taking a stance for or against cannabis use, the book:

- suggests we employ strategies similar to those used in alcohol control to create a solid foundation of policy and best practices;
- focuses on how we can best regulate a complex substance.

APHA PRESS
AN IMPRINT OF AMERICAN PUBLIC HEALTH ASSOCIATION

Built Environment and Public Health: More Than 20 Years of Progress

Kimberly A. Rollings, PhD, MS, Andrew L. Dannenberg, MD, MPH, Howard Frumkin, DrPH, MD, MPH, and Richard J. Jackson, MD, MPH

ABOUT THE AUTHORS

Kimberly A. Rollings is with the Health & Design Research Fellowship Program, University of Michigan Medical School, the Institute for Healthcare Policy and Innovation, and the Institute for Social Research, University of Michigan, Ann Arbor. Andrew L. Dannenberg is with the Department of Environmental and Occupational Health Sciences, School of Public Health, and the Department of Urban Design and Planning, College of Built Environments, University of Washington, Seattle. Howard Frumkin is with the Department of Environmental and Occupational Health Sciences, School of Public Health, University of Washington, and the Land and People Lab, Trust for Public Land, San Francisco, CA. Richard J. Jackson is with the Department of Environmental Health Sciences, Fielding School of Public Health, University of California, Los Angeles.

Fall 2023 marked 20 years since the *AJPH* "Built Environment and Health" (BEH) special issue.[1] The issue highlighted the reengagement of health and design professions and growing interest in the built environment's potential to improve health. Public health and urban planning linkages were not new. Late 19th- and early 20th-century efforts to improve air, water, food, and housing quality; sanitation; and workplace safety contributed to better quality of life and increased life expectancy (Table G, reference 1, available as a supplement to the online version of this article at http://www.ajph.org). The sectors became isolated over time, with little collaboration until recent decades.

The anniversary of the special issue offers an opportunity to inventory progress in BEH: combined perspectives from public health, urban planning, architecture, transportation, and related fields on how the physical components of where we live, work, learn, and play influence health. The following sections contain an overview of BEH progress in research, practice, education, and policy, as well as current context and future priorities.

RESEARCH

BEH research increased dramatically from 2003 to 2022. Figure 1 and Table C (available as a supplement to the online version of this article at http://www.ajph.org; see also Table A, available as a supplement to the online version of this article at http://www.ajph.org) demonstrate this trend based on Web of Science, Scopus, PubMed, and CINAHL (nursing and allied health) database searches for peer-reviewed "built environment" and "health" articles. PsycInfo (social and behavioral sciences), TRID (transportation), and JSTOR-Architecture database searches also indicated modest increases (Table C). Additional increases in research on specific BEH topics according to PubMed were found, including research on health and climate change, nature, land use, parks, architecture, and active transportation (Figure 2 and Table D, available as a supplement to the online version of this article at http://www.ajph.org; see also Table B, available as a supplement to the online version of this article at http://www.ajph.org).

Early BEH research addressed influences of toxic environmental exposures, zoning laws, building codes, and healthy housing and communities on asthma, injury, violence, healthy and unhealthy food consumption, mental health, social capital, and health inequities.[1] Awareness increased regarding the benefits of denser, more walkable, and less automobile-dependent settings, as well as the accessibility, mobility, and livability needs of the growing aging population. Later research emphasized environmental sustainability and healthy settings within the context of climate change, resilience, and the green building movement. Recognition of the importance of nature, greenspace, and parks significantly increased over time, especially during the COVID-19 pandemic (Table G, reference 2).[2]

A substantial body of BEH research focused on the built environment and physical activity within the context of the obesity epidemic. Work on automobile dependence, traffic safety, walking and biking, commuting, and sedentary time was primarily driven by the Robert Wood Johnson Foundation's Active Living Research initiative to promote active living via environment, policy, and practice improvements.[3,4] Research linked specific building and community features to health outcomes, enabling more effective interventions such as appealing stairways, ample sidewalks, and vibrant activity centers.[5]

The business case for health-promoting, walkable places was

AJPH January 2024, Vol. 114, No. 1

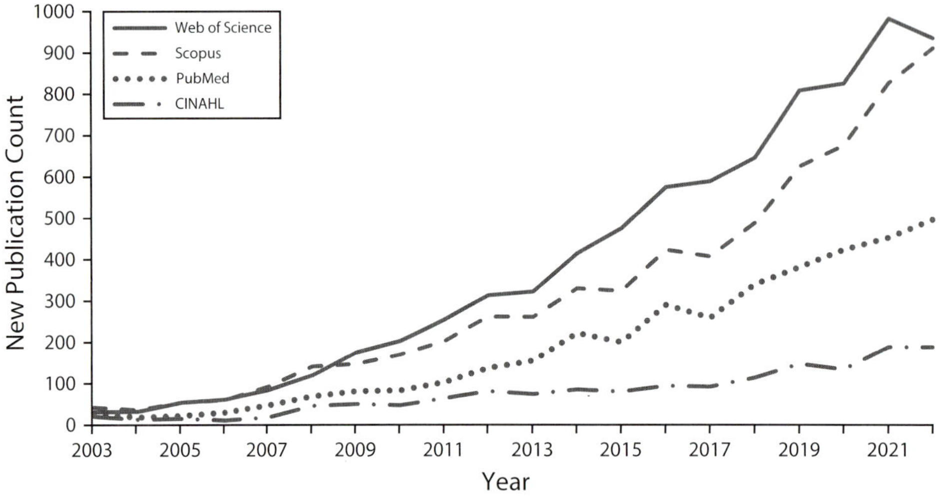

FIGURE 1— Built Environment and Health Articles Indexed by Four Databases, 2003–2022

Note. CINAHL = Cumulated Index to Nursing and Allied Health Literature. Database search expressions are available in Supplemental Table A (available as a supplement to the online version of this article at https://www.ajph.org).

documented.[6] Unintended consequences, including gentrification and displacement, of interventions aimed at improving health among people from racial and ethnic minority groups and of lower incomes were increasingly recognized, resulting in more research focused on how to mitigate these risks.[7] The history of structural racism, segregation, redlining, neighborhood disinvestment, health inequities, and disparities in walkability, housing, and

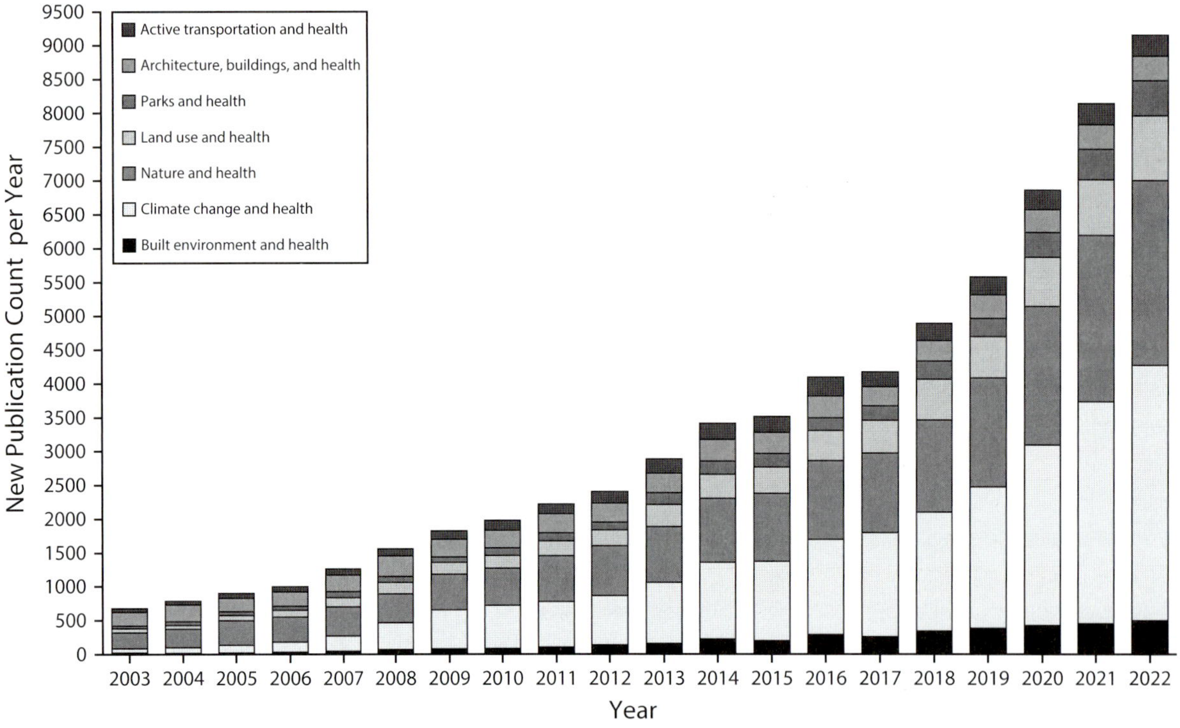

FIGURE 2— Built Environment and Health Topics Indexed by PubMed, 2003–2022

Note. Database search expressions are available in Supplemental Table B (available as a supplement to the online version of this article at https://www.ajph.org).

greenspace access was only recently widely acknowledged.[8]

Numerous books (Table E, available as a supplement to the online version of this article at http://www.ajph.org) and dozens of BEH measures (e.g., walkability [https://www.walkscore.com], access to parks [https://www.tpl.org/ParkScore], livability [http://www.livabilityIndex.AARP.org], and brain health [https://cognability.isr.umich.edu]) were also published, reflecting the growth and maturation of the field. In addition, new data sources, analytic techniques, and technologies emerged. New data sources were created to support research, inform policy, and promote equity (e.g., City Health Dashboard [https://www.cityhealthdashboard.com], National Zoning Atlas [https://www.zoningatlas.org], ParkServe [https://www.tpl.org/parkserve], and Urban Displacement Project [https://www.urbandisplacement.org]). New analytic techniques associated with geospatial mapping, satellite imagery, sensors, drones, Google Street View, social media text and Web scraping, and artificial intelligence enabled advanced study of BEH linkages.[9]

Technological advancements facilitated the development of micromobility (e.g., e-bikes, e-scooters), rideshares (e.g., Lyft, Uber), shared lodging (e.g., Airbnb, VRBO), and electric and autonomous vehicles. The effects of these evolving technologies on land use, housing, economic and community development, traffic patterns, transportation planning and infrastructure, air quality, and associated health outcomes require further research and evaluation (Table G, reference 3).[10]

PRACTICE

Professional organizations across disciplines established BEH committees and working groups (Table F, available as a supplement to the online version of this article at http://www.ajph.org), promoting healthy building and community design through conferences, reports, training, and advocacy (e.g., https://www.15minutecity.com). Health impact assessments (HIAs) were used to consider potential health impacts of proposed projects and programs and identify disproportionately affected populations as well as how to mitigate adverse effects.[9,11,12] HIAs improved collaboration, amplified community member voices, increased awareness of health issues, and informed decision makers, but the time and resources required to complete HIAs limited their success.[12]

Cross-disciplinary public health, planning, policy, real estate, architecture, engineering, transportation, and public–private partnership efforts, along with Complete Streets approaches (https://highways.dot.gov/complete-streets), improved pedestrian infrastructure and safety. The adoption of Walk Score by real estate marketing groups reflected the value renters and homeowners placed on walkability. Local governments hired chief innovation officers who used data-driven approaches, human-centered and participatory design, and behavioral research to improve operations, including access to social and behavioral health services, healthy food, and vaccines (Table G, reference 4).

Design professionals (e.g., urban planners, architects, landscape architects, and developers) also paid more attention to BEH and synergies with environmental sustainability (Table G, reference 5).[9,13,14] Fitwel (https://www.fitwel.org) and WELL Building Certification (https://www.wellcertified.com) programs promoted occupant safety, physical activity, nutrition, and well-being via building design, operations, and maintenance. Sustainable building rating systems, such as the Living Building Challenge (https://living-future.org/lbc), added criteria for water, health, happiness, and equity (Table G, reference 6). Enterprise Green Communities (https://www.GreenCommunitiesonline.org), a national green building certification program for affordable housing, outlined "healthy living environment" criteria for indoor environmental quality, active design, universal design, and healing-centered design. Other Enterprise Communities initiatives engaged public health professionals to address resident health before and after occupancy.

EDUCATION AND TRAINING

New higher education coursework, concurrent degree programs, and training opportunities introduced healthy design principles in public health, planning, and architecture programs, although accreditation requirements continue to exclude BEH criteria. As of 2022, 15 institutions offered concurrent masters of public health–urban planning degree programs (https://bephc.org/tier-4). Several accredited architecture and design programs increased available BEH-related coursework, programming, and research opportunities, as well as concentrations and certificates focused on health, beyond health care. Outcomes of these nascent programs require tracking and evaluation.

POLICY

Renewed interest in BEH informed policy across multiple government levels.[9] The Centers for Disease Control and Prevention (CDC) Community Guide (https://thecommunityguide.org)

identified evidence, gaps, resources, presentation and communications materials, and successful implementation stories related to population health and the built environment. The 2013 "Health in All Policies" approach promoted by the CDC, the American Public Health Association, and the World Health Organization aimed to improve population health and health equity by focusing on the health implications of decisions and building synergies across sectors.

In 2015, the United States adopted the United Nations' 2030 Agenda for Sustainable Development. The agenda established 17 Sustainable Development Goals, all of which related to determinants of health and 11 of which related to building and construction (Table G, reference 7). The 2021 US Bipartisan Infrastructure Law (https://www.whitehouse.gov/build) recognized that significant federal government investment was necessary to upgrade outdated infrastructure, address vacant buildings, and relocate roadways that divided communities, among other health-related built environment interventions.[15]

Several states incorporated healthy housing criteria into their Low-Income Housing Tax Credit program allocation processes (Table G, reference 8). This program is the largest federal funding source for affordable multifamily rental housing. City Health Rankings (https://www.cityhealth.org) inventoried 17 healthy city policies (eight of which were BEH relevant) in 49 US cities between 2017 and 2022. The Americans with Disabilities Act continued to prompt local sidewalk and other accessibility improvements.

In addition, innovative tax policies and financing that incentivized healthy community development and protected affordable housing (e.g., Community Land Trusts) were implemented. Hundreds of municipalities replaced conventional zoning codes with "form-based codes" that emphasized more pedestrian-friendly, compact, mixed-use, and transit-oriented development with various housing types (Table G, reference 9). Some policies and resulting built environment improvements had unintended consequences with adverse impacts on health, including inequitable distribution, gentrification, and displacement among community members and businesses, especially when meaningful community input was lacking.[16,17]

CURRENT CONTEXT

The built environment is now widely recognized as a determinant of health and equity. BEH is often integrated into strategies addressing major societal challenges such as racism, COVID-19, and the climate crisis. Despite increased acknowledgment and understanding of structural racism and resulting inequities, especially those exacerbated by COVID-19, government strategies to reduce systemic inequities have yet to be widely implemented or evaluated.[9,11]

The recent Justice40 Initiative (https://www.whitehouse.gov/environmentaljustice/justice40) aims to direct 40% of federal climate change–related investment benefits (e.g., clean water, energy, and transit; affordable, sustainable housing; pollution remediation) to communities that are marginalized and overburdened by pollution. New York City's Where We Live NYC Plan, a fair housing plan, and Local Law 78 require that certain development applicants submit racial equity reports. These reports contain analyses of demographic conditions, quality of life, access to opportunity, housing security, and displacement risk (https://EquitableExplorer.Planning.NYC.gov/map/drm/nta) using the Equitable Development Data Explorer (https://www.nyc.gov/site/planning/data-maps/edde/edde-overview.page). Although not exclusively motivated by health, establishment of racial equity frameworks and health equity teams, among other displacement mitigation and prevention measures, offers potential strategies to advance health equity.[11,18]

The COVID-19 pandemic demonstrated the built environment's potential to exacerbate or mitigate the spread and impact of infectious diseases. Many conventional building ventilation systems were not equipped to provide ample air exchanges. Crowded microenvironments, including restaurants, bars, and transit vehicles, were loci of disease transmission, especially for people with low incomes and few alternatives. On the positive side, the importance of parks and outdoor spaces was highlighted. Vehicular traffic was reduced where streets were repurposed for walking, cycling, shopping, dining, and outdoor classes, creating inspiring models of human-centered urban space utilization. The pandemic diverted people from public transport toward automobiles—an unhealthy shift over time—and increased working from home, with unknown long-term consequences for business district vitality, urban sprawl, and health. Our understanding of the lasting effects of COVID-19 related to BEH, including effects on loneliness and isolation,[19] is still evolving.[2,9]

The intensifying climate crisis stresses the urgency with which planning, policy, and resilient housing and infrastructure are required to reduce existing and prevent anticipated adverse health consequences.[9,20,21] More extreme weather events; rising temperatures, pollution, sea levels, and carbon dioxide levels; and loss of biodiversity will contribute to population migration, crowding, infectious diseases, and other negative health consequences, especially for populations at higher risk. Solutions will require improvements to land use; protection of natural areas; housing; heating, cooling, and ventilation systems; transportation; and infrastructure (Table G, reference 10).[22–25] The built environment will play an essential role in both mitigating and adapting to climate change and improving health, equity, and resilience.

FUTURE PRIORITIES

Addressing challenges associated with health inequities and racism, lasting effects of the COVID-19 pandemic, and the intensifying climate crisis requires careful study, redesign, and rebuilding of environments with health and equity as priorities. First, future interdisciplinary research agendas[9] and cross-sector action plans—focused on health equity, resilience to climate change, and understanding BEH effects across populations and contexts—are needed for widespread translation to best practices and policy. The following domains can organize future interdisciplinary BEH work[9]; effective solutions will depend on good governance, intersectoral problem solving, citizen participation, and prioritizing equity:

1. Safe, healthy, and affordable housing and aging in place
2. Food security, health, and nutrition
3. Active living assets and facilities
4. Vacant property reclamation and urban greening
5. Neighborhood and community design
6. Regional and local infrastructure, especially related to transportation and energy
7. Disaster resilience, including preparedness for large-scale migration

Design practitioners require evidence-based approaches to expand priorities from energy efficiency, capital costs, and life-cycle costs to encompass health and equity in building and infrastructure projects. Further research to support the business case for healthier built environments is critical to these market-driven professions and to attracting large-scale investment and policymaker attention. Zoning and building code reforms for health and equity, beyond minimal health, safety, and accessibility requirements, are necessary to make healthy building and equitable community development routine practice.[11] Such codes inform professional education requirements, program accreditation, licensing, and standard professional practices. Approaches that recognize how the framing of BEH communications influences reception of research, policy, and advocacy are vital to facilitating action and implementation.[14] Improved translation and dissemination may also attract more resources to support underfunded BEH research and translation efforts.

Second, effective training of future leadership and the workforce to solve complex societal challenges requires BEH components.[9] There is a mismatch between the knowledge and skills required of health and design professionals and available training opportunities. Effective education and training rely on the following:

1. Identifying discipline-specific standardized competencies
2. Updating curricular requirements to include BEH coursework reflective of standardized competencies by accreditation agencies (Council on Education for Public Health, Planning Accreditation Board, National Architectural Accrediting Board, Landscape Architectural Accreditation Board, Council for Interior Design Accreditation, Accreditation Board for Engineering and Technology)
3. Adding BEH content to professional licensing criteria and continuing education requirements
4. Emphasizing the field's interdisciplinary nature and the importance of cross-disciplinary collaboration, maximizing impact, health equity, and environmental justice[14]
5. Strengthening career preparation via degree, certification, and training programs that offer discipline-specific practical applications, real-world experiences, and internships
6. Defining career pathways and aligning education and training with real-world needs by tracking program graduates and partnering with employers
7. Increasing continuing education and training opportunities for professionals requiring BEH skills (e.g., in urban planning and public health departments)
8. Focusing attention on diversity, equity, and inclusion in program content, participants, and instructors as well as pathways for recruiting

Third, a fundamental shift in how built environment policy and design are used to promote health is required.[11,21] Federal, state, and local incentives, regulations, and decision making must consider health and equity. Priorities often focus on up-front costs, short-term benefits, or the prevalence of a single disease.[11] Governments can incentivize longer-term thinking and more equitable distribution of opportunities, economic resources, and healthy environments in several ways, including by prioritizing maintenance and upkeep rather than only new growth. New approaches should be considered that achieve a better balance between profit as a primary driver of development, environmental sustainability, and social priorities including health and equity.

Such shifts in policy and decision making will require transparent processes, power shifts toward communities, ongoing evaluations, and course corrections, especially when making decisions under time and resource pressures. Engaging communities and learning from lived experiences, especially those of individuals experiencing systemic racism and neighborhood disinvestment, are essential to build trust between affected populations and decision makers.[14] Engagement ensures that design and implementation of policies, programs, and interventions account for unique community needs, are culturally competent, and build on community assets.[11]

CONCLUSION

In summary, BEH is now an established field with more than 20 years of substantial growth in research, education, practice, and policy.[9] Public health approaches to the built environment have broadened; research, practice, and policy have been informed by new evidence and methodologies; cross-disciplinary work has increased; and the importance of community engagement and equity has been emphasized. A strong foundation of evidence now exists to inform future work. Inequity and racism, pandemics, and climate change represent some of the greatest current global challenges and require careful study, redesign, and rebuilding of environments with health and equity as priorities. Although these challenges have the potential to permanently alter the planet and severely threaten population health without immediate and appropriate action,[14] they also present historic opportunities to create and redevelop more equitable, sustainable, resilient, and healthy built environments. AJPH

CORRESPONDENCE

Correspondence should be sent to Kimberly A. Rollings, PhD, MS, Institute for Healthcare Policy and Innovation, North Campus Research Complex, 2800 Plymouth Rd, Building #14, Room G100-22, Ann Arbor, MI 48109-2800 (e-mail: kirollin@umich.edu). Reprints can be ordered at http://www.ajph.org by clicking the "Reprints" link.

PUBLICATION INFORMATION

Full Citation: Rollings KA, Dannenberg AL, Frumkin H, Jackson RJ. Built environment and public health: more than 20 years of progress. *Am J Public Health*. 2024;114(1):27–33.

Acceptance Date: September 9, 2023.

DOI: https://doi.org/10.2105/AJPH.2023.307451

CONTRIBUTORS

All of the authors contributed to the conception of the article and revised subsequent drafts. K. A. Rollings led the writing, research, and literature review.

ACKNOWLEDGMENTS

Kimberly A. Rollings was supported by the University of Michigan Health & Design Research Fellowship Program.

We thank the researchers, educators, practitioners, policymakers, community partners, and students who contribute to built environment and health work.

CONFLICTS OF INTEREST

The authors report that they have no conflicts of interest.

REFERENCES

1. Jackson RJ. The impact of the built environment on health: an emerging field. *Am J Public Health*. 2003;93(9):1382–1384. https://doi.org/10.2105/AJPH.93.9.1382
2. Frumkin H. COVID-19, the built environment, and health. *Environ Health Perspect*. 2021;129(7):075001. https://doi.org/10.1289/EHP8888
3. Sallis JF, Linton LS, Kraft MK, et al. The Active Living Research program: six years of grantmaking. *Am J Prev Med*. 2009;36(2):S10–S21. https://doi.org/10.1016/j.amepre.2008.10.007
4. Barker D, Gutman M. Evaluation of Active Living Research: ten years of progress in building a new field. *Am J Prev Med*. 2014;46(2):208–215. https://doi.org/10.1016/j.amepre.2013.10.003
5. Feng J, Glass T, Curriero F, Stewart W, Schwartz B. The built environment and obesity: a systematic review of the epidemiologic evidence. *Health Place*. 2010;16(2):175–190. https://doi.org/10.1016/j.healthplace.2009.09.008
6. Hack G. Business performance in walkable shopping areas. Available at: https://activelivingresearch.org/sites/activelivingresearch.org/files/BusinessPerformanceWalkableShoppingAreas_Nov2013.pdf. Accessed August 11, 2023.
7. Newman K, Wyly E. The right to stay put, revisited: gentrification and resistance to displacement in New York City. *Urban Stud*. 2006;43(1):23–57. https://doi.org/10.1080/00420980500388710
8. Nardone A, Chiang J, Corburn J. Historic redlining and urban health today in U.S. cities. *Environ Justice*. 2020;13(4):109–119. https://doi.org/10.1089/env.2020.0011
9. Botchwey N, Dannenberg AL, Frumkin H, eds. *Making Healthy Places: Designing and Building for Well-Being, Equity, and Sustainability*. 2nd ed. Washington, DC: Island Press; 2022.
10. Rojas-Rueda D, Nieuwenhuijsen M, Khreis H, Frumkin H. Autonomous vehicles and public health. *Annu Rev Public Health*. 2020;41:329–345. https://doi.org/10.1146/annurev-publhealth-040119-094035
11. Fedorowicz M, Schilling J, Bramhall E, Bieretz B, Su Y, Brown S. Leveraging the built environment for health equity. Available at: https://www.urban.org/sites/default/files/publication/102557/leveraging-the-built-environment-for-health-equity.pdf. Accessed August 11, 2023.
12. Dannenberg AL. Effectiveness of health impact assessments: a synthesis of data from five impact evaluation reports. *Prev Chronic Dis*. 2016;13:150559. https://doi.org/10.5888/pcd13.150559
13. Dannenberg AL, Burpee H. Architecture for health is not just for healthcare architects. *HERD*. 2018;11(2):8–12. https://doi.org/10.1177/1937586718772955
14. Association of Schools and Programs of Public Health. Responding to the climate change and health crisis: a framework for academic public health. Available at: https://aspph-prod-web-assets.s3.amazonaws.com/CCH-Framework-Summary.pdf. Accessed August 11, 2023.
15. Jain B, Bajaj SS, Stanford FC. All infrastructure is health infrastructure. *Am J Public Health*. 2022;112(1):24–26. https://doi.org/10.2105/AJPH.2021.306595
16. Tagtachian DA, Barefoot NN, Harreveld AL. Building by right: social equity implications of transitioning to form-based code. Available at: https://repository.law.miami.edu/cgi/viewcontent.cgi?article=1735&context=fac_articles. Accessed August 11, 2023.
17. Schnake-Mahl AS, Jahn JL, Subramanian S, Waters MC, Arcaya M. Gentrification, neighborhood change, and population health: a systematic review. *J Urban Health*. 2020;97(1):1–25. https://doi.org/10.1007/s11524-019-00400-1
18. Serrano N, Realmuto L, Graff KA, et al. Healthy community design, anti-displacement, and equity strategies in the USA: a scoping review. *J Urban*

Health. 2023;100(1):151–180. https://doi.org/10.1007/s11524-022-00698-4

19. U.S. Department of Health and Human Services, Office of the Surgeon General. Our epidemic of loneliness and isolation: the U.S. surgeon general's advisory on the healing effects of social connection and community. Available at: https://www.hhs.gov/sites/default/files/surgeon-general-social-connection-advisory.pdf. Accessed August 11, 2023.
20. Wang H, Horton R. Tackling climate change: the greatest opportunity for global health. *Lancet*. 2015;386(10006):1798–1799. https://doi.org/10.1016/S0140-6736(15)60931-X
21. No public health without planetary health. *Lancet Public Health*. 2022;7(4):e291. https://doi.org/10.1016/S2468-2667(22)00068-8
22. Hernández D. Climate justice starts at home: building resilient housing to reduce disparate impacts from climate change in residential settings. *Am J Public Health*. 2022;112(1):66–68. https://doi.org/10.2105/AJPH.2021.306611
23. Lin BB, Ossola A, Alberti M, et al. Integrating solutions to adapt cities for climate change. *Lancet Planet Health*. 2021;5(7):e479–e486. https://doi.org/10.1016/S2542-5196(21)00135-2
24. Santos MM, Lanzinha JC, Ferreira AV. Review on urbanism and climate change. *Cities*. 2021;114:103176. https://doi.org/10.1016/j.cities.2021.103176
25. Hsu D, Andrews CJ, Han AT, Loh CG, Osland AC, Zegras CP. Planning the built environment and land use towards deep decarbonization of the United States. *J Plann Lit*. 38(3):088541222210979. https://doi.org/10.1177/08854122221097977

is your organization
an **APHA** member?

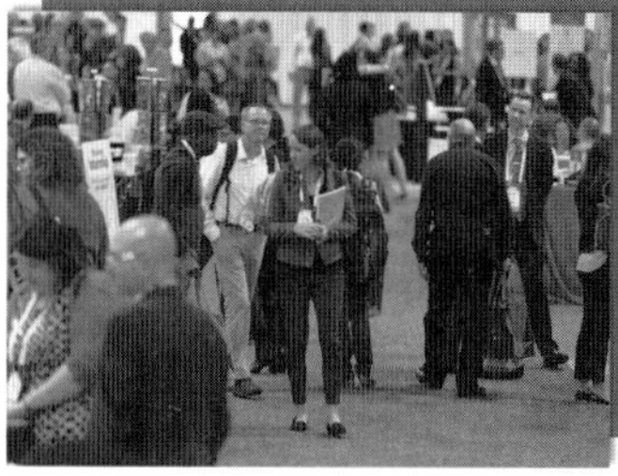

Nonprofits, government agencies and educational institutions play an important role in public health. But did you know they can also be members of APHA?

As an APHA agency member, you get discounts on ads in APHA publications and job postings on Public Health CareerMart.

And your employees receive registration discounts for APHA's Annual Meeting and Expo and savings of up to $150 on individual APHA membership.

Become an APHA agency member today!

For details, call **202-777-3914**
or visit **www.apha.org/membership**.

APHA
AMERICAN PUBLIC HEALTH ASSOCIATION

Wastewater-Informed Digital Advertising as a COVID-19 Geotargeted Neighborhood Intervention: Jefferson County, Kentucky, 2021–2022

Lauren B. Anderson, MPA, Heather D. Ness, MPH, Rochelle H. Holm, PhD, and Ted Smith, PhD

We sought to deliver a geotargeted digital health advertising intervention. We assessed risk of community infection through an integrated public health and wastewater rubric and delivered advertisements between November 2021 and April 2022 in Louisville, Kentucky. The average daily click-through rates for the campaigns were 0.19%, 0.15%, and 0.13%. Results show potential for digital public health interventions that are geographically anchored to subcity sewersheds and community interest and willingness to engage with targeted wastewater-themed public health messaging. (*Am J Public Health*. 2024;114(1):34–37. https://doi.org/10.2105/AJPH.2023.307439)

AJPH January 2024, Vol. 114, No. 1

Geotargeting identifies the location of electronic devices (e.g., smartphones, tablets, and desktop computers) using Wi-Fi, GPS, and Bluetooth to deliver online digital content through an Internet protocol geographic region. Geotargeting is a valuable tool in steering audiences; a benefit is allowing digital ad content to be adapted to the local context to increase the message's relevance, including as a public health tool.[1] Our goal was a logic-based approach to use severe acute respiratory syndrome coronavirus 2 (SARS-CoV-2) wastewater concentration alongside clinical data in developing community messaging promoting COVID-19 testing and vaccination to specific at-risk areas within Jefferson County, Kentucky. Although the COVID-19 pandemic required adapting established norms in health data collection,[2] there are not many examples of using these data to inform subcity interventions. To our knowledge, this is the first effort to employ a blended wastewater and clinical data rubric to guide a geographically targeted delivery of an online public health intervention.

INTERVENTION AND IMPLEMENTATION

We developed a risk rubric inclusive of the concentration of SARS-CoV-2 RNA in sewers across Louisville[3–5] paired with administratively reported vaccination and case data to develop risk scores among 17 sewer zones. Higher scores indicated an increased risk because of high or rising viral wastewater concentrations, high or increasing clinical cases, and low vaccine uptake. Three neighborhoods earned comparatively high risk scores and were selected to receive interventions. Next, we worked with two vendors, CoPilot LLC (Louisville, KY) and El Toro LLC (Louisville, KY), to develop digital wastewater-themed advertisements in campaigns pushed to specific sewer zones via Internet-using device geotargeting, lasting for 30 consecutive days (Table A, available as a supplement to the online version of this article at http://www.ajph.org).

Three campaigns delivered a total of 2 678 547 ad impressions to 86 185 residents living in western, southeastern, and southern Jefferson County and earned 4325 clicks. Advertisement messaging informed residents that their area was experiencing a high risk for COVID-19 infection and included images of the wastewater research process, local leaders, or local landmarks (Figure 1). When residents clicked on the advertisements, they were directed to learn more through a call-to-action

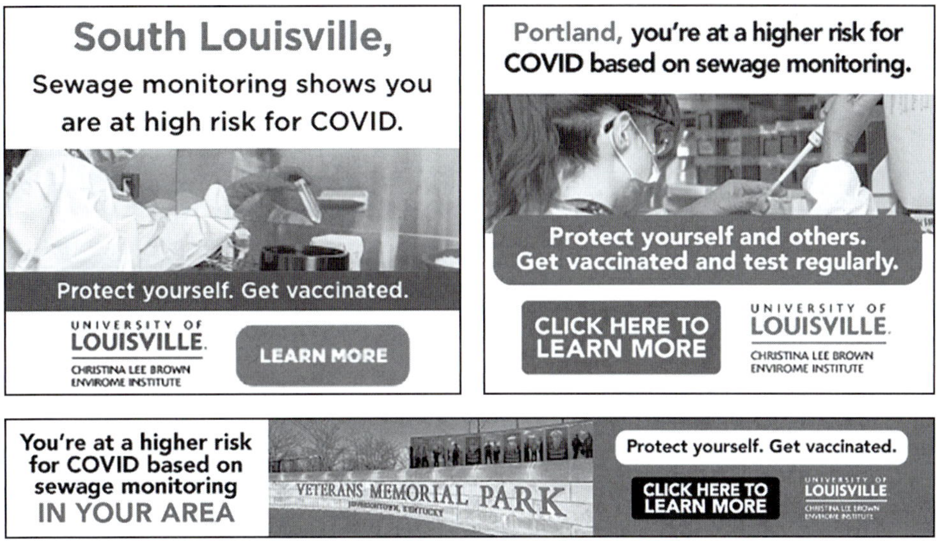

FIGURE 1— Example Digital Advertisements Used for COVID-19 Geotargeted Neighborhood Intervention Campaigns: Louisville, KY, November 2021–April 2022

custom intervention website that contained information about testing or vaccination and links to schedule appointments.

PLACE, TIME, AND PERSONS

Campaign A ran in western Jefferson County from November 19, 2021, through February 11, 2022, and earned a click-through rate of 0.19% against a population of 7820 (Figure B, available as a supplement to the online version of this article at http://www.ajph.org). This campaign occurred during two periods, one before and one after the 2021 holiday season, because seasonal constraints prevented the ad company from delivering impressions on the intervention schedule. The research team recruited two community champions to guide advertisement development for this campaign. These individuals represented two different Black-led nonprofits and demonstrated deep knowledge of their areas, and the city and residents viewed them as influential community leaders. Researchers presented the risk rubric score in their area compared with other countywide areas. Researchers asked the champions what types of health messages would resonate well, be culturally appropriate, and not create stigma. Both community champions advised to emphasize the positive impact testing and vaccination has to reduce COVID-19 spread and to feature leaders involved in direct service to their community, landmarks, and events in the Campaign A advertisements.

Campaign B ran in southeastern Jefferson County from February 14, 2022, through April 14, 2022, and earned a click-through rate of 0.15% against a population of 55 928 (Figure B, available as a supplement to the online version of this article at http://www.ajph.org). No community champions were recruited to assist with advertising development although connections with six trusted nonprofit organizations were made through the Louisville Metro City Council. Nonprofit representatives declined to participate citing fear that perceived political bias could harm their reputation and local fundraising ability.

Campaign C in southern Jefferson County ran from March 1 to 31, 2022, and earned a click-through rate of 0.13% against a population of 22 437 (Figure B, available as a supplement to the online version of this article at http://www.ajph.org). Because of the lessons learned in campaign B, we instead approached small businesses as prospective community champions through the local economic development office: a hardware store, two restaurants, and a barbershop. Again, no community champions were recruited. Business owners declined participation stating they did not want customers to feel unwelcome if they were not vaccinated or not participating in masking or testing practices.

PURPOSE

We aimed to use wastewater concentration in combination with case and vaccination data to identify portions of the county where a geotargeted media campaign intervention promoting testing and vaccination would be delivered. Previous online health marketing initiatives have occurred for nutrition, physical activity, smoking cessation, disease, and dental interventions.[1,6–8] Comparatively, the online Zika awareness campaign earned a click-through rate of 0.60% and a dental clinic awareness campaign earned a click-through rate of 0.09%.[7,8]

EVALUATION AND ADVERSE EFFECTS

The click-through rate was the primary metric of success in this intervention (Box 1). Additional outcome measures, such as testing and vaccination rates, could be considered. However, for this study, insufficient data were available to perform that analysis. Anecdotally, researchers noted that the three campaigns did not move the needle much. The average daily click-through rates for each campaign were 0.19%, 0.15%, and 0.13%, respectively, which is within the same range of other digital health campaigns.[7,8] There are no known adverse effects attributable to this intervention. A limitation of the geofencing approach is that ads are pushed to devices when individuals are active within certain geographic boundaries. A nonresident could receive advertisement impressions if they were in the area for work, school, or other activities.

SUSTAINABILITY

We demonstrate the feasibility of using wastewater monitoring to passively select neighborhoods for a geotargeted digital public health advertising intervention. But it is expensive; each campaign had a base cost of $10 000 plus an hourly rate to develop the ad creative, which averaged $2000 per campaign. Future opportunities exist around other targets able to be informed by wastewater: early detection of seasonal pathogens (e.g., influenza or respiratory syncytial virus) before clinical cases to guide school vaccination clinics; where there is policy change such as removing the personal belief exemption for measles, mumps, and rubella school immunization requirement[10]; or using population-level hormone monitoring to guide mental health campaigns.[11] Further research is required to assess whether click-through rate and behavior change are associated and whether the intervention works better with some diseases over others, and across other cities.

Place could have a significant effect on outcome measures and intervention sustainability. Rural residents had stronger negative sentiments around COVID-19 vaccination.[12] In addition, our study showed political concern cited by individuals who declined to participate as highly localized within the same county. Finally, disparities in universal highspeed Internet access may limit outcome measures.

PUBLIC HEALTH SIGNIFICANCE

Combining wastewater and clinical data into one rubric provides an improved

BOX 1— Implementation and Outcome Measure Challenges and Lessons Learned From Geotargeted Public Health Digital Advertising Intervention: Louisville, KY, November 2021–April 2022

Challenge	Lesson Learned
Split impression delivery schedule because of holiday period affecting click-through rates	Campaign A had two launch dates, and an approximately three-week gap of no intervention delivery because of prioritized digital holiday sales ads. Observed click-through rates were highest in the initial days of each campaign; the unintended split schedule of campaign A could explain why it earned the highest click-through rate of the three campaigns.
Available digital advertising space	During the December holiday season, available digital advertising space was limited because of high demand. It was unanticipated to have this gap in the intervention timing.
No community champions recruited	For campaigns B and C, residents did not have an opportunity to see influential local community champions in images and messages for their digital ads. This is a challenge with geotargeted advertising whereby in a smaller area, more local connections and identifiability is important but also a challenge in a public health context that had turned quite political. As such, the ads created for these two areas may not resonate as strongly with residents, and this could explain fewer ad clicks for these campaigns.
Influential champions and their engagement in complementary active partnerships	To avoid concerns about political bias or negative implications of participating, a lesson learned is to focus on community champion organizations and individuals who are already engaged in similar public health efforts. The influential community champions in images and messages for the digital ads successfully recruited for campaign A were already in active partnerships with the local health department on other complementary public health issues. The influential community individuals approached unsuccessfully for inclusion in campaigns B and C did not have these complementary partnerships.
Clinical data as rubric metric	Throughout the COVID-19 pandemic, clinical data were known to underreport, especially for communities of color.[9]

approach for selecting subcity intervention areas, based on county-level sewer zones, for public health interventions. To our knowledge, this is the first and only public health geotargeted ad intervention driven by wastewater monitoring data and zones, providing initial proof of concept for an alternative to city-wide interventions for other pathogens of interest. AJPH

ABOUT THE AUTHORS

Lauren B. Anderson, Heather D. Ness, Rochelle H. Holm, and Ted Smith are with the Christina Lee Brown Envirome Institute, School of Medicine, University of Louisville, Louisville, KY. L. B. Anderson is also with the Department of Urban and Public Affairs, College of Arts and Sciences, University of Louisville. H. D. Ness is also with the Department of Health Promotion and Behavioral Sciences, School of Public Health and Information Sciences, University of Louisville.

CORRESPONDENCE

Correspondence should be sent to Rochelle H. Holm, Christina Lee Brown Envirome Institute, School of Medicine, University of Louisville, 302 E Muhammad Ali Blvd, Louisville, KY 40202 (e-mail: rochelle.holm@louisville.edu). Reprints can be ordered at https://ajph.org by clicking the "Reprints" link.

PUBLICATION INFORMATION

Full Citation: Anderson LB, Ness HD, Holm RH, Smith T. Wastewater-informed digital advertising as a COVID-19 geotargeted neighborhood intervention: Jefferson County, Kentucky, 2021–2022. *Am J Public Health*. 2024;114(1):34–37.

Acceptance Date: September 4, 2023.

DOI: https://doi.org/10.2105/AJPH.2023.307439

CONTRIBUTORS

T. Smith designed the study. T. Smith and L. B. Anderson conducted the study. H. D. Ness conducted data analyses. L. B. Anderson and R. H. Holm drafted the article. All authors edited and approved the final article.

ACKNOWLEDGMENTS

This work was supported by a contract from the Louisville–Jefferson County Metro Government and a grant from the Rockefeller Foundation. The ad impressions and click data were provided by Co-Pilot LLC and El Toro LLC.

Note. The funding sources had no role in the study design; data collection; administration of the interventions; analysis, interpretation, or reporting of data; or decision to submit findings for publication.

CONFLICTS OF INTEREST

The authors report no relevant competing interests.

HUMAN PARTICIPANT PROTECTION

The University of Louisville institutional review board classified wastewater data as non–human participant research (reference: 717950). The testing and vaccine data were provided by Louisville Metro Department of Public Health and Wellness under a data transfer agreement, and the University of Louisville institutional review board (IRB) approved this as human participant research (IRB: 20.0393).

REFERENCES

1. Graham A, Milner P, Saul J, Pfaff L. Online advertising as a public health and recruitment tool: comparison of different media campaigns to increase demand for smoking cessation interventions [erratum in *J Med Internet Res*. 2009;11(1):e1212]. *J Med Internet Res*. 2008;10(5):e50. https://doi.org/10.2196/jmir.1212
2. Paulose-Ram R, Graber JE, Woodwell D, Ahluwalia N. The National Health and Nutrition Examination Survey (NHANES), 2021–2022: adapting data collection in a COVID-19 environment. *Am J Public Health*. 2021;111(12):2149–2156. https://doi.org/10.2105/AJPH.2021.306517
3. Yeager R, Holm RH, Saurabh K, et al. Wastewater sample site selection to estimate geographically resolved community prevalence of COVID-19: a sampling protocol perspective. *Geohealth*. 2021;5(7):e2021GH000420. https://doi.org/10.1029/2021GH000420
4. Holm RH, Mukherjee A, Rai JP, et al. SARS-CoV-2 RNA abundance in wastewater as a function of distinct urban sewershed size. *Environ Sci Water Res Technol*. 2022;8(4):807–819. https://doi.org/10.1039/D1EW00672J
5. Rouchka EC, Chariker JH, Saurabh K, et al. The rapid assessment of aggregated wastewater samples for genomic surveillance of SARS-CoV-2 on a city-wide scale. *Pathogens*. 2021;10(10):1271. https://doi.org/10.3390/pathogens10101271
6. Gordon R, McDermott L, Stead M, Angus K. The effectiveness of social marketing interventions for health improvement: what's the evidence? *Public Health*. 2006;120(12):1133–1139. https://doi.org/10.1016/j.puhe.2006.10.008
7. Powell R, Rosenthal J, August EM, et al. *Ante La Duda, Pregunta*: a social marketing campaign to improve contraceptive access during a public health emergency. *Health Commun*. 2022;37(2):177–184. https://doi.org/10.1080/10410236.2020.1828534
8. Wright WG, Rafferty AP, Winterbauer N, Locklear K, Tucker-McLaughlin M. Geofencing: mobile technology as a health promotion tool to raise awareness of a dental clinic in rural North Carolina. *J Rural Health*. 2021;37(3):667–674. https://doi.org/10.1111/jrh.12501
9. Keith RJ, Holm RH, Amraotkar AR, et al. Stratified simple random sampling versus volunteer community-wide sampling for estimates of COVID-19 prevalence. *Am J Public Health*. 2023;113(7):768–777. https://doi.org/10.2105/AJPH.2023.307303
10. Moore TP, Bennett JC, Graff K, et al. State policy removing the personal belief exemption for measles, mumps, and rubella (MMR) school immunization requirement, Washington State, 2014–2022. *Am J Public Health*. 2023;113(7):795–804. https://doi.org/10.2105/AJPH.2023.307285
11. Driver EM, Gushgari AJ, Steele JC, Bowes DA, Halden RU. Assessing population-level stress through glucocorticoid hormone monitoring in wastewater. *Sci Total Environ*. 2022;838(pt 2):155961. https://doi.org/10.1016/j.scitotenv.2022.155961
12. Liu Y, Yin Z, Ni C, Yan C, Wan Z, Malin B. Examining rural and urban sentiment difference in COVID-19-related topics on Twitter: word embedding-based retrospective study. *J Med Internet Res*. 2023;25:e42985. https://doi.org/10.2196/42985

Evaluation of the Ontario Mandatory Working-at-Heights Training Requirement in Construction, 2012–2019

Lynda S. Robson, PhD, Victoria Landsman, PhD, Peter M. Smith, PhD, MPH, and Cameron A. Mustard, ScD

The province of Ontario, Canada, implemented mandatory day-long training for construction workers required to use fall-protection equipment. More than 400 000 training sessions were completed by 2017 when the requirement took full effect. The lost-time workers' compensation claim incidence rate attributable to falls targeted by the training was 19% lower in 2017–2019 than in 2012–2014. Rates for two comparator injuries increased or stayed the same. The decline in targeted fall claim incidence rate of the other Canadian provinces was 6%. (*Am J Public Health*. 2024;114(1):38–41. https://doi.org/10.2105/AJPH.2023.307440)

AJPH January 2024, Vol. 114, No. 1

Injuries are a major human health concern, representing 10% of the total economic burden of illness.[1] Among working age adults, 29% of medically treated injuries and 15% of injuries treated in emergency departments have occurred at work.[2,3] Construction remains one of the most hazardous industrial sectors, with falls from heights accounting for 36% of fatal injuries and 14% of nonfatal injuries.[4]

INTERVENTION AND IMPLEMENTATION

In 2014, a new working-at-heights training requirement for construction workers was announced in the province of Ontario, Canada. Implementation began in 2015, with amendments to regulations under the provincial Occupational Health and Safety Act, R.S.O. 1990, which applies to most workers in the province. Employers needed to ensure that all affected workers had successfully completed a specified day-long working-at-heights (WAH) training course. Furthermore, the course and its provider needed accreditation by the Ministry of Labour, Immigration, Training, and Skills Development as meeting, respectively, WAH program[5] and provider[6] standards. Development of these standards had been overseen by a labor-management committee.

The course has both theoretical and hands-on components, with the latter requiring in-person delivery. To pass, learners need to show knowledge achievement through a test and correct demonstration of putting on fall-arrest equipment, inspecting equipment, and maintaining tie-off during transfer of anchor points. The new WAH training requirements were widely communicated within the occupational health and safety and the construction communities, including through a media campaign. By the time requirements were in full effect, 160 training providers had been accredited and 418 000 training sessions successfully completed.[7] Surveyed training providers confirmed the training they were providing had changed substantially as a result of the standard.[7]

PLACE, TIME, AND PERSONS

Following a transition period from April 2015, the regulatory changes came into full effect in October 2017. They applied to all Ontario-regulated workers on construction projects who should use fall-protection systems, estimated as 480 000, the number of workers in the construction sector residing in Ontario in 2016.[8] More precise estimates would exclude anyone who never worked at heights or always worked in sectors under federal jurisdiction, such as transportation, and would include anyone in nonconstruction sectors who worked on construction projects.

PURPOSE

Since 2001, fall-protection training had been required for Ontario construction workers who used personal fall-protection equipment. However, until the regulatory changes, the content and delivery method of that training had not been specified, so training was sometimes very brief and not always hands-on.

EVALUATION AND ADVERSE EFFECTS

We have reported in more detail on an initial comprehensive evaluation of the WAH training initiative, which validated its theory of change.[7,9] The present report strengthens the earlier evaluation by adding two years of follow-up observation of (1) provincial workers' compensation (WC) claims and (2) the WAH knowledge and self-reported work practices of a cohort of trainees. As well, a comparison of the WC claim experience of Ontario with that of the other nine Canadian provinces has been added to control for Canadian-wide secular trends and usual provincial fall-prevention activity.

As before, a quasi-experimental analysis of incidences of lost-time WC claims has been undertaken, comparing claims for injuries targeted by the training (e.g., falls from roofs) to comparator injury claims in two categories. The first comparator is injuries from falls not targeted by the training (e.g., falls down stairs or on the same level); the second is acute traumatic injuries arising from events other than falls. The comparators help control for nonspecific changes over time, unrelated to the intervention, which could impact the WC claim incidence (e.g., changes in work intensity).

Figure 1 shows the incidence rate of targeted fall claims decreased over time in Ontario, contrasting with the trends for the two claims comparators. As shown in Figure 2, the claim incidence rate attributable to targeted falls in 2017–2019 was 19% lower than in 2012–2014 (incidence rate ratio [IRR] = 0.81; 95% confidence interval [CI] = 0.75, 0.87). By contrast, the claim incidence attributable to untargeted falls increased (IRR = 1.12; 95% CI = 1.06, 1.19) and that for all other acute traumatic injuries was unchanged (IRR = 1.00; 95% CI = 0.96, 1.04). The differences between the targeted IRR and each comparator IRR are highly significant statistically ($P < .001$). Though small numbers prevent a robust assessment of changes in the incidence of fatalities targeted by the training, they declined at a similar rate to injuries (IRR = 0.82; 95% CI = 0.45, 1.50).

Figure 2 also compares the Ontario data with that from the other Canadian provinces over the same time periods. The other provinces showed a smaller reduction in targeted fall claim incidence of 6% (IRR = 0.94; 95% CI = 0.90, 0.98) and smaller differences between the targeted fall claim IRR and each of the IRRs for the comparator injuries. This suggests that something beyond usual provincial fall-prevention activity took place in Ontario coincident with the implementation of the WAH initiative.

Alternative plausible explanations for the findings in Ontario were not confirmed. Interviews with labor inspectors revealed that, both before and after intervention implementation, they ensured those working at heights had documented training.[7] Close examination of the claim statistics did not suggest a change in coding practice. There was a contextual factor of note: periodic news media reports during 2012–2018 of the criminal prosecution of a manager responsible for a multiple fall fatality event in 2009.

As described in detail in the Appendix (available as a supplement to the online version of this article at https://ajph.org),

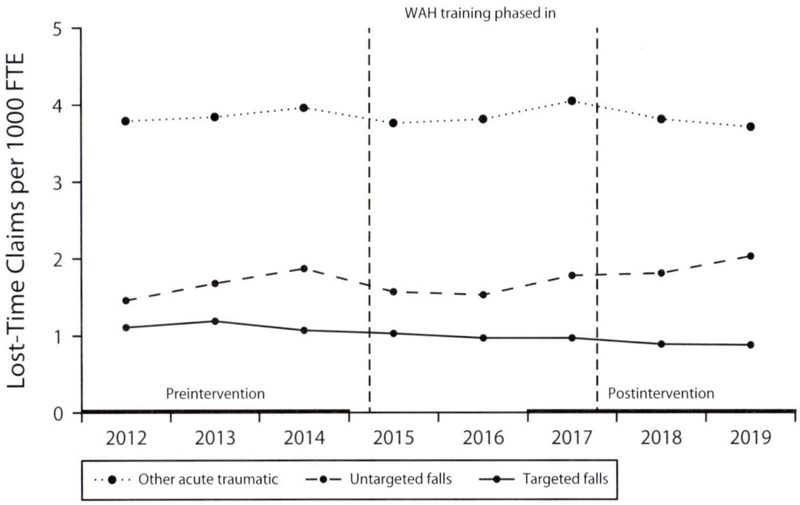

FIGURE 1— Lost-Time Workers' Compensation Injury Claim Incidence Rates in Construction for Three Categories of Injuries: Ontario, Canada, 2012–2019

Note. FTE = full-time equivalent. The working-at-heights (WAH) training standard was phased in April 2015 to October 2017. "Targeted falls" refers to injury claims attributed to events targeted for prevention by the WAH training. The other two injury claim categories are comparators. Annual incidence rates were calculated using claims data from the Association of Workers' Compensation Boards of Canada, information on hours worked in the construction sector,[10] and the assumption that one FTE employee equals 2000 hours.

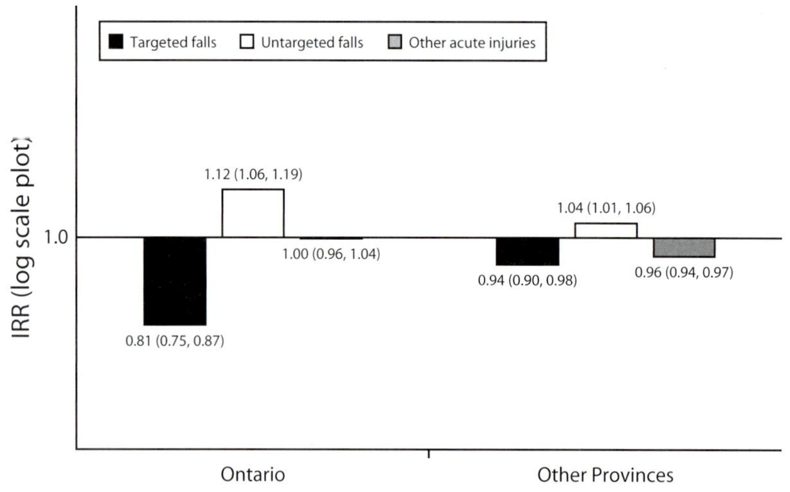

FIGURE 2— Incidence Rate Ratio (IRR) for Lost-Time Workers' Compensation Claim Rates in Construction for Three Categories of Injuries: Ontario, Canada, and in the Remaining Canadian Provinces, 2017–2019 and 2012–2014

follow-up of a cohort of WAH learners (n = 633), first surveyed in fall 2017, showed that the initial gain in WAH safety knowledge, attributable to the training, had eroded after two years, from a score of 9.6 (out of 10) to 7.5 (P < .001), although it remained higher than the pretraining score of 6.8 (P < .001). By contrast, the frequencies of 10 self-reported WAH safety practices, which had also increased following the training, showed no statistically significant erosion over the two-year period.

Adverse effects arising from the intervention were assessed by asking construction employers about "downsides or negative impacts on safety of the WAH training" in a survey.[7(p122)] Of 306 employers with WAH-trained employees, five said that the "ropes" recommended in the training were a tripping hazard, particularly on roofs.

SUSTAINABILITY

Sustainability over the longer term will need to be assessed. Factors supporting sustainability include ongoing enforcement of the training requirement by the inspectorate, promotion of it by training providers, adoption of it by the industry, and, for anyone who took the initial training, a mandatory half-day refresher training every three years.

PUBLIC HEALTH SIGNIFICANCE

As reviewed elsewhere,[9] there are few evaluations of mandatory occupational training standards. Evaluation of the Ontario WAH initiative suggests that a training standard and accreditation program, in the context of enforcement of the requirement by public authorities, can contribute to the prevention of workplace-related traumatic injuries targeted by the training. The 19% decline in the incidence of targeted injuries observed here is relatively modest, but in keeping with workplace-based occupational health and safety training research,[11] despite there being less control in a nonresearch setting. Additional interventions, especially those based higher in the hierarchy of occupational health and safety risk controls (thus, potentially more effective), such as engineering, substitution, or elimination, also have a role to play in addressing falls from heights in construction, as well as workplace-related traumatic injuries more generally. Nevertheless, if the fall-to-lower-level occupational injury incidence in the United States in 2020[12] had been 19% lower, there would have been 2050 fewer nonfatal (often severe) injuries and 67 fewer deaths. AJPH

ABOUT THE AUTHORS

All authors are with the Institute for Work and Health (IWH), Toronto, ON, Canada. Lynda S. Robson is also with Toronto Metropolitan University, Toronto, Canada. Victoria Landsman, Peter M. Smith, and Cameron A. Mustard are also with the Dalla Lana School of Public Health, University of Toronto.

CORRESPONDENCE

Correspondence should be sent to Lynda S. Robson, Institute for Work and Health, 400 University Ave, Suite 1800, Toronto, Ontario, M5G 1S5, Canada (e-mail: lrobson@iwh.on.ca). Reprints can be ordered at https://doi.org by clicking the "Reprints" link.

PUBLICATION INFORMATION

Full Citation: Robson LS, Landsman V, Smith PM, Mustard CA. Evaluation of the Ontario mandatory working-at-heights training requirement in construction, 2012–2019. *Am J Public Health*. 2024; 114(1):38–41.

Acceptance Date: September 4, 2023.

DOI: https://doi.org/10.2105/AJPH.2023.307440

CONTRIBUTORS

L. S. Robson conceptualized this follow-up study and drafted the article. L. S. Robson, P. M. Smith, and C. A. Mustard designed the study. L. S. Robson led the statistical analysis of workers' compensation injury claims; V. Landsman led the statistical analysis for the survey of trainees. All authors were involved in interpretation, providing critical feedback on draft content, and reviewing the final version of the article.

ACKNOWLEDGMENTS

The research was supported through funding to the IWH from the Ontario's Ministry of Labour, Immigration, Training, and Skills Development.

The authors note with appreciation the earlier contributions of Benjamin Amick and Hyunmi Lee to the initial working-at-heights training evaluation study, which has been reported on separately. As well, the authors thank Lyudmila Mansurova for masterfully administering the follow-up survey, and Fran Copelli for her adept administrative assistance in preparing the article. Many thanks to the Infrastructure Health and Safety Association who went above and beyond as collaborating WAH training partner.

Note. The Ministry played no role in the design or conduct of the research; nor in the collection, analysis, or interpretation of the data; nor in the preparation, review, or approval of the publication.

CONFLICTS OF INTEREST

All authors work for the IWH, which is supported through funding from Ontario's Ministry of Labour, Immigration, Training and Skills Development.

HUMAN PARTICIPANT PROTECTION

The study protocol was approved by the University of Toronto Health Sciences Research Ethics Board.

REFERENCES

1. Public Health Agency of Canada. Economic burden of illness in Canada, 2010. Ottawa, ON, Canada: Government of Canada; 2018.
2. Chambers A, Ibrahim S, Etches J, Mustard C. Diverging trends in the incidence of occupational and nonoccupational injury in Ontario, 2004–2011. *Am J Public Health.* 2015;105(2):338–343. https://doi.org/10.2105/AJPH.2014.302223
3. Smith GS, Wellman HM, Sorock GS, et al. Injuries at work in the US adult population: contributions to the total injury burden. *Am J Public Health.* 2005;95(7):1213–1219. https://doi.org/10.2105/AJPH.2004.049338
4. *The Construction Chart Book: The US Construction Industry and Its Workers.* 6th ed. Center for Construction Research and Training. 2018. Available at: https://www.cpwr.com/wp-content/uploads/publications/The_6th_Edition_Construction_eChart_Book.pdf. Accessed July 22, 2023.
5. Ministry of Labour, Immigration, Training, and Skills Development of Ontario. Program standard for working at heights training. Government of Ontario. April 27, 2023. Available at: https://www.ontario.ca/page/program-standard-working-heights-training. Accessed July 22, 2023.
6. Ministry of Labour, Immigration, Training, and Skills Development of Ontario. Provider standard for working at heights training. Government of Ontario. April 27, 2023. Available at: https://www.ontario.ca/page/provider-standard-working-heights-training. Accessed July 22, 2023.
7. Robson L, Mustard C. Implementation and effectiveness of the Ontario Working at Heights Training Standard – final report. Institute for Work and Health. 2019. Available at: https://www.iwh.on.ca/scientific-reports/evaluation-of-implementation-and-effectiveness-of-ontario-working-at-heights-training-standard-final-report. Accessed July 11, 2023.
8. Census profile, 2016 Census. Statistics Canada. June 18, 2019. Available at: https://www12.statcan.gc.ca/census-recensement/2016/dp-pd/prof/index.cfm?Lang=E. Accessed July 22, 2023.
9. Robson LS, Lee H, Amick BC III, Landsman V, Smith PM, Mustard CA. Preventing fall-from-height injuries in construction: effectiveness of a regulatory training standard. *J Safety Res.* 2020;74:271–278. https://doi.org/10.1016/j.jsr.2020.06.007
10. Statistics Canada. Table 14-10-0037-01 Actual hours worked by industry, annual. Available at: https://www150.statcan.gc.ca/t1/tbl1/en/tv.action?pid=1410003701. Accessed January 24, 2022.
11. Burke MJ, Sarpy SA, Smith-Crowe K, Chan-Serafin S, Salvador RO, Islam G. Relative effectiveness of worker safety and health training methods. *Am J Public Health.* 2006;96(2):315–324. https://doi.org/10.2105/AJPH.2004.059840
12. US Bureau of Labour Statistics. Injuries, illnesses, and fatalities. US Department of Labour. Available at: https://www.bls.gov/iif. Accessed July 19, 2023.

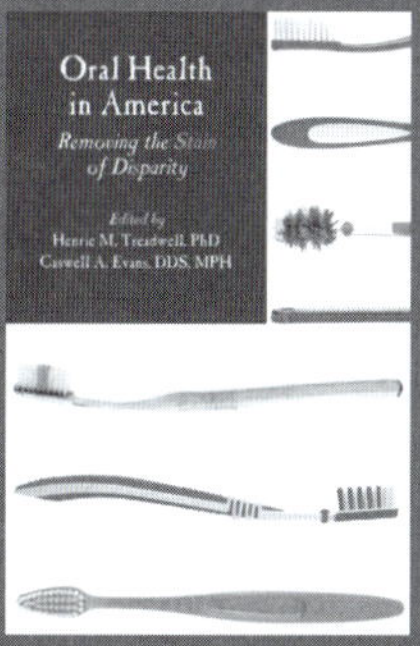

Oral Health in America: Removing the Stain of Disparity

Edited by: Henrie M. Treadwell, PhD and Caswell A. Evans, DDS, MPH

Oral Health in America details inequities to an oral health care system that disproportionately affects the poor, those without insurance, underrepresented and underserved communities, the disabled, and senior citizens. This book addresses issues in workforce development including the use of dental therapists, the rationale for the development of racially/ethnically diverse providers, and the lack of public support through Medicaid, which would guarantee access and also provide a rationale for building a system, one that takes into account the impact of a lack of visionary and inclusive leadership on the nation's ability to insure health justice for all.

Place orders at **aphabookstore.org**. Email **bookstoreservices@apha.org** to request exam copy for classroom use.

ISBN: 978-087553-3056 2019, Softcover List Price: $30 APHA Member Price: $21

APHA PRESS
AN IMPRINT OF AMERICAN PUBLIC HEALTH ASSOCIATION

Public Health Workforce: Retention, Enumeration, and Safety

Alfredo Morabia, MD, PhD

ABOUT THE AUTHOR

Alfredo Morabia is the editor-in-chief of AJPH.

See also Kirkland et al., p. 44, Krasna et al., p. 48, and Stephan-Recaido et al., p. 57.

The US public health workforce crisis is at the heart of public health's future. Our field has lost thousands of jobs since 2010 and has not recuperated yet.[1] It needs to be reinforced by at least double the number of jobs lost, approximately 80 000 (https://bit.ly/46UvgqD), most likely more.

AJPH has been tracking the evolution of the public health workforce and has published data showing both the grim[2,3] and positive[4] trends, identifying causes and solutions.[5,6] In this issue, three articles illustrate some of the key weaknesses of the current situation: threats to community health worker (CHW) retention, lack of appropriate job classifications to enumerate the workforce, and the often neglected issue of chemical exposure.

Kirkland et al. (p. 44) describe factors affecting CHW retention in the public health workforce, using data from the Public Health Workforce Interest and Needs Survey (PH WINS), an essential source of information (https://bit.ly/49pde1o). CHWs are frontline public health workers, a core component of public health community engagement.[7] According to the US Bureau of Labor Statistics (BLS), there were 67 200 CHWs in 2022, with an expected growth of 14% (or 9400 jobs) from 2022 to 2032 (https://bit.ly/3ssX4Df); their median salary is $46 190 per year ($22.21 per hour). Despite the expected upward trend, no public health workforce sector will be immune to demoralization and burnout if work conditions worsen.[8] This new assessment of PH WINS by Kirkland et al. reinforces previous observations,[9] showing that, besides the lack of higher wages and better training, the insecurity related to the prevalent grant-based and short-term funding motivates CHWs to seek more stable jobs elsewhere.

A shocking deficiency in the federal management of the public health workforce is the absence of a common lexicon and standardized system for enumerating the public health workforce, such as the BLS's Standard Occupational Classification (SOC) system. Currently, the BLS cannot count the members of the public health workforce, identify hiring gaps, or guide recruitment and training.[10] This is illustrated by Krasna et al. (p. 48), who matched the job titles reported by 26 516 respondents to the 2021 PH WINS with existing SOC codes. Occupational titles such as disease intervention specialist, policy analyst, program manager, grants or contracts specialist, and peer counselor do not align well with any existing SOC codes. Public health/preventive medicine physician and environmental health worker also align poorly with available SOCs. Public health nurses matched well with registered nurse but, as discussed by Kneipp et al.,[11] the classifications do not provide enough detail to include functions of broader population-level determinants that differ between registered nurses in general and public health nurses in particular.

Assessments of public health workforce needs often fail to consider the health and safety dimension of the jobs.[12] Workers employed in hospitals, health clinics, universities, laboratories, and schools often use chemicals to ensure the cleanliness and hygiene of their buildings or to run their laboratories. Because of these potentially toxic exposures, building maintenance workers, janitors, housekeepers, and lab workers may suffer from occupational ailments ranging from respiratory problems to cancer and endocrine-disrupting exposures. Overall, cleaning and antimicrobial agents are used by 22.5 million workers in the United States, of which more than 10 million are racialized and ethnic minoritized groups (https://bit.ly/3QTAltL). This inequal exposure to toxic agents is documented in this issue by Stephan-Recaido et al. (p. 57), who show that marginalized sociodemographic groups bear the greatest burden of occupational chemical exposure. More generally, equity and diversity should be integral to all considerations related to the public health workforce.

These three articles on public health workforce retention, enumeration, and safety stress the magnitude of the challenges facing the public health workforce but also indicate that, first, the accomplishments of public health during the COVID-19 pandemic have created an opportunity to vitalize the workforce and, second, there are solutions for building up, to use the terms of a recent White House report, a "robust, well-trained, well-compensated public health workforce" (https://bit.ly/46UvgqD). AJPH

CORRESPONDENCE

Correspondence should be sent to Alfredo Morabia, MD, PhD, Barry Commoner Center for Health and the Environment, Queens College, CUNY, 65-30 Kissena Blvd, Flushing, NY 11367 (e-mail: amorabia@qc.cuny.edu). Reprints can be ordered at http://www.ajph.org by clicking the "Reprints" link.

PUBLICATION INFORMATION

Full Citation: Morabia A. Public health workforce: retention, enumeration, and safety. *Am J Public Health*. 2024;114(1):42–43.

Acceptance Date: November 2, 2023.

DOI: https://doi.org/10.2105/AJPH.2023.307524

CONFLICTS OF INTEREST

The author has no conflicts of interest to declare.

REFERENCES

1. Leider JP, Yeager VA, Kirkland C, Krasna H, Hare Bork R, Resnick B. The state of the US public health workforce: ongoing challenges and future directions. *Annu Rev Public Health*. 2023;44:323–341. https://doi.org/10.1146/annurev-publhealth-071421-032830
2. Sellers K, Leider JP, Gould E, et al. The state of the US governmental public health workforce, 2014–2017. *Am J Public Health*. 2019;109(5):674–680. https://doi.org/10.2105/AJPH.2019.305011
3. Wigington CJ, Colman LT, Sobelson RK, Young AC. Tracking public health workforce retention: observations from CDC's public health associate program. *Am J Public Health*. 2019;109(9):1202–1204. https://doi.org/10.2105/AJPH.2019.305156
4. Erwin PC, Beck AJ, Yeager VA, Leider JP. Public health undergraduates in the workforce: a trickle, soon a wave? *Am J Public Health*. 2019;109(5):685–687. https://doi.org/10.2105/AJPH.2019.305004
5. Kett PM, Bekemeier B, Patterson DG, Schaffer K. Competencies, training needs, and turnover among rural compared with urban local public health practitioners: 2021 Public Health Workforce Interests and Needs Survey. *Am J Public Health*. 2023;113(6):689–699. https://doi.org/10.2105/AJPH.2023.307273
6. Gerding JA, Brooks BW, Landeen E, et al. Identifying needs for advancing the profession and workforce in environmental health. *Am J Public Health*. 2020;110(3):288–294. https://doi.org/10.2105/AJPH.2019.305441
7. Sabo S, Allen CG, Sutkowi K, Wennerstrom A. Community health workers in the United States: challenges in identifying, surveying, and supporting the workforce. *Am J Public Health*. 2017;107(12):1964–1969. https://doi.org/10.2105/AJPH.2017.304096
8. Jones TM, Jeung C, Schulte A, Lewis CM, Maddox PJ. Hourly wages and turnover of community health workers according to US state certification policy and Medicaid reimbursement, 2010–2021. *Am J Public Health*. 2022;112(10):1480–1488. https://doi.org/10.2105/AJPH.2022.306965
9. Leider JP, Harper E, Shon JW, Sellers K, Castrucci BC. Job satisfaction and expected turnover among federal, state, and local public health practitioners. *Am J Public Health*. 2016;106(10):1782–1788. https://doi.org/10.2105/AJPH.2016.303305
10. Gebbie KM, Raziano A, Elliott S. Public health workforce enumeration. *Am J Public Health*. 2009;99(5):786–787. https://doi.org/10.2105/AJPH.2008.137539
11. Kneipp SM, Edmonds JK, Cooper J, Campbell LA, Little SH, Mix AK. Enumeration of public health nurses in the United States: limits of current standards. *Am J Public Health*. 2022;112(suppl 3):S292–S297. https://doi.org/10.2105/AJPH.2022.306782
12. Michaels D, Barab J. The occupational safety and health administration at 50: protecting workers in a changing economy. *Am J Public Health*. 2020;110(5):631–635. https://doi.org/10.2105/AJPH.2020.305597

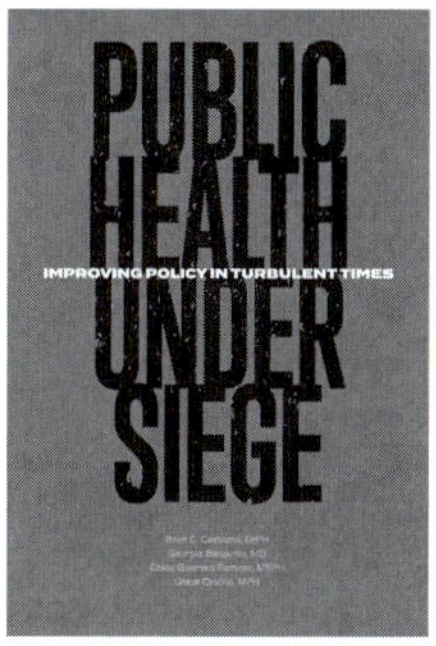

2021, SOFTCOVER, 250 PP
ISBN: 978-0-87553-319-3

APHABOOKSTORE.ORG

Public Health Under Siege: Improving Policy in Turbulent Times

Edited by: Brian C. Castrucci, DrPH, Georges C. Benjamin, MD, Grace Guerrero Ramirez, MSPH, Grace Castillo, MPH

This new book focuses on the importance of health policy through a variety of perspectives, and addresses how policy benefits society, evidently through increased life expectancy and improved health. The book describes how detrimental social determinants can be to the overall population health and emphasizes how the nation is centered on policy change to create equal health care opportunities for all sectors of health.

APHA PRESS
AN IMPRINT OF AMERICAN PUBLIC HEALTH ASSOCIATION

Retention of Community Health Workers in the Public Health Workforce: Public Health Workforce Interests and Needs Survey, 2017 and 2021

Chelsey Kirkland, PhD, MPH, CHW, Janette S. Dill, PhD, MPH, MA, and Harshada Karnik, PhD, MS, MPP

See also Public Health Workforce, pp. 38–67.

Objectives. To investigate the organizational factors contributing to the intent of community health workers (CHWs) to quit their jobs in local and state health departments in the United States.

Methods. We used the 2017 (n = 844) and 2021 (n = 1014) Public Health Workforce Interests and Needs Survey data sets to predict CHWs' intent to leave with Stata 17 balanced repeated replication survey estimations.

Results. CHWs dissatisfied with organizational support, pay, or job security had high probabilities of reporting an intent to leave (50%, $P < .01$; 39%, $P < .01$; and 42%, $P < .01$, respectively) relative to satisfied or neutral workers (24%, $P < .01$; 21%, $P < .01$; and 26%, $P < .01$, respectively).

Conclusions. Improving organizational support, pay satisfaction, and job security satisfaction in public health agencies can significantly improve CHW retention, potentially lowering overall organizational costs, enhancing organizational morale, and promoting community health.

Public Health Implications. Our findings shed light on actionable ways to improve CHW retention, including assessing training needs; prioritizing diversity, equity, and inclusion; and improving communication between management and workers. (*Am J Public Health*. 2024;114(1):44–47. https://doi.org/10.2105/AJPH.2023.307462)

AJPH January 2024, Vol. 114, No. 1

Community health workers (CHWs) are frontline public health workers who usually engage with underserved communities and are often members of or have a close connection to and understanding of the communities they serve.[1] As a proportion of the public health workforce, CHWs have steadily increased in recent years.[2] A primary reason for CHW importance in local health departments is that they often share the same cultural background (ethnicity and language), socioeconomic status, and life experiences as members of underserved communities and are thus able to gain their trust.[3]

CHWs are a diverse group, with about 40% of CHWs across the United States being non-White,[4] although retention issues disproportionately affect people of color within public health agencies.[5] As a professional group, CHWs face several challenges related to their occupation, including limited visibility, low compensation, and work-related stressors contributing to burnout.[6,7] Previous studies have demonstrated that organizational support (e.g., resources for performing work, autonomy, career advancement), satisfaction with pay, and job security are important predictors of retention among the public health workforce,[8–10] but little is known about employment intentions and retention among CHWs, especially in the public health context.[4]

This study expands on past research by exploring the organizational factors that contribute to CHWs' intent to leave their jobs within local and state health departments in the United States. Specifically, we examined (1) characteristics of the CHW workforce in local health departments and how they changed from 2017 to 2021 and (2) key factors associated with CHWs' intent to leave their positions.

METHODS

We analyzed data for CHWs included in the Public Health Workforce Interests and Needs Survey (PH WINS) 2017 (n = 844) and 2021 (n = 1014) data sets with the built-in Stata 17 balanced repeated replication survey estimations. The PH WINS methodology has been described elsewhere.[11]

The dependent variable in this study was intent to leave, which indicates that individuals intend to leave their position in the next 5 years. We had 3 key independent variables: organizational support, pay satisfaction, and job security satisfaction. To create the organizational support variable, we conducted exploratory factor analyses with all of the environmental factors in the PH WINS data set; 9 items with a correlation of 0.92 were retained for organizational support (Appendix A, available as a supplement to the online version of this article at http://www.ajph.org). Control variables included gender, age, race, perceptions of being bullied or threatened, number of posttraumatic stress disorder factors, tenure in public health practice, and type of agency. Appendix A includes a full list of survey items, the response categories included in each measure, and how response categories were developed.

First, we compared descriptive statistics for the CHW workforce between 2017 and 2021. Second, we used stepwise logistic regression models to examine predictors of intent to leave among CHWs. Importantly, only 2021 data were included in the stepwise logistic regression; the reason was that some covariates were collected only in that year, including the bullied or threatened and posttraumatic stress disorder variables. We then used the postestimation margins command (model 3 in Appendix B, available as a supplement to the online version of this article at http://www.ajph.org) to calculate the predicted probability of intent to leave across the 3 key independent variables (organizational support, pay satisfaction, and job security satisfaction).

RESULTS

The estimated number of CHWs within health departments increased from 3359 in 2017 to 4649 in 2021 (Appendix B). The CHW workforce was also younger and more diverse in 2021 than in 2017, and CHWs' intent to leave increased from 25% (2017) to 28% (2021). Organizational support and job security dissatisfaction experienced by CHWs decreased from 2017 to 2021 (from 19% to 16%).

Our logistic stepwise regression analyses (Appendix B) demonstrated that CHWs were most likely to intend to leave if they were dissatisfied with their organizational support ($P < .001$), pay ($P < .001$), or job security ($P < .001$). We also found that workers who perceived that they were being bullied or threatened were significantly more likely to indicate an intent to leave ($P < .05$).

We examined the predicted probability of CHWs indicating an intent to leave (Figure 1) and found that workers who were dissatisfied with organizational support, pay, or job security had higher probabilities of reporting that they intended to leave (50%, $P < .01$; 39%, $P < .01$; and 42%, $P < .01$, respectively) than satisfied or neutral workers (24%, $P < .01$; 21%, $P < .01$; and 26%, $P < .01$; respectively).

DISCUSSION

The size of the CHW workforce in both clinical health care and public health settings has increased.[2] However, because the CHW position is an emerging role within health-related agencies,

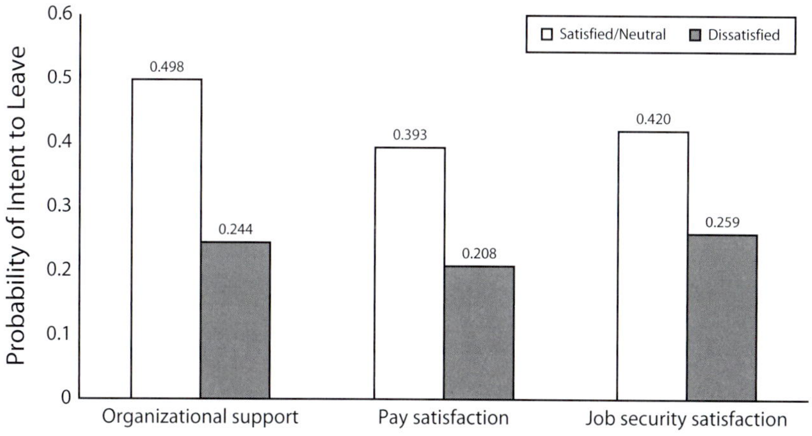

FIGURE 1— Percentage Likelihood That CHWs Will Indicate an Intent to Leave Their Position on the Basis of Experienced Organizational Support, Pay Satisfaction, and Job Security Satisfaction: United States, 2017 and 2021

Note. CHW = community health worker. There were 806 observations; the estimated population size was 3893.

especially public health, little research has been conducted on CHW recruitment and retention strategies. In this study, we estimated the size of the CHW workforce in public health agencies, changes in its size and composition between 2017 and 2021, and key factors associated with employment intentions of CHWs within public health agencies.

Our analysis of predictors of employment intentions allowed us to explore factors promoting retention of CHWs. Dissatisfaction with organizational support, pay, or job security was a strong predictor of employment intentions among CHWs in our study. Our measure of organizational support contained many actionable items for public health agencies (Appendix A).

First, CHWs clearly value having the resources they need to do their work. Our organizational support survey items indicated that CHWs appreciate having their training needs assessed and having sufficient training to use required workplace technology. Second, a few of the items in our measure of organizational support indicated a need for career opportunity and professional development. Finally, one of our organizational support survey items was "My organization prioritizes diversity, equity, and inclusion." This can be improved through prioritizing hiring racially minoritized, disabled, or other workers with lived experiences; providing training around diversity, equity, and inclusion; and targeting health equity programs toward historically marginalized communities.

Finally, satisfaction with pay and satisfaction with job security are important predictors of CHW retention. CHW positions are often grant funded, and short-term funding may lead CHWs to perceive their position as insecure and ultimately leave.[12] Thus, our study findings reiterate the importance of sustainable funding for CHWs such as leveraging braided funding (i.e., multiple funding streams), converting soft dollars to hard dollars, and engaging in legislative work to obtain Medicaid reimbursement.

This study involves some limitations. First, our primary dependent variable was intent to leave an organization, which is not an exact proxy for CHW retention. Second, our regression analysis did not reflect change over time as we restricted our sample to 1 year because some measures were collected only in 2021. Finally, PH WINS does not include data from some small and rural public health departments, so our analysis is limited to larger public health departments.

PUBLIC HEALTH SIGNIFICANCE

Our study provides a description of the CHW workforce in public health departments in the United States and offers valuable and actionable information for public health agencies seeking to retain a diverse CHW workforce. Improving organizational support, satisfaction with pay, and job security can significantly improve CHW retention, which may lower overall organizational costs from hiring and training, enhance organizational morale, and promote community health through continued trust and relationships between CHWs and community members. AJPH

ABOUT THE AUTHORS

The authors are with the Center for Public Health Systems, University of Minnesota School of Public Health, Minneapolis.

CORRESPONDENCE

Correspondence should be sent to Chelsey Kirkland, PhD, MPH, CHW, 420 Delaware St SE, MMC 729, Minneapolis, MN 55455 (e-mail: ckirk@umn.edu). Reprints can be ordered at http://www.ajph.org by clicking the "Reprints" link.

PUBLICATION INFORMATION

Full Citation: Kirkland C, Dill JS, Karnik H. Retention of community health workers in the public health workforce: Public Health Workforce Interests and Needs Survey, 2017 and 2021. *Am J Public Health*. 2024;114(1):44–47.

Acceptance Date: September 15, 2023.

DOI: https://doi.org/10.2105/AJPH.2023.307462

CONTRIBUTORS

All of the authors conceptualized and designed the study and drafted and edited the article. C. Kirkland analyzed the data and interpreted the results.

ACKNOWLEDGMENTS

The Public Health Workforce Interests and Needs Survey was funded by the de Beaumont Foundation.

CONFLICTS OF INTEREST

The authors declare no conflicts of interest.

HUMAN PARTICIPANT PROTECTION

This study was determined to be exempt by the University of Chicago institutional review board.

REFERENCES

1. Love MB, Gardner K, Legion V. Community health workers: who they are and what they do. *Health Educ Behav*. 2016;24(4):510–522. https://doi.org/10.1177/109019819702400409
2. US Bureau of Labor Statistics. Health education specialists and community health workers: Occupational Outlook Handbook. Available at: https://www.bls.gov/ooh/community-and-social-service/health-educators.htm. Accessed August 20, 2023.
3. Gold RB. 'I am who I serve'—community health workers in family planning programs. *Guttmacher Policy Rev*. 2010;13(3):8–13.
4. Jones TM, Jeung C, Schulte A, Lewis CM, Maddox PJ. Hourly wages and turnover of community health workers according to US state certification policy and Medicaid reimbursement, 2010–2021. *Am J Public Health*. 2022;112(10):1480–1488. https://doi.org/10.2105/AJPH.2022.306965
5. Coronado F, Beck AJ, Shah G, Young JL, Sellers K, Leider JP. Understanding the dynamics of diversity in the public health workforce. *J Public Health Manag Pract*. 2020;26(4):389–392. https://doi.org/10.1097/PHH.0000000000001075
6. Jaskiewicz W, Tulenko K. Increasing community health worker productivity and effectiveness: a review of the influence of the work environment. *Hum Resour Health*. 2012;10(1):38. https://doi.org/10.1186/1478-4491-10-38
7. Orpinas P, Matthew RA, Alvarez-Hernandez LR, Calva A, Bermudez JM. Promotoras voice their challenges in fulfilling their role as community health workers. *Health Promot Pract*. 2021;22(4):502–511. https://doi.org/10.1177/1524839920921189
8. Leider JP, Harper E, Shon JW, Sellers K, Castrucci BC. Job satisfaction and expected turnover among federal, state, and local public health

practitioners. *Am J Public Health*. 2016;106(10): 1782–1788. https://doi.org/10.2105/AJPH.2016.303305

9. Liss-Levinson R, Bharthapudi K, Leider JP, Sellers K. Loving and leaving public health: predictors of intentions to quit among state health agency workers. *J Public Health Manag Pract*. 2015; 21(suppl 6):S91–S101. https://doi.org/10.1097/PHH.0000000000000317
10. Pourshaban D, Basurto-Davila R, Shih M. Building and sustaining strong public health agencies: determinants of workforce turnover. *J Public Health Manag Pract*. 2015;21(suppl 6):S80–S90. https://doi.org/10.1097/PHH.0000000000000311
11. Leider JP, Bharthapudi K, Pineau V, Liu L, Harper E. The methods behind PH WINS. *J Public Health Manag Pract*. 2015;21(suppl 6):S28–S35. https://doi.org/10.1097/PHH.0000000000000285
12. Schmit CD, Washburn DJ, LaFleur M, Martinez D, Thompson E, Callaghan T. Community health worker sustainability: funding, payment, and reimbursement laws in the United States. *Public Health Rep*. 2022;137(3):597–603. https://doi.org/10.1177/00333549211006072

Our Communities Our Sexual Health

Awareness and Prevention for African Americans

Edited By: Madeline Sutton, MD, MPH;
Jo A. Valentine, MSW; and
William C. Jenkins, PhD, MS, MPH

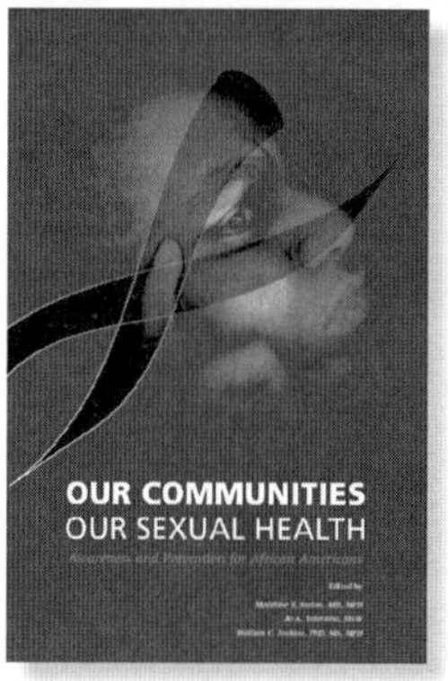

This groundbreaking book provides a comprehensive historical prospective of the disproportionate burden of HIV and other sexually transmitted infections (STIs) among African Americans.Chapters that follow explore the context of HIV and STIs in African American communities and include discussions of sexuality and the roles of faith and spirituality in HIV and STI prevention efforts. Additional chapters provide insight into strategies, e.g., HIV testing, condom distribution and marketing campaigns, parent-child communication, effective clinical care and support, and partnerships, for addressing HIV and other STI-related health disparities within these communities. The book is a valuable resource for practitioners, scholars, clinicians, educators, providers, policy makers and students.

2016, 283 pp., soft cover
ISBN: 978-0-87553-275-2
Order Online at
www.aphabookstore.org

APHA PRESS
AN IMPRINT OF AMERICAN PUBLIC HEALTH ASSOCIATION

Standard Occupational Classification Codes: Gaps in Federal Data on the Public Health Workforce

Heather Krasna, PhD, EdM, MS, Malvika Venkataraman, MS, Moriah Robins, MPH, Isabella Patino, BA, and Jonathon P. Leider, PhD

See also Public Health Workforce, pp. 38–67.

Objectives. To determine whether US Department of Labor standard occupational classification (SOC) codes can be used for public health workforce research.

Methods. We reviewed past attempts at SOC matching for public health occupations and then used the National Institute for Occupational Safety and Health Industry and Occupation Computerized Coding System (NIOCCS) to match the actual job titles for 26 516 respondents to the 2021 Public Health Workforce Interests and Needs Survey (PH WINS) with SOC codes, grouped by respondents' choice of job category in PH WINS. We assessed the accuracy of the NIOCCS matches and excluded matches under a cutpoint using the Youden Index. We assessed the percentage of SOC matches with insufficient information and diversity of SOC matches per PH WINS category using the Herfindahl–Hirschman Index.

Results. Several key public health occupations do not have a SOC code, including disease intervention specialist, public health nurse, policy analyst, program manager, grants or contracts specialist, and peer counselor.

Conclusions. Without valid SOC matches and detailed data on local and state government health departments, the US Department of Labor's data cannot be used for public health workforce enumeration. (*Am J Public Health*. 2024;114(1):48–56. https://doi.org/10.2105/AJPH.2023.307463)

AJPH January 2024, Vol. 114, No. 1

The local, state, and Tribal government public health workforce is the backbone of the US public health infrastructure, providing services crucial to health, safety, and national biosecurity. The workforce serves as frontline responders to public health emergencies, ensures clean water and air, controls infectious disease outbreaks, prevents chronic disease and injury, and maintains vital statistics such as birth and death certificates.[1] Building and maintaining this workforce is 1 of the 10 essential public health services[2] and is essential for providing foundational public health services.[1] To determine whether the workforce can provide needed services, we must understand how many individuals are in this workforce, what they do, how much they get paid, and what training they have. Without this basic information, researchers, policymakers, and the public cannot determine whether there are workforce or funding shortages.

An essential aspect of workforce research is an occupational taxonomy that categorizes the unique job functions of different workers. The US Department of Labor Bureau of Labor Statistics (BLS) is charged with collecting, analyzing, and publishing data on the US workforce. It tracks 867 detailed occupations using the standard occupational classification (SOC) system categories.[3] Examples of SOCs include such specific positions as denturists, shampooers, and braille transcribers, as well as subspecialists such as nurse anesthetists and advanced practice psychiatric nurses. BLS uses surveys such as the Occupational Requirements Survey, the National Compensation Survey, Employment Projections, and the Occupational Employment and Wage Statistics (OEWS) program to collect data on working conditions, education, training, and experience as well as salaries and benefits.

Another key classification used in workforce research is the North American Industry Classification System (NAICS), used to classify business establishments by industry or sector.[4] Using SOC codes in conjunction with NAICS codes allows detailed enumeration, categorization, and salary information for workers in a specific industry. Like SOC codes, NAICS codes have broader categories (e.g., category 62, "Health Care and Social Assistance") with detailed subcategories ("621310 Offices of Chiropractors"), allowing us to know, for example, how many accountants work in chiropractors' offices.[5] However, although the NAICS code, "923120 Administration of Public Health Programs," exists, the OEWS uses only broader NAICS codes, "Local Government, excluding schools and hospitals" and "State Government, excluding schools and hospitals," perhaps because BLS does not prioritize gathering detailed employment data on government agencies.

The 1997 report "The Public Health Workforce: An Agenda for the 21st Century" (Appendix C)[6] recommended the development of a standard taxonomy to characterize the public health workforce, specifically one linked to SOC codes. However, it has been noted repeatedly since then[7–13] that SOC codes do not match well with several public health occupations, creating challenges in researching the workforce. "The Public Health Work Force: Enumeration 2000 Report" (Appendix C, part 3) reiterated the need for public health SOCs,[14] but many of the recommended SOC codes were never established. A 2023 report by the President's Council of Advisors on Science and Technology again recommended new SOCs for public health and recommended that they "include the public health workforce in . . . the next revision of the SOC manual."[15(p23)]

Public health workforce researchers, in an attempt to better categorize the workforce, established a public health workforce occupational taxonomy, imperfectly connected to SOC codes, in the "Enumeration 2000 Report."[16] A workforce taxonomy was revised in 2014[17,18] and then adapted for research such as the Public Health Workforce Interests and Needs Survey (PH WINS),[19] but matching with SOC codes was not an explicit aspect of the 2014 taxonomy or PH WINS.

PH WINS is the largest national source of data on individual state and local governmental public health workers.[20,21] Respondents select their job function from a list of 70 job categories. Matching these categories with SOC codes could improve workforce research, allow salary benchmarking, and contribute to workforce enumeration. We sought to determine which public health job titles clearly match to a SOC code and where there are gaps between SOC codes and public health occupations.

METHODS

Our fundamental approach to answering our project's research questions was to use a federally supported machine learning system that autocodes industry and occupation data into SOC code standards. This allowed us to (1) compare administrative and civil service data on job titles from PH WINS fielding, which was not previously available to researchers; and (2) examine where SOC codes do not capture the occupations of public health workers.

We conducted a literature review on past schema-matching efforts. The National Institute for Occupational Safety and Health's Industry and Occupation Computerized Coding System (NIOCCS)[22] matched the job titles with SOC codes, giving a probability of the match being correct, with some titles coded as "insufficient information." We manually assessed the validity of the NIOCCS matches for the 200 most common civil service job titles, coded the matches as correct or incorrect using a receiver operating characteristic (ROC), and determined a cutpoint using the Youden Index, a statistic that conveys the performance of dichotomous diagnostic tests. We then excluded SOC matches with a predicted SOC probability below the threshold. Finally, we analyzed each PH WINS job category to assess which had the largest proportion of "insufficient information" instead of clear matches, which had lower SOC-matching probability and had the most diversity in SOC matches using the Herfindahl–Hirschman Index (HHI)—a metric that expresses how evenly dispersed a group is throughout a selection of states—to determine which PH WINS categories had the least clear SOC matches.

Past Schema-Matching Efforts

A 2021 study[23] attempted to match PH WINS titles with SOC codes. First, the study's authors used the SOC codes from the Enumeration 2000 public health workforce taxonomy[14] and connected them to the 2014 taxonomy[17]; second, they used machine-learning software developed by the National Institutes of Health to match the job descriptions in the 2014 taxonomy with SOC codes[24]; and, finally, they validated the matches with a coauthor of the 2014 taxonomy. Additionally, the authors analyzed a data set of 38 533 full job descriptions from the Burning Glass database, in both government and nongovernment organizations, for which employers sought public health degree candidates. The Burning Glass system used machine learning to match these job descriptions with SOC codes, allowing an analysis of which organizations compete to hire public health graduates, as well as which occupations in the public health workforce require public health degrees. We used the taxonomy matching from the 2021 as a framework to begin the SOC to PH WINS matching process in our study.

Code Matching With NIOCCS

We accessed administrative data used to field 2021 PH WINS, specifically the survey recipients' actual job titles (referred to in this article as "civil service job titles"), and linked these job titles with respondents' choice of job category from the list of 70 categories in the PH WINS instrument. There were 108 044 records from the PH WINS 2021 distribution. Of these, 65 115 were nonresponders to PH WINS, so we excluded them; 16 413 respondents to PH WINS did not have a job title (or the title was a string of numbers with no text), so we excluded them as well. We analyzed the remaining 26 516 PH WINS respondents who also had a civil service job title. We then cleaned the job title data so that it could be coded by NIOCCS, which matches job titles with the 2018 (latest) SOC codes using machine learning.[22] Data cleaning examples are provided in Appendix A (available as a supplement to the online version of this article at http://www.ajph.org).

ROC Curve and Cutoff Value

Although NIOCCS provides a match probability, we wanted to establish an independent threshold for confidence in the system's ability to assign occupation codes. To find the most valid SOC code matches for each PH WINS job category, we reviewed the SOC matches of the NIOCCS for the 200 most common civil service titles (representing 13 257 of 26 497 respondents).

The lead researcher (H. K.) identified whether NIOCCS had matched the job titles to a correct SOC code and made observations of patterns in the code matching (Appendix B, available as a supplement to the online version of this article at http://www.ajph.org). When it was unclear whether NIOCCS had matched to the correct SOC code, we looked up the civil service title using O*NetOnline, which draws from SOC codes but also contains multiple alternative job titles per occupation.[25] In some cases, we also searched for the civil service job titles in job boards, including Indeed.com, to review currently posted job descriptions.

We looked at performance using both a ROC curve[26] and a Youden Index.[27]

ROC classes:

(1) $y = 1$ if NIOCCS probability ≥ 0.5

(2) $y = 0$ if NIOCCS probability < 0.5

The ROC curve is a probability curve that plots the true positive rate versus false positive rate at various cutpoint values.[28]

The ideal cutpoint for the Youden Index is the one that maximizes the Youden function, which represents the difference between the true positive rate and the false positive rate among all plausible cutpoint values. The formula for the index is shown as

$$J_{max} = \max_t\{\text{sensitivity}(t) + \text{specificity}(t) - 1\}, \quad (3)$$

where t denotes the classification cutpoint for which J is maximal, with values for J ranging between 0 and 1.[28]

We used the cutpoint function in R version 4.2.2 (R Foundation for Statistical Computing, Vienna, Austria) to fit an ROC curve on the NIOCCS coder–predicted SOC probabilities and our determined actual value (1 = predicted correctly, 0 = predicted improperly). The coder had a fair predictive ability with an area under the curve of 0.8072. The optimal cutpoint using the Youden Index was 0.4811. We used the Youden Index to determine the cutpoint, as it conceptually allowed us to balance sensitivity and specificity. We excluded all rows with a NIOCCS-predicted SOC probability less than this value in the subsequent analysis (Appendix C, available as a supplement to the online version of this article at http://www.ajph.org).

Analysis

We analyzed the SOC codes for respondents, grouped by the PH WINS job category they selected, to determine which titles had the largest proportion of insufficient information instead of a SOC code match, the lowest SOC probability, and an examined distribution of SOC codes per PH WINS category using the HHI. We also examined which, if any, had insufficient SOC matches. We conducted these analyses using SAS on Demand for Academics, 2023 (SAS Institute, Cary, NC).

Herfindahl–Hirschman Index

We used the HHI[29] in this analysis to assess the diversity of SOC codes per PH WINS category. In Equation 4, s_i is the proportion of SOC title guesses for each PH WINS title i. A higher HHI implies that the SOC occupation "guesses" are less diverse, and a lower HHI implies that the SOC occupation guesses are more diverse.

$$H = \sum_{i=1}^{N} s_i^2 \quad (4)$$

For each PH WINS title, we calculated s_i by dividing the count of each SOC title guess by the sum of all SOC titles guesses; we then squared and summed up s_i to get the final HHI.

RESULTS

Our analysis allowed us to identify which occupations within health departments were well matched to SOCs, and which were poorly matched.

Occupations With No or Poorly Matched SOCs

Business support roles and those with clinical titles were well matched by NIOCCS to an accurate SOC code. Epidemiologist matched well, as did health educator, nutritionist or dietitian, pharmacist, dentist, attorney, and economist.

However, certain critical public health occupations had insufficient information as the most frequent SOC response or had SOC matches that are clearly incorrect, indicating that they have no SOC code. Others matched a SOC code, but the description of the SOC occupation did not accurately describe the job tasks for public health professionals in that occupation. In particular, we found the following:

- Disease intervention specialist had insufficient information as the most frequent match result. Titles including "disease intervention specialist" and "communicable disease investigator" matched "epidemiologist." "Contact tracer" matched "community health worker." "Case investigator" matched "social workers, all other." "Disease investigator" or "public health investigator" matched "private investigator" (although these matches had low certainty so we excluded them after ROC analysis). We excluded 28% of PH WINS responders who selected disease intervention specialist as their classification under the ROC cutpoint, and it had a low HHI of 0.146. This lack of SOC code is consistent with the recent 2021 taxonomy matching article, which found "private investigators" as a common SOC code for contact tracers or disease intervention specialist.[23]
- Policy analyst matched operations research analysts, software developers, "managers, all other," or management analysts, whereas the correct match using O*NetOnline is political scientist. We excluded 26.3% of PH WINS respondents in this classification, and the role had a low HHI of 0.13.
- Public health agency director (HHI 0.29), department/bureau director (HHI 0.22), deputy director (HHI 0.21), health officer (0.14), program director (0.2), and program manager (0.25) all match the very broad SOC title "managers, all other" or "general and operations managers," with some matching "medical and health services managers" or "social and community services managers."
- Public health nurse and other nurse titles matched well with registered nurse and had high HHIs and low percentages of insufficient data, but the job duties of registered nurses are different from those of public health nurses. Public health nurses have their own certification in certain states, their own professional association, their own competency instrument, and unique job functions.[30]
- Grants or contracts specialist matched "managers, all other" or "office and administrative support workers, all other." No other SOC clearly aligns with the role of a grants or contracts specialist in a government agency. The title had a very low HHI of 0.075, and we excluded 31% of titles under the ROC curve.
- Peer counselor matched "counselors, all other," an incorrect match because counselors require credentialling and peer counselors are typically paraprofessionals.
- Program evaluator had insufficient information as the highest match followed by "managers, all other" and had a low HHI of 0.086.
- Public health informatics specialist had an HHI of 0.09 and insufficient information as the top match, and information systems manager had an HHI of 0.09.
- Vital records staff had an HHI of 0.07 and insufficient information as the top match.
- Inspector/compliance roles: licensure/regulation/enforcement worker, quality improvement, sanitarian or inspector, and nurse appear to have some of the same civil service job titles relating to compliance. Licensure/regulation/enforcement matched registered nurses, perhaps because health facilities inspectors are often nurses.
- Quality improvement worker had a low HHI of 0.085 and did not match a SOC clearly.

Because the PH WINS study did not have a goal of matching with specific SOC codes, certain job categories in PH

WINS were too vague to match with particular SOC codes. Examples include "other business support services," "other (please specify)," "other program staff." Similarly, certain PH WINS job classifications did not match SOCs clearly because they encompassed diverse occupations, such as "behavioral health professional" (HHI of 0.1, matching social workers, medical and health services managers, substance abuse counselors etc.); "data or research analyst" (HHI of 0.07, with insufficient information as the highest match). "Implementation specialist" (47% insufficient information), and "population specialist" did not have consistent civil service job titles, and the civil service titles rarely included these terms.

We created a table (Appendix D, available as a supplement to the online version of this article at http://www.ajph.org) illustrating the most common civil service titles, and SOC code matches, by PH WINS title. To our knowledge this crosswalking between the PH WINS titles (and the previous public health workforce taxonomy) is the first evidence-based taxonomy mapping between public health titles and SOC codes since 1997. When the SOC matches are inadequate, this is noted in Table 1.

Insufficient Information

To show which PH WINS job categories had a higher percentage of insufficient information SOC titles (i.e., could not match) as well as the diversity of SOC matches per category, we created Table 1. This table contains the PH WINS job category, total number respondents per job category in the PH WINS 2021 data subset used in this research, the percentage of responses excluded below the cutpoint, the percentage of titles resulting in an insufficient information SOC match, and the HHI. It also lists the median and interquartile range for NIOCCS-reported SOC match probability and the total number of unique SOC matches per PH WINS category.

The positions with the largest percentage of insufficient information rather than an estimated SOC code include student, implementation specialist, emergency medical services worker, laboratory aide or assistant, emergency medical technician/advanced emergency medical technician/paramedic, physical/occupational/rehabilitation therapist, and disease intervention specialist/contact tracer.

DISCUSSION

BLS maintains SOC coding guidelines, which state, "Each occupation is assigned to only one occupational category at the most detailed level of the classification" and "Occupations are classified based on work performed and, in some cases, on the skills, education and/or training needed to perform the work."[3(p24)] From our analyses, it is clear that although certain public health occupations have a SOC match, many important public health occupations do not.

Several public health occupations, such as disease intervention specialist and public health nurse, have job task analyses,[30,31] professional associations, and even certifications, attributes that denote a clearly defined occupation. Many of these roles, such as public health nurse, "public health program specialist," and "infection control/disease investigator" were requested as new SOCs in the Enumeration 2000 study.[6,14] Certain roles without clear SOCs, such as policy analyst and grant manager, are common across government agencies and nonprofit organizations; creating a clear SOC for them could improve workforce research beyond health departments. In the 2018 update to the SOCs, several new occupations or revisions for occupations in the public health workforce were requested,[32] but most were denied. SOC codes are typically updated every 10 years. Public health researchers, collaborating with relevant professional associations, must take the next opportunity to document how their occupations differ from existing SOC occupations and present a case for new codes to the interagency SOC Policy Committee when it convenes.

An important, related challenge to public health workforce research is the lack of specificity in NAICS codes. The OEWS survey provides occupational and salary information by NAICS industry for many detailed industries. Even though an "administration of public health programs" NAICS code exists,[33] it is not used in OEWS; only "local government, excluding schools and hospitals" and "state government, excluding schools and hospitals" are used.

This is especially problematic for public health leadership and program management roles, most of which match "managers, all other," a SOC too vague to capture the specialist nature of these roles. Without the use of the public health NAICS code, OEWS cannot currently be used for enumeration of the public health workforce, especially for vague SOC occupations (e.g., "managers, all other") or occupations that could exist in many local or state government departments, such as social workers or nutritionists.

Limitations

The PH WINS survey asked respondents to select job categories, but the

TABLE 1— PH WINS Job Categories With Percentages Excluded, Percentages of Insufficient Information, and HHI: United States, 2021

PH WINS Job Category (2021)	Total Respondents in PH WINS 2021 Data Subset[a]	% Excluded After Youden Removed[b]	% Insufficient Information SOC Match[c]	HHI[d]	NIOCCS-Reported SOC Match Probability,[e] Median (IQR)	Total Unique SOC Matches[f]
Animal control worker	18	55.6	25.0	0.25	0.90 (0.72–0.99)	5
Attorney or legal counsel	110	12.7	2.1	0.43	0.61 (0.94–0.99)	13
Behavioral health professional	230	29.6	8.6	0.10	0.76 (0.96–0.97)	32
Business support–accountant/fiscal	822	14.6	8.0	0.14	0.74 (0.96–1.00)	36
Business support services–administrator	385	18.7	12.5	0.09	0.68 (0.87–0.97)	41
Business support services–coordinator	232	19.0	11.7	0.13	0.73 (0.88–0.96)	33
Clerical personnel–administrative assistant	1650	11.8	7.4	0.17	0.67 (0.82–0.96)	62
Clerical personnel–secretary	403	12.9	7.4	0.18	0.74 (0.97–1.00)	37
Community health worker	574	17.9	8.1	0.14	0.64 (0.80–0.97)	52
Custodian	22	0.0	13.7	0.33	0.83 (0.90–1.00)	8
Customer service/support professional	597	13.9	10.5	0.18	0.83 (0.98–1.00)	63
Data or research analyst	848	21.5	14.9	0.07	0.71 (0.81–0.95)	59
Department/bureau director	414	13.8	6.2	0.22	0.64 (0.80–0.93)	31
Deputy director	170	13.5	11.6	0.21	0.72 (0.80–0.94)	16
Disability claims/benefits examiner or adjudicator	25	20.0	0.0	0.17	0.55 (0.97–1.00)	10
Disease intervention specialist/contact tracer	806	28.0	25.5	0.15	0.60 (0.83–0.97)	38
Economist	5	20.0	0.0	0.63	0.94 (0.94–0.97)	2
Emergency medical services worker	18	16.7	40.0	0.26	0.60 (0.83–0.95)	6
Emergency medical technician/advanced emergency medical technician/paramedic	22	9.1	35.0	0.18	0.77 (0.95–0.99)	10
Emergency preparedness/management worker	410	22.4	13.5	0.09	0.76 (0.88–0.97)	40
Engineer	119	20.2	11.6	0.15	0.77 (0.96–0.98)	21
Environmental health worker	1056	12.6	1137.6	0.21	0.70 (0.78–0.88)	48
Epidemiologist	1350	9.1	9.5	0.44	0.86 (1.00–1.00)	38
Grants or contracts specialist	382	31.2	12.2	0.08	0.73 (0.85–0.96)	33
Health educator	911	17.1	12.2	0.27	0.73 (0.95–0.97)	48
Health navigator	55	12.7	10.4	0.09	0.64 (0.94–0.99)	17
Health officer	158	26.6	9.5	0.14	0.69 (0.78–0.91)	26
Human resources personnel	235	11.1	6.7	0.10	0.80 (0.91–0.98)	29
Implementation specialist	56	35.7	47.2	0.27	0.61 (0.82–0.94)	11
Information systems manager/information technology specialist	468	14.1	12.2	0.09	0.75 (0.94–0.99)	42
Laboratory aide or assistant	52	36.5	39.4	0.20	0.65 (0.96–0.98)	13
Laboratory quality control worker	31	3.2	13.3	0.12	0.77 (0.93–0.99)	14

Continued

TABLE 1— Continued

PH WINS Job Category (2021)	Total Respondents in PH WINS 2021 Data Subset[a]	% Excluded After Youden Removed[b]	% Insufficient Information SOC Match[c]	HHI[d]	NIOCCS-Reported SOC Match Probability,[e] Median (IQR)	Total Unique SOC Matches[f]
Laboratory scientist/medical technologist	712	12.6	10.0	0.15	0.64 (0.85–0.99)	22
Laboratory technician	188	18.6	9.2	0.18	0.56 (0.68–0.97)	17
Licensed practical or vocational nurse	91	4.4	6.9	0.59	0.99 (1.00–1.00)	8
Licensure/regulation/enforcement worker	629	29.3	15.5	0.08	0.65 (0.86–0.97)	54
Medical examiner	42	4.8	0.0	0.14	0.61 (0.94–1.00)	13
Medical/vital records staff	194	23.7	16.5	0.07	0.67 (0.89–0.98)	35
Nurse practitioner	111	9.0	4.0	0.49	0.93 (0.99–0.99)	10
Nursing and home health aide	120	5.0	3.5	0.51	0.92 (0.99–1.00)	13
Nutritionist or dietitian	633	9.5	5.2	0.41	0.75 (0.98–1.00)	24
Other (please specify)	573	24.4	15.5	0.05	0.71 (0.88–0.97)	86
Other business support services	333	17.7	17.9	0.06	0.72 (0.92–0.98)	59
Other facilities or operations worker	138	19.6	9.0	0.05	0.68 (0.84–0.96)	40
Other health professional/clinical support staff	506	20.8	16.2	0.05	0.68 (0.93–0.99)	64
Other Nurse–clinical services	137	5.8	2.3	0.44	0.86 (0.99–0.99)	14
Other oral health professional	84	14.3	15.3	0.20	0.85 (0.99–1.00)	14
Other program staff	1296	31.8	20.4	0.09	0.66 (0.82–0.95)	69
Peer counselor	85	22.4	4.5	0.40	0.94 (0.97–0.97)	14
Pharmacist	47	19.2	7.9	0.53	0.97 (1.00–1.00)	6
Physical/occupational/rehabilitation therapist	147	15.7	34.7	0.25	0.89 (0.97–0.98)	11
Physician assistant	9	11.1	12.5	0.31	0.78 (0.81–0.99)	5
Policy analyst	224	26.3	7.3	0.13	0.70 (0.90–0.97)	25
Population health specialist	99	44.4	20.0	0.14	0.57 (0.80–0.91)	17
Program director	589	16.5	6.9	0.20	0.70 (0.80–0.94)	40
Program evaluator	144	23.6	18.2	0.09	0.71 (0.83–0.94)	29
Public health agency director	90	8.9	3.7	0.29	0.72 (0.80–0.92)	11
Public health dentist	19	10.5	5.9	0.46	0.72 (0.85–0.85)	5
Public health informatics specialist	189	23.3	23.5	0.09	0.68 (0.91–0.97)	37
Public health manager or program manager	1611	18.7	8.4	0.25	0.67 (0.80–0.94)	65
Public health veterinarian	18	11.1	0.0	0.38	0.79 (0.80–0.82)	5
Public health/preventive medicine physician	100	18.0	14.6	0.13	0.58 (0.74–0.95)	11
Public information specialist	217	26.8	16.9	0.12	0.65 (0.87–0.95)	40
Quality improvement worker	179	23.5	13.1	0.08	0.67 (0.82–0.96)	30
Registered nurse–public health or community health nurse	2086	4.8	5.9	0.70	0.97 (0.99–1.00)	31
Registered nurse–unspecified	519	9.6	7.3	0.52	0.82 (0.98–1.00)	18
Sanitarian or inspector	736	10.3	7.0	0.43	0.77 (0.87–0.97)	37

Continued

TABLE 1— Continued

PH WINS Job Category (2021)	Total Respondents in PH WINS 2021 Data Subset[a]	% Excluded After Youden Removed[b]	% Insufficient Information SOC Match[c]	HHI[d]	NIOCCS-Reported SOC Match Probability,[e] Median (IQR)	Total Unique SOC Matches[f]
Social worker/social services professional	671	18.6	19.4	0.18	0.78 (0.91–0.95)	34
Statistician	44	13.6	5.3	0.19	0.60 (0.78–0.97)	11
Student, professional or scientific	51	23.5	53.9	0.31	0.77 (0.85–0.92)	14

Note. HHI = Herfindahl-Hirschman Index; IQR = interquartile range; NIOCCS = NIOSH's Industry and Occupation Computerized Coding System; NIOSH = National Institute for Occupational Safety and Health; PH WINS = Public Health Workforce Interests and Needs Survey; SOC = standard occupational classification.
[a]Total number of PH WINS respondents who selected this job category and who also had a civil service job title.
[b]% responses after excluding inaccurate matches via receiver operating characteristic matching.
[c]% of civil service job titles that the NIOCCS could not match to any SOC code.
[d]A lower number indicates more diverse SOC matches.
[e]The NIOCCS-reported probability of a correct match between titles in this PH WINS category and a SOC category. This includes median, first quartile, and third quartile.
[f]The total number of unique SOC codes that matched to the job titles in each PH WINS category.

survey instrument did not include descriptions of each category, leaving the survey respondents to self-identify without detailed guidance. There is also always a chance of survey responder error.

Some mismatches are attributable to generic civil service job titles used in government, such as "research scientist," which mismatched with the SOC for "physical scientist," and "health services consultant," which mismatched with "health technologists and technicians, all other." Some mismatches reflect the challenge of cleaning the job titles and removing abbreviations. Certain job titles have the name of the program in the title (e.g., tuberculosis epidemiologist or maternal/child health program manager), which may make NIOCCS matching more challenging. We had access only to job titles, not full job descriptions; full descriptions might have matched more accurately.

Occupations with fewer responses may have had skewed high HHI's because of the lower number of responses.

Public Health Implications

Because of a lack of accurate, public health–specific SOC codes and lack of the use of NAICS codes specific to health departments, the US Department of Labor does not provide data that can be used to enumerate the entire public health workforce. As a result, the crucial task of public health workforce enumeration has been left primarily to professional associations or philanthropically funded efforts, and a full workforce enumeration has not been conducted since 2014.[34] If BLS used appropriately detailed NAICS codes for OEWS, the federal government would enumerate the public health workforce at least every 3 years.

Future research could use the SOC codes we identified within the constraints of the excessive breadth of NAICS codes to contrast salaries of public health occupations in government versus competitor organizations or contrast education or experience levels between workers in government compared with other sectors.

Without clear SOC codes, the public health workforce—the backbone of our nation's biodefense—will lack data on workforce shortages and recruitment challenges, and our nation—and our nation's public health systems—will be less healthy as a result. AJPH

ABOUT THE AUTHORS

Heather Krasna, Malvika Venkataraman, and Isabella Patino are with Columbia University Mailman School of Public Health, New York, NY. Moriah Robins is with the de Beaumont Foundation, Bethesda, MD. Jonathon P. Leider is with the School of Public Health, University of Minnesota, Minneapolis.

CORRESPONDENCE

Correspondence should be sent to Heather Krasna, 722 W 168 St, New York, NY 10032 (e-mail: hk2778@cumc.columbia.edu). Reprints can be ordered at http://www.ajph.org by clicking the "Reprints" link.

PUBLICATION INFORMATION

Full Citation: Krasna H, Venkataraman M, Robins M, Patino I, Leider JP. Standard occupational classification codes: gaps in federal data on the public health workforce. *Am J Public Health*. 2024;114(1): 48–56.

Acceptance Date: September 15, 2023.

DOI: https://doi.org/10.2105/AJPH.2023.307463

CONTRIBUTORS

H. Krasna conceptualized the study, wrote the article, and conducted the coding, data cleaning, and schema matching. M. Venkataraman conducted statistical analysis, coding, writing, and data visualizations. M. Robins reviewed the article and provided input regarding Public Health Workforce Interests and Needs Survey (PH WINS) data. I. Patino provided additional data analysis and review. J. P. Leider provided guidance on statistical approaches and reviewed, edited, and cowrote the article.

ACKNOWLEDGMENTS

This project was supported by the Centers for Diseases Control and Prevention and the Health Resources and Services Administration (awards U81HP47167 and UR2HP47371).

The de Beaumont Foundation and the Association of State and Territorial Health Officials developed PH WINS to understand the interests and needs of the state and local governmental public health workforce in the United States. PH WINS was fielded in 2014, 2017, and 2021. For more information, visit phwins.org.

We would like to dedicate this article to the memory of Kristine Gebbie, DrPH.

CONFLICTS OF INTEREST

The authors have no conflicts of interest to declare.

HUMAN PARTICIPANT PROTECTION

The study was deemed to not involve human participants under 45 CFR 46 by Columbia University's institutional review board (IRB-AAAU3962).

REFERENCES

1. Public Health National Center for Innovations. Foundational Public Health Services (FPHS): building a strong foundation of public health infrastructure. Available at: https://phnci.org/transformation/fphs#:~:text=The%20FPHS%20framework%20outlines%20the,activities%3B%20and%20justify%20funding%20needs. Accessed December 25, 2020.
2. Centers for Disease Control and Prevention. 10 essential public health services. Available at: https://www.cdc.gov/publichealthgateway/publichealthservices/essentialhealthservices.html. Accessed November 17, 2019.
3. US Bureau of Labor Statistics. 2018 standard occupational classification user guide. November 2017. Available at: https://www.bls.gov/soc/2018/soc_2018_user_guide.pdf. Accessed November 24, 2023.
4. US Census Bureau. North American Industry Classification System. Available at: https://www.census.gov/naics. Accessed April 16, 2023.
5. US Bureau of Labor Statistics. Occupational employment and wage statistics. May 2022. Available at: https://www.bls.gov/oes/current/naics5_621310.htm. Accessed May 2, 2023.
6. US Department of Health and Human Services. The public health workforce: an agenda for the 21st century. Available at: https://www.govinfo.gov/content/pkg/GOVPUB-HE20-PURL-LPS46996/pdf/GOVPUB-HE20-PURL-LPS46996.pdf. Accessed November 24, 2023.
7. Chauvin SW, Anderson AC, Bowdish BE. Assessing the professional development needs of public health professionals. *J Public Health Manag Pract.* 2001;7(4):23–37. https://doi.org/10.1097/00124784-200107040-00005
8. Fraser MR. The local public health agency workforce: research needs and practice realities. *J Public Health Manag Pract.* 2003;9(6):496–499. https://doi.org/10.1097/00124784-200311000-00009
9. Gebbie K, Merrill J, Sanders L, Gebbie EN, Chen DW. Public health workforce enumeration: beware the "quick fix." *J Public Health Manag Pract.* 2007;13(1):72–79. https://doi.org/10.1097/00124784-200701000-00012
10. Sumaya CV. Enumeration and composition of the public health workforce: challenges and strategies. *Am J Public Health.* 2012;102(3):469–474. https://doi.org/10.2105/AJPH.2011.300388
11. American Public Health Association. Advancing efforts to enumerate and characterize the nation's public health workforce. November 5, 2013. Available at: https://www.apha.org/policies-and-advocacy/public-health-policy-statements/policy-database/2014/07/08/07/50/advancing-efforts-to-enumerate-and-characterize-the-nations-public-health-workforce. Accessed April 6, 2023.
12. Montes JH, Webb SC. The Affordable Care Act's implications for a public health workforce agenda: taxonomy, enumeration, and the standard occupational classification system. *J Public Health Manag Pract.* 2015;21(1):69–79. https://doi.org/10.1097/PHH.0000000000000085
13. Czabanowska K, Middleton J. Professionalism of the public health workforce—how to make it happen? *J Public Health (Oxf).* 2022;44(suppl 1):i54–i59. https://doi.org/10.1093/pubmed/fdac091
14. Gebbie KM. *The Public Health Work Force: Enumeration 2000.* Washington, DC: US Department of Health and Human Services; 2000.
15. President's Council of Advisors on Science and Technology. Report to the president: supporting the US public health workforce. May 2023. Available at: https://www.whitehouse.gov/wp-content/uploads/2023/04/PCAST_Public-Health-Report_May2023.pdf. Accessed November 22, 2023.
16. Tilson H, Gebbie KM. The public health workforce. *Annu Rev Public Health.* 2004;25:341–356. https://doi.org/10.1146/annurev.publhealth.25.102802.124357
17. Boulton ML, Beck AJ, Coronado F, et al. Public health workforce taxonomy. *Am J Prev Med.* 2014;47(5 suppl 3):S314–S323. https://doi.org/10.1016/j.amepre.2014.07.015
18. Beck AJ, Coronado F, Boulton ML, Merrill JA; Public Health Enumeration Working Group. The public health workforce taxonomy: revisions and recommendations for implementation. *J Public Health Manag Pract.* 2018;24(5):E1–E11. https://doi.org/10.1097/PHH.0000000000000690
19. Leider JP, Bharthapudi K, Pineau V, Liu L, Harper E. The methods behind PH WINS. *J Public Health Manag Pract.* 2015;21(suppl 6):S28–S35. https://doi.org/10.1097/PHH.0000000000000285
20. Sellers K, Leider JP, Harper E, et al. The Public Health Workforce Interests and Needs Survey: the first national survey of state health agency employees. *J Public Health Manag Pract.* 2015;21(suppl 6):S13–S27. https://doi.org/10.1097/PHH.0000000000000331
21. Robins M, Leider JP, Schaffer K, Gambatese M, Allen E, Hare Bork R. PH WINS 2021 methodology report. *J Public Health Manag Pract.* 2023;29(suppl 1):S35–S44. https://doi.org/10.1097/PHH.0000000000001632
22. Centers for Disease Control and Prevention. NIOSH Industry and Occupation Computerized Coding System (NIOCCS). December 13, 2022. Available at: https://csams.cdc.gov/nioccs. Accessed July 21, 2021.
23. Krasna H, Czabanowska K, Beck A, Cushman LF, Leider JP. Labour market competition for public health graduates in the United States: a comparison of workforce taxonomies with job postings before and during the COVID-19 pandemic. *Int J Health Plann Manage.* 2021;36(suppl 1):151–167. https://doi.org/10.1002/hpm.3128
24. Russ DE, Ho KY, Colt JS, et al. Computer-based coding of free-text job descriptions to efficiently identify occupations in epidemiological studies. *Occup Environ Med.* 2016;73(6):417–424. https://doi.org/10.1136/oemed-2015-103152
25. National Center for O*NET Development. O*NET OnLine. Available at: https://www.onetonline.org. Accessed August 21, 2020.
26. James G, Witten D, Hastie T, Tibshirani R. *An Introduction to Statistical Learning: With Applications in R.* 2nd ed. New York, NY: Springer; 2021. https://doi.org/10.1007/978-1-0716-1418-1
27. Fluss R, Faraggi D, Reiser B. Estimation of the Youden Index and its associated cutoff point. *Biom J.* 2005;47(4):458–472. https://doi.org/10.1002/bimj.200410135
28. Unal I. Defining an optimal cut-point value in ROC analysis: an alternative approach. *Comput Math Methods Med.* 2017;2017:3762651. https://doi.org/10.1155/2017/3762651
29. Watts RD, Bowles DC, Fisher C, Li IW. What do public health graduates do and where do they go? An analysis of job destinations and mismatch in Australian public health graduates. *Int J Environ Res Public Health.* 2021;18(14):7504. https://doi.org/10.3390/ijerph18147504
30. Krasna H, Kulik PKG, Karnik H, Leider JP. Recruiting new talent for public health jobs with evidence-based job descriptions and attractive job postings. *J Public Health Manag Pract.* 2023;29(5):E162–E168. https://doi.org/10.1097/PHH.0000000000000177
31. Public Health Accreditation Board. *Disease Intervention Specialist Certification Project: Final Report to the Centers for Disease Control and Prevention.* June 2017. Available at: https://phaboard.org/wp-content/uploads/PHAB-DIS-Full-Report.pdf. Accessed April 20, 2022.
32. US Bureau of Labor Statistics. Standard occupational classification. September 19, 2017. Available at: https://www.bls.gov/soc/2018/soc_responses_July_2016.htm. Accessed March 5, 2023.
33. NAICS Association. 923120—administration of public health programs. Available at: https://www.naics.com/naics-code-description/?code=923120. Accessed April 16, 2023.
34. Beck AJ, Boulton ML, Coronado F. Enumeration of the governmental public health workforce, 2014. *Am J Prev Med.* 2014;47(5 suppl 3):S306–S313. https://doi.org/10.1016/j.amepre.2014.07.018

Characterizing the Burden of Occupational Chemical Exposures by Sociodemographic Groups in the United States, 2021

Shelley C. Stephan-Recaido, MS, Trevor K. Peckham, PhD, Jérôme Lavoué, PhD, and Marissa G. Baker, PhD

See also Public Health Workforce, pp. 38–67.

Objectives. To estimate the number and prevalence of workers in the United States exposed to chemical hazards available in the Canadian job-exposure matrix (CANJEM) database and examine exposure disparities across sociodemographic groups.

Methods. We merged US worker demographic data from the Current Population Survey with CANJEM to characterize the burden and sociodemographic distribution of 244 chemical exposures in the United States in 2021. An interactive version of the full data set is available online (https://deohs.washington.edu/us-exposure-burden).

Results. Of the chemical exposures examined, the most prevalent were cleaning and antimicrobial agents (14.7% of workforce estimated exposed), engine emissions (12.8%), organic solvents (12.1%), polycyclic aromatic hydrocarbons (10.1%), and diesel engine emissions (8.3%). Racial and ethnic minoritized groups, persons with lower educational attainment, foreign-born noncitizens, and males were generally overrepresented in exposure to work-related chemical hazards.

Conclusions. In the United States, marginalized sociodemographic groups are estimated to experience an inequitable burden to many chemical exposures because of occupational segregation. Data from this analysis can inform occupational and public health research, policy, and interventions aimed at reducing the burden of disease and health inequities in the United States. (*Am J Public Health*. 2024;114(1):57–67. https://doi.org/10.2105/AJPH.2023.307461)

AJPH January 2024, Vol. 114, No. 1

Each year, hazardous work-related exposures are responsible for thousands of deaths and millions of injuries and illnesses in the United States.[1] Yet, occupational health surveillance, a key component of public health prevention, remains limited in the United States.[2] Occupational health surveillance is the ongoing systematic collection, analysis, interpretation, and dissemination of data related to occupational hazards and health outcomes.[2–4] Current occupational health surveillance systems primarily focus on the collection of health outcome data[2] and are known to undercount injuries and illnesses,[2,5] especially latent and chronic diseases.[4,5] Surveillance of occupational exposures has historically been limited in the United States, but was identified as a top priority in the 2018 National Academies of Sciences, Engineering, and Medicine report, "Developing a Smarter National Surveillance System for Occupational Safety and Health in the 21st Century."[2] Exposure surveillance can address gaps in current health surveillance efforts, especially identifying opportunities for intervention before work-related injuries and illnesses occur.[2–4]

In addition to characterizing the burden of workplace exposures, it is also important to consider how they are distributed across working populations—another need highlighted in the report.[2] This is critical because the US workforce remains heavily segregated across sociodemographic strata,[6] resulting in the uneven distribution of work-related exposures, which may influence health and contribute to health disparities.[2,7–10] Although previous research has documented occupational health disparities in the United States, with workers from marginalized groups generally experiencing worse health outcomes,[7,11,12] a lack of empirical information on the social distribution of work-related exposures remains.

Identification of at-risk working populations is particularly important considering that many groups have been underrepresented or excluded from public health policies, research, and interventions. The primary governmental agency responsible for worker health and safety in the United States is the Occupational Safety and Health Administration (OSHA), which was shaped largely by lobbying of labor unions that historically represented White male workers in goods-producing industries.[13] While OSHA has been successful in reducing exposures to certain widely recognized hazards, many working populations and hazards have long been excluded from OSHA protections, such as domestic workers who are predominantly female and from racial and ethnic minoritized (REM) groups.[14] Since its inception, OSHA has faced challenges in updating existing standards, as well as introducing new standards that may be more relevant to a more diverse American workforce that is largely employed in services-providing industries.[15] Exposure surveillance can help us understand who is most at risk, a critical step toward prevention and achieving occupational health equity.

Population-level exposure surveillance is considerably challenging, due largely to limited accurate exposure information for a wide variety of hazards and work settings. The last large-scale exposure surveillance effort in the United States was the National Occupational Exposure Survey, a nationwide observational survey conducted in the early 1980s.[2] While the survey addressed the need for general working population exposure surveillance, it was highly resource-intensive, and the data are now considered outdated and of limited use.[2] More recent exposure surveillance efforts, such as the Occupational Health Supplements in the National Health Interview Survey, have been more narrow in scope, focusing on a limited set of exposures or work settings.[2] One approach that can address the need for population-level exposure surveillance takes advantage of existing data in the form of a job-exposure matrix (JEM). JEMs are data sources that link individual job titles to exposure indices and have been used for decades in occupational epidemiology research.[16] Though JEMs are not without limitations, they are highly efficient and low cost to use,[16] making them an attractive and powerful source of exposure information when individual worker-level data are unavailable.

Few multihazard JEMs covering a wide span of work settings exist in the world, and fewer are applicable to a North American population. Arguably, the most comprehensive JEM available for developing population-level estimates of work-related chemical exposures in the US context is the Canadian job-exposure matrix (CANJEM).[17] CANJEM provides exposure prevalence, intensity, and frequency estimates for more than 250 occupational agents based on data from jobs held in the Montreal, Quebec, area between 1930 and 2005.[17,18] CANJEM's strengths lie in its wide coverage of work settings and chemical exposures, semiquantification of frequency and intensity of exposure, and expert assessment of exposures from worker interviews. CARcinogen EXposure (CAREX) Canada is another JEM providing exposure prevalence and level estimates for multiple occupational agents across a wide span of work settings in Canada in 2016; however, this database is limited to select carcinogens.[19]

Although not a JEM, other researchers have used the Occupational Information Network (O*NET) as a source of occupational exposure information.[20] O*NET is a public database providing detailed occupational characteristic information for hundreds of occupations, which can be used to estimate a variety of occupational exposures. However, O*NET lacks coverage of chemical exposures and is reliant on self-report. While obtaining exposure information represents a considerable challenge, CANJEM is one of the few exposure information systems in the world with data on multiple agents spanning a wide range of work settings.

Previous US studies have used JEMs to estimate the prevalence of occupational exposures at the population level.[21,22] However, these studies were limited in the scope of chemical exposures, geographical area, or working populations investigated and did not look comprehensively at sociodemographic differences in exposure burden. In this study, we combined US employment and workforce demographic data with exposure data from CANJEM to characterize the burden and sociodemographic distribution of 244 chemical exposures in US workplaces. Identifying prevalent exposures and at-risk working populations can inform future interventions to improve worker health and reduce health inequities.

TABLE 1— Average Employment Estimates in the United States by Sociodemographic Group: 2021 Current Population Survey

Sociodemographic Group	Employee Count (% of Workforce)
Race/ethnicity[a]	
AI/AN	1 674 000 (1.1)
Asian	10 017 000 (6.6)
Black or African American	18 726 000 (12.3)
Multiracial	3 203 000 (2.1)
NH/PI	670 000 (0.4)
White	118 291 000 (77.5)
Non-Hispanic White	93 983 000 (61.6)
Hispanic White	24 308 000 (15.9)
Hispanic or Latino, any race	27 429 000 (18.0)
Not Hispanic or Latino, any race	125 152 000 (82.0)
Racial and ethnic minoritized groups[b]	58 597 000 (38.4)
Sex	
Female	71 752 000 (47.0)
Male	80 829 000 (53.0)
Education level	
< High-school diploma	11 438 000 (7.5)
High-school diploma or equivalent	39 006 000 (25.6)
Some college or associate degree	40 278 000 (26.4)
≥ Bachelor's degree	61 858 000 (40.5)
Nativity and citizenship status	
Native-born	126 177 000 (82.7)
Foreign-born, citizen	13 354 000 (8.8)
Foreign-born, noncitizen	13 049 000 (8.6)
Total	152 581 000 (100)

Note. AI/AN = American Indian/Alaska Native; NH/PI = Native Hawaiian/Pacific Islander. Employee counts are rounded to the nearest thousand.
[a]Persons of Hispanic or Latino ethnicity are of any race and are also counted in their preferred race category.
[b]Racial and ethnic minoritized groups include persons identifying as AI/AN, Asian, Black/African American, multiracial, NH/PI, or Hispanic/Latino.

METHODS

We used two sources of data in this analysis, which are described in more detail here.

Data Sources

Current Population Survey. We obtained 2021 employment and worker demographic data using the Employed Labor Force query system developed by the National Institute for Occupational Safety and Health, which generates workforce estimates based on the US Census Bureau and US Bureau of Labor Statistics Current Population Survey (CPS).[23] We obtained employment counts by 2018 Census occupation codes and sociodemographic groups describing race and ethnicity, sex, education, and nativity and citizenship (Table 1). These categories represent axes of social and health inequity and allow us to examine how occupational segregation across sociodemographic characteristics may contribute to unequal occupational exposure burdens.

For race and ethnicity categories, persons within each race category are of any ethnicity, except for persons who identify as non-Hispanic White, and persons of Hispanic/Latino ethnicity are also counted in their preferred race category. American Indian/Alaska Native, Asian, Black/African American, multiracial, Native Hawaiian/Pacific Islander, and Hispanic/Latino persons were aggregated into an additional category of all REM groups. Employment estimates less than 1000 are considered unstable within the Employed Labor Force query system. Although their contribution to the overall burden estimates is minor, we have purposefully included these estimates to maximize our representation of small populations often left out of occupational health research.

Canadian Job-Exposure Matrix. CANJEM is a general-population JEM providing semiquantitative exposure information for 258 occupational agents—mainly chemical—by industry or occupation.[17,18] CANJEM was built from the accumulation of more than 40 person-years of expert assessment of occupational exposures from detailed worker interviews completed in 4 case–control cancer studies conducted between 1979 and 2004 in Canada. Collectively, more than 30 000 jobs from 1930 to 2005 held by nearly 9000 participants comprising a largely urban population in the greater Montreal region were evaluated. Details regarding the development and validity of CANJEM have been previously described.[17,18] CANJEM represents a uniquely large and extensive database of exposure information collected from a North American population into the early 21st century.

To develop the JEM data, a team of experts assessed each job for potential exposure to approximately 300 occupational agents. The experts considered a job to be exposed to an agent if it was present in the workplace above background levels found in the general population. For each job thought to be exposed, the experts assigned exposure characteristics of intensity (low, medium, high), frequency (hours per week), and degree of confidence that the exposure occurred (possible, probable, definite). For each coded occupation, CANJEM provides a probability of exposure for each occupational agent. An additional exposure metric, frequency-weighted intensity (FWI) is also provided, which is a continuous measure of intensity of exposure averaged over a 40-hour workweek (FWI = exposure intensity*frequency of exposure in hours worked per week/40 hours).

As informed by Sauvé et al.,[18] we calculated probability of exposure as the proportion of jobs exposed to an agent with a frequency of exposure of at least 30 minutes per week, a "possible" or higher degree of confidence that the exposure occurred, and an FWI of at least 0.05 (corresponding to low exposure for 2 hours/week). We used versions of CANJEM coded into 3-, 5-, and 6-digit 2010 Standard Occupational Classification codes that summarized data collected from jobs held between 1985 and 2005 (closest to present day) and included occupations with a sample size of 5 or more jobs from 5 or more participants. We included 244 chemical agents from CANJEM, including specific chemicals, mixtures, families, or groups based on use. While the chemical agents vary in toxicity and health effects, all the evaluated exposures have some health risk to workers, and we did not conduct any risk assessment or weigh the exposures by toxicity in reporting our results.

Analytic Approach

We used R statistical software version 4.3.0 to merge and analyze the data.[24] We merged the data sets by 2018 Census codes at the specific (most granular) occupation level using crosswalks provided by the Bureau of Labor Statistics.[25] The final matrix included exposure information on 229 Census occupation codes based on 6220 jobs from CANJEM.

Exposure burden estimates. We estimated the number of US workers exposed for each occupational agent by multiplying the number of workers in each occupation by the agent–occupation specific probability of exposure and summing the estimated numbers across all occupations. We calculated the prevalence of exposed workers by dividing the estimated number of workers exposed by the total number of workers in the United States. We assumed workers employed in occupations without exposure information to have no exposure and included them in the denominator for the prevalence calculations. We calculated count and prevalence estimates for all workers and separately by sociodemographic group.

Exposure disproportionality estimates. Estimates of exposure disproportionality reflect the extent to which sociodemographic groups are over- or underrepresented in exposure burden. We calculated these estimates by finding the absolute and relative differences between the estimated number of exposed workers in a sociodemographic group and the number of workers expected to be exposed based on their overall proportion in the total workforce. We considered a group to be overrepresented if the estimated number of exposed workers in a particular sociodemographic group was in excess of the expected value.

Sensitivity analyses. We conducted 3 sensitivity analyses to examine the robustness of our results to alternative methodological decisions: (1) using a more stringent level of experts' confidence of exposure when developing the JEM data, (2) excluding workers employed in specific Census occupation codes without exposure information from our calculations, and (3) using JEM data based on broader occupational categories, which improved coverage of workers with exposure information. Detailed methods are presented in Appendix A (available as a supplement to the online version of this article at https://ajph.org).

RESULTS

In 2021, the US workforce comprised approximately 152.6 million workers per CPS estimates. Average employment estimates by sociodemographic group are presented in Table 1. CANJEM exposure information meeting temporal and sample size selection criteria covered 229 of 525 (43.6%) 2018 US Census codes with employment data in the CPS, representing approximately 116.8 million of the 152.6 million (76.5%) workers counted in the 2021 US workforce (Appendix B Table A). Workers for whom exposure information was available were somewhat more likely to be male or from historically marginalized sociodemographic groups (Appendix B Table B). These workers were also more

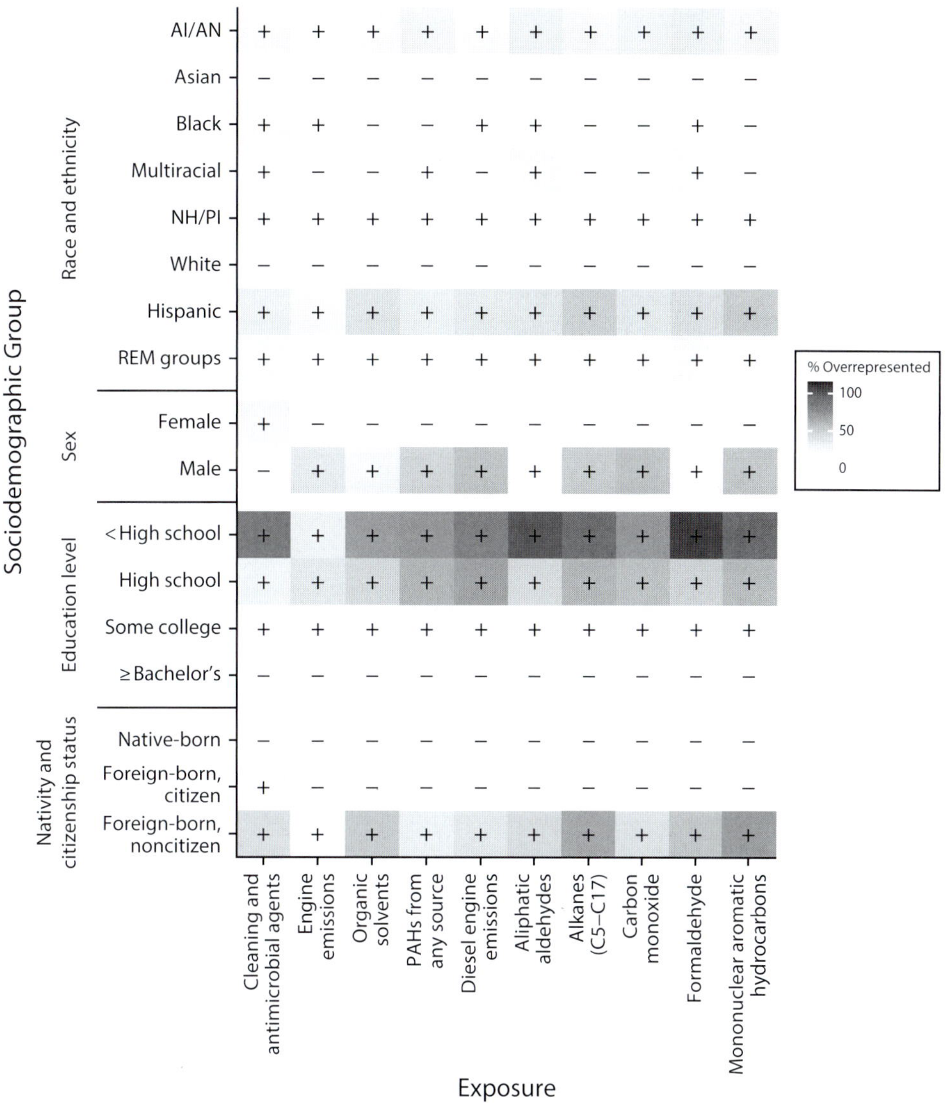

FIGURE 1— Magnitude of US Workers by Sociodemographic Group Overrepresented in Exposure to the 10 Most Prevalent Chemical Agents in CANJEM, 2021

Note. AI/AN = American Indian/Alaska Native; Black = Black/African American; CANJEM = Canadian job-exposure matrix; Hispanic = Hispanic/Latino; NH/PI = Native Hawaiian/Pacific Islander; PAHs = polycyclic aromatic hydrocarbons; REM groups = racial and ethnic minoritized groups; White = non-Hispanic White. A positive sign indicates overrepresentation of exposure (i.e., the number of workers exposed is in excess of the expected exposed based on the group's share of the total workforce). Darker shades of gray indicate higher percentages of overrepresentation. A negative sign indicates underrepresentation of exposure (i.e., the number of workers exposed is under the expected exposed based on the group's share of the total workforce). Persons within each race category are of any ethnicity, except for persons who identify as non-Hispanic White, and persons of Hispanic/Latino ethnicity are also counted in their preferred race category. REM groups include persons identifying as AI/AN, Asian, Black/African American, multiracial, Native Hawaiian/Pacific Islander, or Hispanic/Latino.

likely to be employed in blue-collar occupations (Appendix B Table C).

Figure 1 shows the estimated number and percentage of US workers exposed to the 10 most-prevalent chemical agents, stratified by sociodemographic group. Among all workers, the most-prevalent exposures were cleaning and antimicrobial agents (22.5 million US workers exposed; 14.7% of total workforce), engine emissions (19.5 million; 12.8%), organic solvents (18.5 million; 12.1%), polycyclic aromatic hydrocarbons (15.4 million; 10.1%), and diesel engine emissions (12.7 million; 8.3%). The prevalence of exposures varied across sociodemographic groups. Figure 2 shows the total number of exposures in which each sociodemographic group was disproportionately exposed. For both the 10 most prevalent agents and all agents combined, American Indian/Alaska Native, Hispanic/Latino,

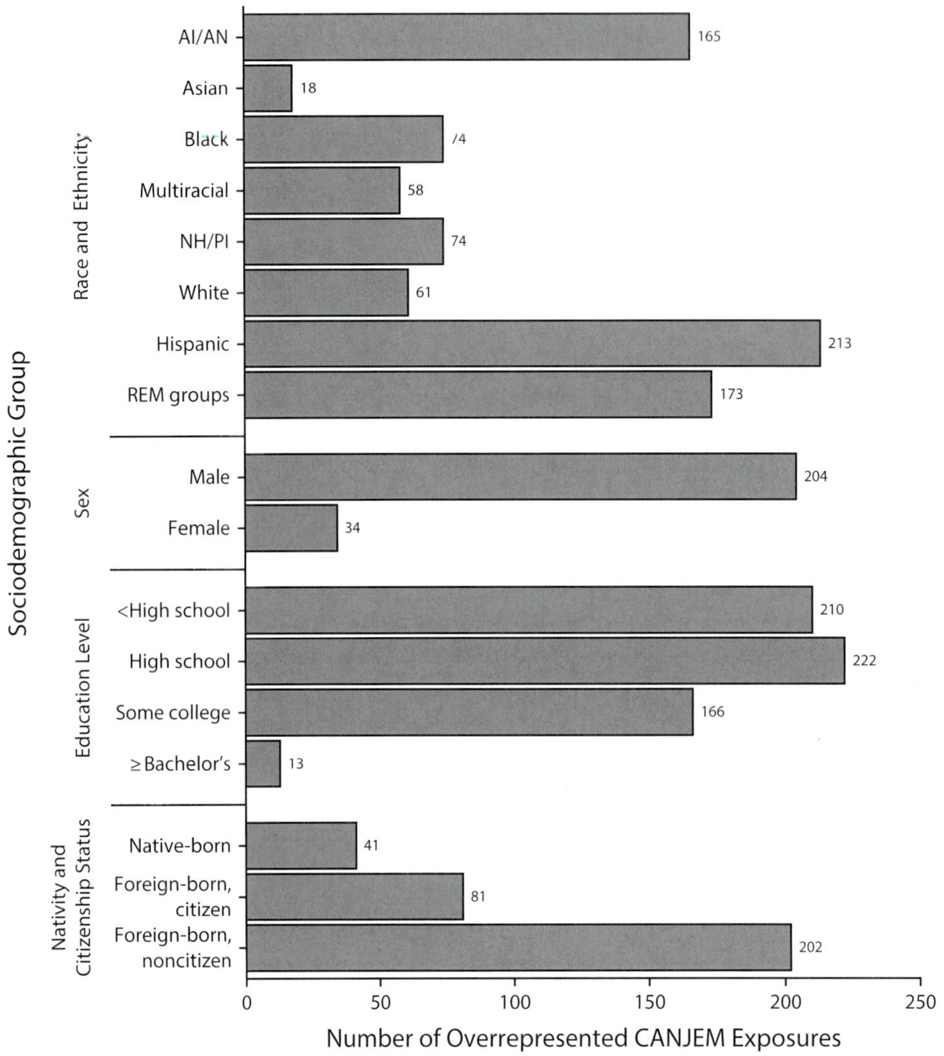

FIGURE 2— Total Number of Overrepresented Chemical CANJEM Exposures by Sociodemographic Group in the United States, 2021

Note. AI/AN = American Indian/Alaska Native; Black = Black/African American; CANJEM = Canadian job-exposure matrix; Hispanic = Hispanic/Latino; NH/PI = Native Hawaiian/Pacific Islander; REM groups = racial and ethnic minoritized groups; some college = some college or associate degree; White = non-Hispanic White. Persons within each race category are of any ethnicity, except for persons who identify as non-Hispanic White, and persons of Hispanic/Latino ethnicity are also counted in their preferred race category. REM groups include persons identifying as American Indian/Alaska Native, Asian, Black/African American, multiracial, Native Hawaiian/Pacific Islander, or Hispanic/Latino.

male, and foreign-born noncitizen workers; workers from REM groups as a whole; and workers with lower educational attainment were routinely overrepresented in exposure. Workers from other REM groups were estimated to experience disproportionate exposure to many of the 10 most-prevalent exposures, including Native Hawaiian/Pacific Islander (10 of 10), Black/African American (5 of 10), and multiracial (4 of 10) groups. Table 2 shows the number and percentage of US workers disproportionately exposed to the 10 most prevalent agents. Workers with lower educational attainment generally experienced increasingly greater magnitudes of disproportionate exposure, and Hispanic workers experienced the greatest magnitude of disproportionate exposure among all racial and ethnic groups.

A full interactive version of the data set is available for use by occupational and public health researchers, policymakers, practitioners, and others at https://deohs.washington.edu/us-exposure-burden. The online application allows users to generate tables and figures of the estimates for all agents and sociodemographic groups considered. Users can additionally explore estimates based on high-level

TABLE 2— Number, in Thousands, and Percentage of US Workers by Sociodemographic Group Exposed to the 10 Most Prevalent Chemical CANJEM Exposures, 2021

Sociodemographic Group	No. of Workers Exposed (% of Group Exposed)									
	Cleaning and Antimicrobial Agents	Engine Emissions	Organic Solvents	PAHs From Any Source	Diesel Engine Emissions	Aliphatic Aldehydes	Alkanes (C5–C17)	Carbon Monoxide	Formaldehyde	Mononuclear Aromatic Hydrocarbons
All	22 474 (14.7)	19 479 (12.8)	18 465 (12.1)	15 437 (10.1)	12 706 (8.3)	11 882 (7.8)	11 787 (7.7)	9 862 (6.5)	9 530 (6.2)	9 328 (6.1)
Race/ethnicity[a]										
AI/AN	292 (17.4)[b]	229 (13.7)[b]	238 (14.2)[b]	213 (12.7)[b]	164 (9.8)[b]	170 (10.1)[b]	159 (9.5)[b]	139 (8.3)[b]	137 (8.2)[b]	128 (7.7)[b]
Asian	1 347 (13.4)	800 (8.0)	805 (8.0)	599 (6.0)	453 (4.5)	658 (6.6)	433 (4.3)	379 (3.8)	533 (5.3)	329 (3.3)
Black	3 252 (17.4)[b]	2 642 (14.1)[b]	2 129 (11.4)	1 779 (9.5)	1 699 (9.1)[b]	1 509 (8.1)[b]	1 333 (7.1)	1 154 (6.2)	1 223 (6.5)[b]	964 (5.1)
Multiracial	544 (17.0)[b]	391 (12.2)	381 (11.9)	326 (10.2)[b]	265 (8.3)	304 (9.5)[b]	240 (7.5)	188 (5.9)	238 (7.4)[b]	189 (5.9)
NH/PI	116 (17.2)[b]	90 (13.4)[b]	88 (13.1)[b]	74 (11.1)[b]	61 (9.2)[b]	58 (8.6)[b]	54 (8.1)[b]	47 (6.9)[b]	47 (6.9)[b]	43 (6.5)[b]
White	12 234 (13.0)	11 559 (12.3)	10 642 (11.3)	9 130 (9.7)	7 255 (7.7)	6 566 (7.0)	6 688 (7.1)	5 750 (6.1)	5 174 (5.5)	5 358 (5.7)
Hispanic	5 275 (19.2)[b]	4 188 (15.3)[b]	4 642 (16.9)[b]	3 673 (13.4)[b]	3 109 (11.3)[b]	2 940 (10.7)[b]	3 178 (11.6)[b]	2 436 (8.9)[b]	2 444 (8.9)[b]	2 554 (9.3)[b]
REM groups[c]	10 240 (17.5)[b]	7 920 (13.5)[b]	7 822 (13.3)[b]	6 306 (10.8)[b]	5 452 (9.3)[b]	5 316 (9.1)[b]	5 099 (8.7)[b]	4 112 (7.0)[b]	4 356 (7.4)[b]	3 970 (6.8)[b]
Sex										
Female	12 763 (17.8)[b]	5 573 (7.8)	6 495 (9.1)	3 381 (4.7)	2 230 (3.1)	5 370 (7.5)	2 349 (3.3)	1 693 (2.4)	4157 (5.8)	1 750 (2.4)
Male	9 710 (12.0)	13 906 (17.2)[b]	11 970 (14.8)[b]	12 055 (14.9)[b]	10 477 (13.0)[b]	6 512 (8.1)[b]	9 438 (11.7)[b]	8 168 (10.1)[b]	5 373 (6.6)[b]	7 578 (9.4)[b]
Education level										
< High-school diploma	3 140 (27.5)[b]	1 905 (16.7)[b]	2 361 (20.6)[b]	1 993 (17.4)[b]	1 729 (15.1)[b]	1 796 (15.7)[b]	1 705 (14.9)[b]	1 264 (11.1)[b]	1 542 (13.5)[b]	1 360 (11.9)[b]
High-school diploma or equivalent	7 278 (18.7)[b]	6 754 (17.3)[b]	6 864 (17.6)[b]	6 307 (16.2)[b]	5 427 (13.9)[b]	4 358 (11.2)[b]	4 796 (12.3)[b]	3 942 (10.1)[b]	3 580 (9.2)[b]	3 759 (9.6)[b]
Some college	6 412 (15.9)[b]	5 606 (13.9)[b]	5 229 (13.0)[b]	4 620 (11.5)[b]	3 621 (9.0)[b]	3 559 (8.8)[b]	3 360 (8.3)[b]	2 912 (7.2)[b]	2 802 (7.0)[b]	2 692 (6.7)[b]
≥ Bachelor's degree	5 644 (9.1)	5 214 (8.4)	4 011 (6.5)	2 517 (4.1)	1929 (3.1)	2 170 (3.5)	1 926 (3.1)	1 744 (2.8)	1 606 (2.6)	1 518 (2.5)
Nativity and citizenship status										
Native-born	17 377 (13.8)	15 932 (12.6)	14 452 (11.5)	12 479 (9.9)	10 098 (8.0)	9 380 (7.4)	9 113 (7.2)	7 851 (6.2)	7 432 (5.9)	7 213 (5.7)
Foreign-born, citizen	2 321 (17.4)[b]	1 650 (12.4)	1 591 (11.9)	1 201 (9.0)	1 086 (8.1)	1 014 (7.6)	989 (7.4)	805 (6.0)	828 (6.2)	750 (5.6)
Foreign-born, noncitizen	2 775 (21.3)[b]	1 898 (14.5)[b]	2 422 (18.6)[b]	1 757 (13.5)[b]	1 522 (11.7)[b]	1 488 (11.4)[b]	1 685 (12.9)[b]	1 206 (9.2)[b]	1 270 (9.7)[b]	1 366 (10.5)[b]

Note. AI/AN = American Indian/Alaska Native; ≥ Bachelor's = bachelor's or advanced degree; Black = Black/African American; CANJEM = Canadian job-exposure matrix; Hispanic = Hispanic/Latino, NH/PI = Native Hawaiian/Pacific Islander; PAHs = polycyclic aromatic hydrocarbons; REM groups = racial and ethnic minoritized groups; Some college = some college or associate degree; White = non-Hispanic White.

[a]Persons within each race category are of any ethnicity, except for persons who identify as non-Hispanic White, and persons of Hispanic/Latino ethnicity are also counted in their preferred race category.

[b]Overrepresentation in exposure.

[c]REM groups include persons identifying as American Indian/Alaska Native, Asian, Black/African American, multiracial, Native Hawaiian/Pacific Islander, or Hispanic/Latino.

exposures and different occupational classification levels.

Results from our 3 sensitivity analyses suggest our conclusions are robust to alternative analytic decisions. In each case, the rank order of the most common occupational exposures (i.e., number of workers exposed) and the pattern of exposure disparities across sociodemographic groups were generally similar, resulting in the same conclusions as our primary analysis. The overall prevalence of the occupational exposures did vary in expected ways, with prevalence of exposures generally decreasing in sensitivity analysis 1 and increasing in sensitivity analyses 2 and 3. The full results and discussion of the sensitivity analyses are presented in Appendix A.

DISCUSSION

Our goal was to quantify the number of US workers exposed to a large set of chemical hazards and characterize patterns of exposure by sociodemographic strata. Our estimates suggest that a substantial number of US workers experience exposure to chemical hazards at work. Of the chemical exposures examined, the most common were cleaning and antimicrobial agents, engine emissions, organic solvents, polycyclic aromatic hydrocarbons, and diesel engine emissions. Our results are largely consistent with Doubleday et al.,[22] who applied a subset of the CANJEM data to workers in Federal Region 10 (Alaska, Idaho, Oregon, and Washington State) in 2019. Using a qualitative JEM to estimate cancer-related occupational exposures among California working women, Beckman et al.[21] similarly found cleaning and antimicrobial agents were among the most common exposures. However, there were also some differences in findings—for example, Beckman et al.[21] finding phthalates among the most common exposures, which were not as common in our study. This is likely attributable to the different goals and methods of the studies, the time period in which the exposure data were obtained, and increasing knowledge on the ubiquity of phthalates in occupational settings.

Exposures were found to be unevenly distributed by sociodemographic groups, driven by the occupational segregation of workers. This pattern was observed whether examining the sociodemographic distribution of the 10 most-prevalent exposures or the total number of overrepresented exposures. Particularly stark disparities in occupational exposures were observed across education and nativity, as workers with lower educational attainment and foreign-born (especially noncitizen) workers were disproportionately exposed to a larger number of agents compared with workers with higher educational attainment and native-born workers, respectively. Compared with non-Hispanic White workers, workers from REM groups as a whole, Hispanic/Latino workers, and American Indian/Alaskan Native workers were notably more likely to be disproportionately exposed to the agents examined in this analysis, while Asian workers were less likely to be disproportionately exposed. Though women were largely underrepresented in exposures in this analysis, they were disproportionately exposed to cleaning and antimicrobial agents, which is generally associated with service-providing occupations. In contrast, men were disproportionately exposed to the remaining top exposures, generally associated with goods-producing occupations. When looking at the magnitude of overrepresentation of exposure to the 10 most-prevalent exposures, a stark gradient was found across educational groups in which, generally, the lower the educational attainment level, the greater the degree of overrepresentation. Among all racial and ethnic groups, Hispanic/Latino workers experienced the greatest degree of overrepresentation of exposures.

Although Asian and female workers generally experienced a lower burden of the chemical exposures considered, this should not be interpreted as these populations needing less attention from occupational health practice and policy. There are work settings in which these populations have been documented to experience substantial chemical exposures (e.g., nail salons).[26] Our analysis may also somewhat underestimate their level of exposure because these workers have historically been underrepresented in occupational health research,[27] which may contribute to less knowledge of chemical hazards in jobs in which they are overrepresented. These gaps in historical occupational health knowledge may have affected the types of hazards evaluated and ascertainment of exposure within CANJEM, possibly leading to less or inaccurate information on exposures within occupations that women and Asian workers are overrepresented.

Overall, the sociodemographic groups found to carry the greatest burden of exposures in our analysis are consistent with Krieger's inverse hazard law, which postulates that the "accumulation of health hazards tends to vary inversely with the power and resources of the populations affected."[28(p1971)] Our findings are also generally consistent with earlier research on disparities in occupational health outcomes, in which workers from historically marginalized sociodemographic groups were observed to suffer more work-related injuries and illnesses.[7,11,12] While our study focused upstream on exposures rather than health outcomes, the consistency of findings provides some external validation to our study's results.

The results from our analysis call particular attention to cleaning and antimicrobial agents, identified as the most common exposure based on number of US workers exposed and which disproportionately burden marginalized working populations. Occupational cleaners and some studied cleaning and antimicrobial agents have been associated with various adverse respiratory effects, though specific causal agents and mechanisms of this broad category are still not well understood.[29] Many also do not have specific OSHA regulations, implying less knowledge, awareness, and control in the workplace. Attention to cleaning and antimicrobial agents is especially imperative and timely given enhanced cleaning and disinfecting measures in workplaces because of the COVID-19 pandemic.[30] Overall, our findings suggest that public health research and control efforts for cleaning and antimicrobial agents could be impactful for reducing occupational exposure and health inequities.

Limitations

First, it is important to acknowledge occupational hazards and populations that are not covered in this analysis. Military and institutionalized workers are excluded from the CPS, so these populations were not covered.[23] Approximately a quarter of the counted workforce did not have exposure information because of employment in occupations either missing from CANJEM or excluded on the basis of our selection criteria. The portion of the workforce without CANJEM-provided exposure information was disproportionately employed in white-collar and service occupations (88% employed within white-collar and service occupations; see Appendix B Table C) in which chemical exposures are less likely,[31] and would thus be expected to contribute minimally to the overall burden estimates.

In assuming workers without exposure information had no occupational exposure, we therefore expect that our results may slightly underestimate true exposure prevalence. Furthermore, the portion of the workforce with CANJEM-provided exposure information was slightly more likely to be from historically marginalized groups, including REM groups as a whole; Hispanic/Latino, Black/African American, and foreign-born noncitizen persons; and persons with lower educational attainment (see Appendix B Table B). We therefore expect that our results may slightly overestimate exposure disparities for those groups overrepresented in the sample with CANJEM-provided information. We tested the implications of our methodological decisions for handling workers without exposure information and found that our results and overall conclusions are robust to alternative analytic approaches (see sensitivity analyses 2 and 3 in Appendix A).

Overall, we feel our primary estimates balance adequate coverage of the workforce with valid estimates of exposure and reduced misclassification, while being specific enough to inform future research, practice, and policy. It is still important to consider that workers in some of the excluded occupations likely do experience relevant chemical exposures (e.g., home health aides) and are amenable to intervention efforts. Furthermore, while our analysis includes many chemicals, it does not cover other important occupational hazards, including psychosocial, biological, physical, and other chemical hazards.

In addition, the probabilities of exposures of the CANJEM data are static and based on jobs held by an urban Canadian population between 1985 and 2005, which is geographically and temporally different than the US population in 2021 and may not account for differences in industries, occupations, and regulations between the 2 populations or changes in exposures over time. These limitations could potentially lead to an over- or underestimation of exposures for some agents attributable to, for example, changes in federal and state regulations (e.g., crystalline silica), increased knowledge and awareness of certain occupational hazards (e.g., phthalates), changes in protective technologies (e.g., carbon monoxide), and changes in work practices (e.g., cleaning and antimicrobial agents because of the COVID-19 pandemic[30]). It is therefore important to consider the historical context of these agents when interpreting the study's findings. Despite these limitations, CANJEM is the most comprehensive JEM available for a wide range of occupations and chemical exposures in North America.

Another important limitation is exposure misclassification associated with the use of a JEM.[16] All individuals within an occupation code were assigned the same probability of exposure, and we were therefore unable to account for intraoccupational exposure differences across individuals or groups that may exist because of differences in assigned tasks or other occupational inequities, which have been previously documented.[7] Investigation of sex differences in the underlying CANJEM data by Lacourt et al.[32] found exposures were generally similar between men and women within the same occupation when employed in sufficient number. However, some notable differences in exposures between sexes were found, which could mostly be explained by different suboccupations, industries, or tasks performed within the same occupation. A subsequent investigation by Xu et al.[33] found that CANJEM's applicability to women may vary by agent. These studies suggest that there could be important intraoccupational exposure disparities that we are not able to account for in this analysis. Exposure disparities identified in our analysis can only be attributed to the differential distribution of workers across occupations (i.e., occupational segregation). Misclassification may have also been introduced from the use of crosswalks needed to merge the data sets by a common occupational classification system.[16]

The CPS also has important limitations to consider as our source of employment and demographic information. While we used the most recent year of employment data available, it is important to acknowledge that the US labor market in 2021 was in process of recovering from an economic recession caused by the COVID-19 pandemic in 2020.[34] Accordingly, our estimates are expected to be slightly different than current and future levels. We were also limited by the sociodemographic variables captured in the CPS, as more detailed demographic data would be useful in better identifying exposure disparities in specific populations. Lastly, while we did not investigate intersecting identities, an intersectional approach has been demonstrated to be useful in highlighting important social inequities and could be considered in future studies.[35]

Public Health Implications

To our knowledge, this is the first study to combine a population-based JEM with employment and demographic data to estimate the burden of occupational exposures and characterize exposure disparities by sociodemographic groups in the United States. JEM-based research approaches can help address the pressing need for occupational health surveillance to move upstream and characterize the burden of exposures rather than only health outcomes. Data from this analysis can inform occupational and public health research, policy, and interventions aimed at reducing the burden of disease in the United States. Our incorporation of sociodemographic information can additionally help inform equitable approaches to reduce health inequities and ensure health justice. Continual improvement to occupational exposure surveillance should be made a top priority in the United States as it is vital to the primary prevention of occupational injuries and illnesses and the broader understanding of work as a social determinant of health and health disparities. AJPH

ABOUT THE AUTHORS

Shelley C. Stephan-Recaido and Marissa G. Baker are with the Department of Environmental and Occupational Health Sciences, University of Washington School of Public Health, Seattle. Trevor K. Peckham is with the Hazardous Waste Management Program in King County, Seattle, and the Department of Environmental and Occupational Health Sciences, University of Washington School of Public Health. Jérôme Lavoué is with the University of Montreal Hospital Research Center and the Department of Environmental and Occupational Health, University of Montreal, Montreal, QC, Canada.

CORRESPONDENCE

Correspondence should be sent to Marissa G. Baker, 4225 Roosevelt Way NE, Suite 100, Seattle, WA 98105 (e-mail: bakermg@uw.edu). Reprints can be ordered at https://ajph.org by clicking the "Reprints" link.

PUBLICATION INFORMATION

Full Citation: Stephan-Recaido SC, Peckham TK, Lavoué Jérôme, Baker MG. Characterizing the burden of occupational chemical exposures by sociodemographic groups in the United States, 2021. *Am J Public Health*. 2024;114(1):57–67.

Acceptance Date: September 13, 2023.

DOI: https://doi.org/10.2105/AJPH.2023.307461

CONTRIBUTORS

S. C. Stephan-Recaido led the drafting of the article and led the data management, analysis, and interpretation. M. G. Baker and T. K. Peckham contributed to the conceptualization and design of the work, helped with interpretation of the data, and helped with drafting and reviewing the article for critically important intellectual content. J. Lavoué originated and designed the Canadian job-exposure matrix, contributed to the interpretation and analysis of the data, and reviewed the article for important intellectual content. All authors approved the final version of the article and agree to be held accountable for all aspects of the work and for ensuring questions related to the accuracy or integrity of any part of the work are appropriately investigated and resolved.

ACKNOWLEDGMENTS

This project was supported by the National Institute for Occupational Safety and Health (NIOSH) under federal training grant T42OH008433, and the National Institute of Environmental Health Sciences (NIEHS) under award P30ES00703. Additional funding was provided by the Hazardous Waste Fund, administered by the Hazardous Waste Management Program in King County, Washington.

Note. The content is solely the responsibility of the authors and does not necessarily represent the official views of NIOSH, NIEHS, or King County.

CONFLICTS OF INTEREST

The authors declare no conflicts of interest.

HUMAN PARTICIPANT PROTECTION

As this article was an analysis of de-identified existing secondary data, no human participant review was required.

REFERENCES

1. US Bureau of Labor Statistics. IIF Latest Numbers. November 21, 2022. Available at: https://www.bls.gov/iif/latest-numbers.htm. Accessed August 15, 2023.
2. National Academies of Sciences, Engineering, and Medicine. *A Smarter National Surveillance System for Occupational Safety and Health in the 21st Century*. Washington, DC: The National Academies Press; 2018. https://doi.org/10.17226/24835
3. Greife A, Halperin W, Groce D, et al. Occupational health and safety surveillance: hazard surveillance:

its role in primary prevention of occupational disease and injury. *Appl Occup Environ Hyg.* 1995;10(9):737–742. https://doi.org/10.1080/1047322X.1995.10387678

4. Wegman DH, Froines JR. Surveillance needs for occupational health. *Am J Public Health.* 1985;75(11):1259–1261. https://doi.org/10.2105/AJPH.75.11.1259
5. Azaroff LS, Levenstein C, Wegman DH. Occupational injury and illness surveillance: conceptual filters explain underreporting. *Am J Public Health.* 2002;92(9):1421–1429. https://doi.org/10.2105/AJPH.92.9.1421
6. Alonso-Villar O, del Rio C, Gradin C. The extent of occupational segregation in the United States: differences by race, ethnicity, and gender. *Ind Relat.* 2012;51(2):179–212. https://doi.org/10.1111/j.1468-232X.2012.00674.x
7. Lipscomb HJ, Loomis D, McDonald MA, Argue RA, Wing S. A conceptual model of work and health disparities in the United States. *Int J Health Serv.* 2006;36(1):25–50. https://doi.org/10.2190/BRED-NRJ7-3LV7-2QCG
8. Krieger N. Workers are people too: societal aspects of occupational health disparities—an ecosocial perspective. *Am J Ind Med.* 2010;53(2):104–115. https://doi.org/10.1002/ajim.20759
9. Ahonen EQ, Fujishiro K, Cunningham T, Flynn M. Work as an inclusive part of population health inequities research and prevention. *Am J Public Health.* 2018;108(3):306–311. https://doi.org/10.2105/AJPH.2017.304214
10. Fujishiro K, Hajat A, Landsbergis PA, Meyer JD, Schreiner PJ, Kaufman JD. Explaining racial/ethnic differences in all-cause mortality in the Multi-Ethnic Study of Atherosclerosis (MESA): substantive complexity and hazardous working conditions as mediating factors. *SSM Popul Health.* 2017;3:497–505. https://doi.org/10.1016/j.ssmph.2017.05.010
11. Baron SL, Steege AL, Marsh SM, Menéndez CC, Myers JR. Nonfatal work-related injuries and illnesses—United States, 2010. *MMWR Suppl.* 2013;62(3):35–40.
12. Stanbury M, Rosenman KD. Occupational health disparities: a state public health-based approach. *Am J Ind Med.* 2014;57(5):596–604. https://doi.org/10.1002/ajim.22292
13. Rosner D, Markowitz G. A short history of occupational safety and health in the United States. *Am J Public Health.* 2020;110(5):622–628. https://doi.org/10.2105/AJPH.2020.305581
14. Castro C. Dying to work: OSHA's exclusion of health and safety standards for domestic workers. *The Modern American.* Spring 2008:3–9.
15. Michaels D. Is OSHA working for working people? *New Solut.* 2008;18(3):391–403. https://doi.org/10.2190/NS.18.3.n
16. Peters S. Although a valuable method in occupational epidemiology, job-exposure matrices are no magic fix. *Scand J Work Environ Health.* 2020;46(3):231–234. https://doi.org/10.5271/sjweh.3894
17. Siemiatycki J, Lavoué J. Availability of a new job-exposure matrix (CANJEM) for epidemiologic and occupational medicine purposes. *J Occup Environ Med.* 2018;60(7):e324–e328. https://doi.org/10.1097/JOM.0000000000001335
18. Sauvé JF, Siemiatycki J, Labrèche F, et al. Development of and selected performance characteristics of CANJEM, a general population job-exposure matrix based on past expert assessments of exposure. *Ann Work Expo Health.* 2018;62(7):783–795.
19. Peters CE, Ge CB, Hall AL, Davies HW, Demers PA. CAREX Canada: an enhanced model for assessing occupational carcinogen exposure. *Occup Environ Med.* 2015;72(1):64–71. https://doi.org/10.1136/oemed-2014-102286
20. Cifuentes M, Boyer J, Lombardi DA, Punnett L. Use of O* NET as a job exposure matrix: a literature review. *Am J Ind Med.* 2010;53(9):898–914. https://doi.org/10.1002/ajim.20846
21. Beckman S, Silver E, Weinberg JL, et al. Development of a data visualization tool for occupational exposure to chemicals of concern for breast cancer among California working women, 2010–2014. *New Solut.* 2022;31(4):400–412. https://doi.org/10.1177/10482911211032971
22. Doubleday A, Baker MG, Lavoué J, Siemiatycki J, Seixas NS. Estimating the population prevalence of traditional and novel occupational exposures in federal region X. *Am J Ind Med.* 2019;62(2):111–122. https://doi.org/10.1002/ajim.22931
23. National Institute for Occupational Safety and Health Division of Safety Research. The Employed Labor Force (ELF) query system. Centers for Disease Control and Prevention. December 9, 2021. Available at: https://wwwn.cdc.gov/wisards/cps. Accessed May 13, 2021.
24. R Core Team. R: A language and environment for statistical computing. 2023. Available at: https://www.R-project.org. Accessed April 26, 2023.
25. US Bureau of Labor Statistics. SOC 2010 to 2018 crosswalk. November 2017. Available at: https://www.bls.gov/soc/2018/crosswalks.htm. Accessed November 11, 2021.
26. Leong FTL, Mak S. Occupational health disparities among Asian Americans: a critical review with recommendations. *Asian Am J Psychol.* 2014;5(1):44–52. https://doi.org/10.1037/a0034907
27. Zahm SH, Blair A. Occupational cancer among women: where have we been and where are we going? *Am J Ind Med.* 2003;44(6):565–575. https://doi.org/10.1002/ajim.10270
28. Krieger N, Chen JT, Waterman PD, et al. The inverse hazard law: blood pressure, sexual harassment, racial discrimination, workplace abuse and occupational exposures in US low-income Black, White and Latino workers. *Soc Sci Med.* 2008;67(12):1970–1981. https://doi.org/10.1016/j.socscimed.2008.09.039
29. Archangelidi O, Sathiyajit S, Consonni D, Jarvis D, De Matteis S. Cleaning products and respiratory health outcomes in occupational cleaners: a systematic review and meta-analysis. *Occup Environ Med.* 2020;78(8):604–617. https://doi.org/10.1136/oemed-2020-106776
30. Occupational Safety and Health Administration. Protecting workers: guidance on mitigating and preventing the spread of COVID-19 in the workplace. Available at: https://www.osha.gov/coronavirus/safework. Accessed March 1, 2023.
31. Nguyen VK, Colacino J, Patel CJ, Sartor M, Jolliet O. Identification of occupations susceptible to high exposure and risk associated with multiple toxicants in an observational study: National Health and Nutrition Examination Survey 1999–2014. *Exposome.* 2022;2(1):osac004. https://doi.org/10.1093/exposome/osac004
32. Lacourt A, Labrèche F, Goldberg MS, Siemiatycki J, Lavoué J. Agreement in occupational exposures between men and women using retrospective assessments by expert coders. *Ann Work Expo Health.* 2018;62(9):1159–1170. https://doi.org/10.1093/annweh/wxy074
33. Xu M, Ho V, Lavoué J, Richardson L, Siemiatycki J. Concordance of occupational exposure assessment between the Canadian Job-Exposure Matrix (CANJEM) and expert assessment of jobs held by women. *Ann Work Expo Health.* 2022;66(6):728–740. https://doi.org/10.1093/annweh/wxac008
34. Edwards R, Essien LS, Levinstein MD. US labor market shows improvement in 2021, but the COVID-19 pandemic continues to weigh on the economy. US Bureau of Labor Statistics. June 7, 2022. Available at: https://www.bls.gov/opub/mlr/2022/article/us-labor-market-shows-improvement-in-2021-but-the-covid-19-pandemic-continues-to-weigh-on-the-economy.htm. Accessed March 1, 2023.
35. Andrea SB, Eisenberg-Guyot J, Peckham T, Oddo VM, Hajat A. Intersectional trends in employment quality in older adults in the United States. *SSM Popul Health.* 2021;15:100868. https://doi.org/10.1016/j.ssmph.2021.100868

Preexposure Prophylaxis Uptake Among Spanish-Speaking Transgender Women: A Randomized Controlled Trial in North and South Carolina, 2019–2022

Scott D. Rhodes, PhD, MPH, Jorge Alonzo, JD, Lilli Mann-Jackson, MPH, Lucero Refugio Aviles, Amanda E. Tanner, PhD, MPH, Carla A. Galindo, MPH, Patricia A. Bessler, MPH, Cari Courtenay-Quirk, PhD, Manuel Garcia, Ana D. Sucaldito, PhD, MPH, Benjamin D. Smart, MD, MS, Tamar Goldenberg, PhD, MPH, and Beth A. Reboussin, PhD

AJPH January 2024, Vol. 114, No. 1

Objectives. To evaluate Chicas Creando Acceso a la Salud (Girls Creating Access to Health; ChiCAS), a Spanish-language, small-group intervention designed to increase preexposure prophylaxis (PrEP) use, consistent condom use, and medically supervised gender-affirming hormone therapy use among Spanish-speaking transgender Latinas who have sex with men.

Methods. Participants were 144 HIV-negative Spanish-speaking transgender Latinas, aged 18 to 59 years, living in North and South Carolina. From July 2019 to July 2021, we screened, recruited, and randomized them to the 2-session ChiCAS intervention or the delayed-intervention waitlist control. Participants completed assessments at baseline and 6-month follow-up. Follow-up retention was 94.4%.

Results. At follow-up, relative to control participants, ChiCAS participants reported increased PrEP use (adjusted odds ratio [AOR] = 4.64; 95% confidence interval [CI] = 1.57, 13.7; $P < .006$). However, ChiCAS participants did not report increased use of condoms or medically supervised gender-affirming hormone therapy. ChiCAS participants reported increases in knowledge of HIV ($P < .001$), sexually transmitted infections ($P < .001$), and gender-affirming hormone therapy ($P = .01$); PrEP awareness ($P < .001$), knowledge ($P < .001$), and readiness ($P < .001$); condom use skills ($P < .001$); and community attachment ($P < .001$).

Conclusions. The ChiCAS intervention was efficacious in increasing PrEP use among Spanish-speaking, transgender Latinas in this trial. (*Am J Public Health*. 2024;114(1):68–78. https://doi.org/10.2105/AJPH.2023.307444)

Transgender women are disproportionately affected by HIV. Current estimates indicate that about 14% of transgender women in the United States are living with HIV,[1] fewer than half of whom know their status.[2] Certain subpopulations of transgender women are particularly affected by HIV, including transgender Latinas.[1,3] Evidence-based strategies are needed to prevent HIV transmission through the use of preexposure prophylaxis (PrEP), a critical biomedical strategy to prevent new HIV infections.[4,5] PrEP clinical practice guidelines recommend daily oral combination tenofovir and emtricitabine (brand name Truvada) or tenofovir and alafenamide (brand name Descovy) as safe and effective in reducing the risk of HIV infection in adults and adolescents; injectable intramuscular extended-release cabotegravir as PrEP is also now an option.[6] However, awareness, knowledge, and use of PrEP are low among transgender women, particularly transgender Latinas.[5,7–11]

Transgender Latinas also report little use of medically supervised gender-affirming hormone therapy.[12–14] Many report little access to formal health care and thus may obtain hormones from nonmedical sources (e.g., Latine ["Latine" uses a gender-neutral "e," which replaces the gendered endings "a" and "o" in "Latina" and "Latino" and is similar to "Latinx." This term is increasingly used within Latine LGBTQ+ (lesbian, gay, bisexual, transgender/-sexual, queer or questioning, and all subsects) communities] grocers, the Internet, and countries of origin) and take hormones without medical supervision; instead, they may rely on one another for guidance about dosage, administration, timing, and side effects.[12,13] The use of medically supervised gender-affirming hormone therapy is associated with positive mental health outcomes and behaviors (e.g., lower rates of suicidal ideation and drug and alcohol use), which also shape risk behaviors.[13]

Transgender Latinas using gender-affirming hormone therapy often prioritize the use of hormones over PrEP for HIV prevention because of fears that taking PrEP will interfere with hormone use.[15] Furthermore, medically supervised gender-affirming hormone therapy can be costly and difficult to access with no or insufficient health insurance; some transgender Latinas may obtain gender-affirming hormone therapy from less reliable sources or engage in sex work to pay for gender-affirming hormone therapy.[13,16]

Despite the disproportionate burden of HIV among transgender Latinas, no efficacious evidence-based or evidence-informed intervention for Spanish-speaking transgender Latinas is listed in the *Compendium of Evidence-Based Interventions and Best Practices for HIV Prevention* (https://bit.ly/3SoQwjz). The US Centers for Disease Control and Prevention (CDC) has reiterated calls for scaled-up HIV prevention strategies for transgender women, especially Latinas, given a recent finding that 35% of transgender Latinas tested positive for HIV in a study in 7 major US cities.[3]

Our objective in this intervention trial was to test whether participants randomized to Chicas Creando Acceso a la Salud (Girls Creating Access to Health; ChiCAS) increased their use of PrEP, condoms, and medically supervised gender-affirming hormone therapy compared with participants randomized to a delayed-intervention wait list control.

METHODS

We used community-based participatory research (CBPR) throughout all phases of this trial. CBPR is an effective approach to improving health and well-being, aiding in disease prevention, and promoting health equity and reduce disparities. CBPR blends the perspectives of community members, organization representatives, and academic partners to yield studies that have community buy-in and are authentic to how community members engage, convene, and interact.[17,18] Compared with approaches that do not blend this array of perspectives, CBPR ensures higher recruitment and retention rates, more precise measurement, and more acceptable data collection strategies. Moreover, data analysis and interpretation of findings may be more accurate. CBPR also contributes to the development of interventions that are more likely to be efficacious.[17,19]

Our long-standing CBPR partnership is composed of local Latine community members; representatives from HIV service organizations, public health departments, and other community organizations; federal partners; and academic researchers from multiple universities, and it developed, implemented, and evaluated ChiCAS.[11] The partnership worked collaboratively with a 6-member community steering committee of transgender Latinas that met monthly for the first year of the trial and quarterly thereafter. The steering committee provided guidance to the partnership on all aspects of the trial, including trial design (e.g., intervention and delayed-intervention wait list control); recruitment and retention strategies; inclusion of medically supervised gender-affirming hormone therapy as an intervention focus; development of the intervention logic model and intervention activities, scripts, and materials, including video segments that role modeled seeking care; measurement; and dissemination. They also helped address emergent challenges, such as how to adapt the trial and intervention to the COVID-19 pandemic.[9]

Intervention Development and Enhancement

After obtaining CDC funding in 2016, our CBPR partnership and the trial steering committee enhanced the locally developed ChiCAS intervention, as described elsewhere,[9,11] by developing a logic model (Table A, available as a supplement to the online version of this article at http://www.ajph.org) and an intervention logo; incorporating updated data on HIV burden and context among transgender Latinas; producing a video segment outlining how to access PrEP using transgender Latina role models deciding to obtain PrEP and then seeking care in a local clinic; refining intervention activities and materials; outlining ways to access PrEP, including in the context of lacking health insurance and being undocumented; and carefully scripting intervention delivery. We also reduced the intervention from 4 to 2 sessions.

Based on social cognitive theory[20] and empowerment education,[21] ChiCAS is designed to increase PrEP use, consistent condom use, and use of medically supervised gender-affirming hormone therapy.[11] The intervention addresses critical behavioral determinants, which have been found to be associated with HIV prevention behaviors among transgender Latinas.[11,13,22,23] These determinants include knowledge of HIV and sexually transmitted infections (STIs) and their modes of transmission and prevention strategies, knowledge of PrEP and medically supervised gender-affirming hormone therapy and of eligibility for accessing various services and resources, perceived access to available health care services and self-efficacy to overcome access barriers, communication skills with providers and sexual partners, sociocultural context (e.g., internalized transphobia), and relationships and sense of community among transgender Latinas. We did not provide PrEP in this intervention; rather, we built the skills among participants to seek and successfully obtain PrEP in the community. Building community capacity to reduce health inequities is an important strategy in our CBPR partnership.

Study Design

We used a 2-group, randomized, intervention wait list control design with a 1 to 1 allocation ratio to evaluate the efficacy of ChiCAS. From July 2019 to July 2021, we recruited participants by distributing information about the study (e.g., posters and flyers) at bars and clubs, community colleges, Latine-owned businesses, and community events (e.g., LGBTQ+ pride events and Latine cultural festivals); through the use of social media and networking Web sites, including apps for social and sexual networking used by or designed for members of the LGBTQ+ community (e.g., Facebook and Grindr); and by word of mouth whereby study participants invited friends to participate.

Study participants were eligible if they self-identified as a transgender woman or reported having been assigned male sex at birth and self-identifying as female, self-identified as Hispanic/Latina, were aged 18 years or older, reported sex with at least 1 man in the past 6 months, were HIV-negative (based on self-report and verified by HIV testing during the consent process), spoke fluent Spanish, and provided informed consent. Persons who had participated in any other HIV prevention intervention in the past 12 months were ineligible. The study team referred and linked potential participants who tested positive for HIV during screening to HIV care. Linkage included helping these individuals make appointments for confirmatory HIV tests and subsequent HIV care and accompanying them to initial appointments if desired.

We recruited and enrolled 144 transgender Latinas to the study in 10 waves of approximately 14 participants per wave. Participants completed written informed consent and a baseline assessment, and a block randomization scheme generated with SAS version 9.3 (SAS Institute, Cary, NC) assigned them to ChiCAS (n = 72) or the delayed-intervention wait list control (n = 72; Figure 1). Half of the sample was recruited and participated in the intervention before the onset of the pandemic.

Because of the onset of the COVID-19 pandemic, we adapted the trial as previously described.[9] We gave participants cash as a token of appreciation for completing the baseline assessment ($30), the 2 intervention sessions (before COVID: $40 per session), and the 6-month follow-up assessment ($40). Before the pandemic, sessions were in person and dinner was served at each session. After the onset of the pandemic, we implemented ChiCAS virtually via videoconferencing and dinner was not served. Each participant also received a T-shirt and a bag with the project logo. We provided a graduation ceremony for participants after they completed all ChiCAS sessions, and participants received framed certificates of completion.

Three interventionists delivered the ChiCAS intervention: a native Spanish-speaking transgender Latina woman, a native Spanish-speaking cisgender Latino gay man, and a fluent Spanish-speaking cisgender White woman. These interventionists were experienced in implementing HIV prevention and PrEP promotion interventions in LGBTQ+ communities and were trained in ChiCAS implementation. Before the COVID-19 pandemic, the interventionists delivered ChiCAS in person to participants during 2 sessions lasting 4 hours each on consecutive Sunday evenings in safe and conveniently located community settings. After the onset of the pandemic, we adapted the 2 sessions to last 2 hours each via Zoom, given the challenges of maintaining attention via videoconferencing. Additional adaptations made to the ChiCAS intervention and study delivery are described elsewhere.[9]

Raters provided quality assurance during intervention delivery; they attended each session and documented whether activities were implemented with fidelity.

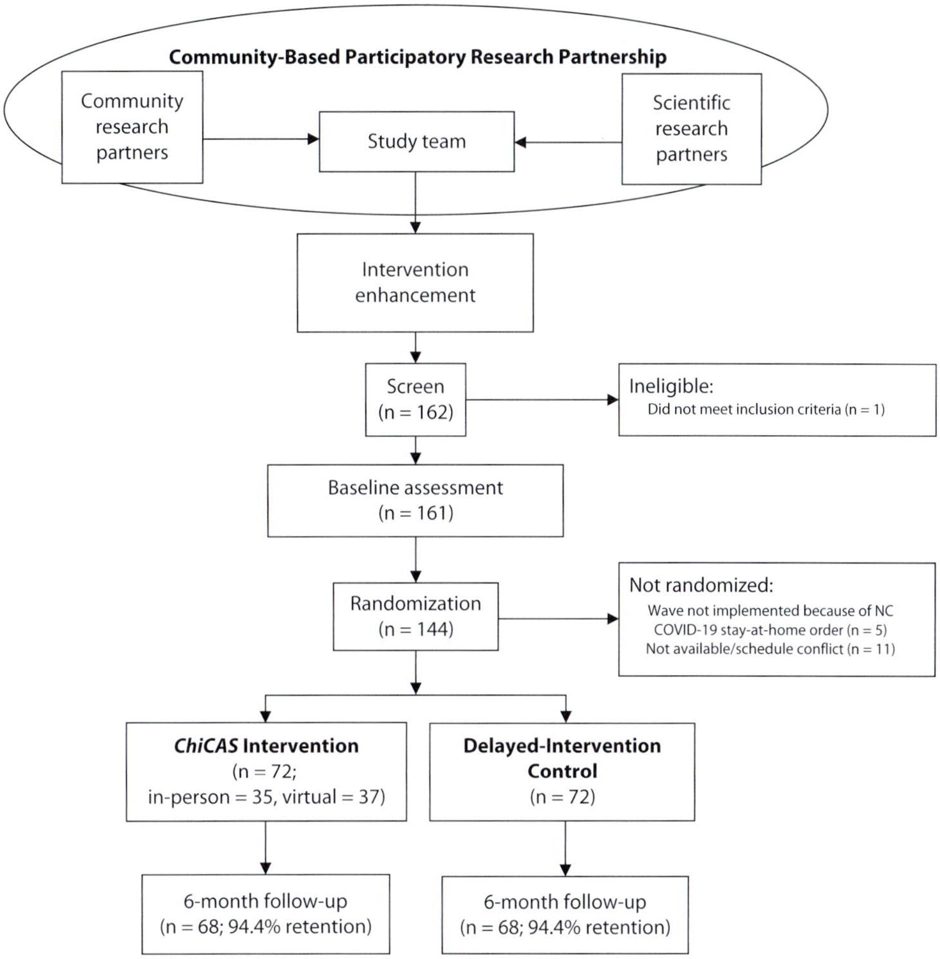

FIGURE 1— Schematic of the Research Design to Test the ChiCAS Intervention for HIV-Negative Spanish-Speaking Transgender Latinas: North and South Carolina, 2019–2022

Note. ChiCAS = Chicas *Creando Acceso a la Salud* (Girls Creating Access to Health).

Outcome Measures

We collected all outcome measures at baseline upon enrollment and then again at a follow-up. We collected outcomes via assessments that a trained interviewer administered in Spanish. PrEP use was a primary outcome because of its demonstrated effectiveness at reducing the risk of sexual HIV transmission. We assessed current PrEP use by asking participants whether they were currently using PrEP. We assessed 2 additional outcomes: consistent condom use and current use of medically supervised gender-affirming hormone therapy. We defined consistent condom use as using condoms during every instance of insertive anal or receptive anal or vaginal sex with men and insertive vaginal or anal sex with women in the 30 days before the baseline and 6-month follow-up assessments. We measured the use of medically supervised gender-affirming hormone therapy by asking whether participants were currently using it and, if so, where they obtained the gender-affirming hormones.

We also measured changes in determinants that ChiCAS was designed to influence. We measured HIV,[24] STI,[25] and gender-affirming hormone therapy knowledge with true–false items. A sample gender-affirming hormone therapy knowledge item included "Only a medical doctor or nurse can determine the appropriate hormone therapy and dose."

We assessed awareness and knowledge of PrEP and readiness to take PrEP. We assessed PrEP awareness using the scale item "On a scale from 0 to 10, with 0 being knowing nothing at all and 10 being knowing a lot, how much would you say you know about PrEP?" Sample PrEP knowledge items included "PrEP can reduce the chances of getting HIV among those without HIV" and

"PrEP interacts with gender-affirming hormones that some transgender persons take or plan to take." We assessed PrEP readiness using the item "How likely is it that you'd use PrEP?" Response options ranged from "not at all likely" (1) to "extremely likely" (5).

We used an adapted version of the Condom-Use Skills Checklist to assess knowledge about correct condom use[25] and condom use intentions.[25,26] We used the 26-item Internalized Transphobia Scale[27] to measure internalized transphobia, the 12-item Multigroup Ethnic Identity Measure[28] to measure ethnic group pride, and an adapted 18-item version of the Index of Sojourner Social Support Scale[29] to measure social support. We measured community attachment using an adapted 3-item scale[30] consisting of "Please indicate how much you feel a part of or connected to . . ." ". . . the transgender community," ". . . the Hispanic/Latino community," and ". . . the Hispanic/Latino transgender community." Response options ranged from "not at all" (0) to "to a great extent" (5).

We measured medical mistrust using a scale that we have successfully used previously with Spanish-speaking populations.[31] Participants ranked on a scale from strongly disagree (1) to strongly agree (4) how much they agree with 5 statements, including "Sometimes doctors care more about what is convenient for them than about their patients' medical needs." We also measured patient activation (i.e., provider communication skills and health management efficacy) using an adapted version of the short form of the Patient Activation Measure. Participants indicated on a scale from strongly disagree (1) to strongly agree (4) how much they agreed with 13 statements, including "I am confident I can tell my health care provider concerns I have even when he or she does not ask."[32]

We also measured barriers to health care.[33] Sample barriers to which participants were asked to respond included, "You didn't have transportation" and "You felt like you would be treated poorly." We measured barriers using yes–no responses and yes responses added together.

We completed reverse coding as warranted, and higher scores for each determinant indicated higher levels of that determinant.

Statistical Analyses

We used an intention-to-treat protocol to analyze participants' outcomes relative to their assigned intervention group, irrespective of the number of sessions they attended.[34] At baseline, we calculated descriptive statistics to summarize sociodemographic characteristics of intervention and delayed-intervention wait list control participants. We assessed differences between the groups at baseline using the Student *t* test for continuous variables and χ^2 for categorical variables.

Our primary data analyses to evaluate ChiCAS efficacy compared proportions of PrEP use, consistent condom use, and use of medically supervised gender-affirming hormone therapy by intervention and delayed-intervention wait list control participants at the 6-month postintervention follow-up while adjusting for baseline rates. Statistical analysis used multivariable random effects logistic regression modeling that adjusted for potential clustering in intervention groups by including a random effect for the intervention group.[35] This adjustment accounted for the possibility that participants in the same study wave and intervention group may exhibit more similar patterns of PrEP use, condom use, and use of gender-affirming hormone therapy at 6-month follow up compared with participants in other study waves. We adjusted models for age, education, employment, country of origin, and whether participants participated in in-person or virtual implementation to obtain adjusted odds ratios (AORs) and computed the 95% confidence intervals (CIs) and corresponding *P* values. We fit models using PROC GLIMMIX in SAS.

In our secondary analysis, we used the *t* test to assess changes in determinants that the ChiCAS intervention addressed. We included the same sociodemographic factors in these analyses that we included in the final outcome models. For each scale, we replaced missing scale items with the person-mean imputed value for each specific scale if 20% or less of scale items responses were missing. If more than 20% was missing, we considered that scale missing and did not use it in our analyses. For each model, we calculated adjusted means and SEs and differences of adjusted means and their corresponding *P* values. We estimated all models in the context of multivariable random effects linear regression modeling using PROC MIXED in SAS. We performed all analyses using SAS/STAT version 9.3.

RESULTS

The average age of the 144 study participants was 33.1 years (SD = 9.4), nearly 50% had less than a high school education or general equivalency diploma equivalent, 65% were employed year round, and 80.1% reported earning less than $2000 per month. The majority of participants were foreign born (88%). Seventy percent of the participants reported speaking only or mostly Spanish. Foreign-born participants had been living in the United States for a mean of 16.4 years. Participants self-identified as female (98%) or transgender (2%). Sexual orientation was reported as heterosexual (81%), bisexual (10%), gay (6%), and "something else" (3%). Three percent of participants reported sex with women in addition to men within the past 6 months. There were no significant differences between sociodemographic characteristics of intervention and control participants (Table 1).

Most participants (69.4%) assigned to the ChiCAS intervention completed both of their assigned intervention sessions; however, attendance rates varied by mode of intervention delivery. Virtual implementation had a higher rate of retention, with 73.0% (27 of 37) attending both sessions; in-person implementation had a retention rate of 65.7% (23 of 35) attending both sessions.

Overall retention for 6-month follow-up assessments across intervention and delayed-intervention wait list control participants was 94.4%. We delivered the intervention with a high degree of fidelity.

Intervention Effects

At 6-month follow-up, ChiCAS participants' reports of current PrEP use significantly increased, from 10.6% at baseline to 31.8% ($P = .002$). PrEP use among delayed-intervention wait list control participants did not significantly change (7.5% at baseline vs 13.4% at 6-month follow-up; $P = .23$). Adjusting for age, education, employment, country of origin, and mode of intervention delivery (i.e., in person or virtual) at 6-month follow-up, ChiCAS participants were 4.64 (95% CI = 1.57, 13.7) times as

TABLE 1— Characteristics of Participants in the ChiCAS Intervention Trial by Intervention Group at Baseline: North and South Carolina, 2019–2022

Characteristic[a]	Intervention Group, No. (%) or Mean ±SD	Delayed-Intervention Wait List Group, No. (%) or Mean ±SD)	P^b
Age, y (n = 143)	33.0 ±9.4	33.2 ±9.4	.93
Years living in US among foreign born (n = 122)	15.9 ±8.5	17.0 ±8.9	.54
Country of origin (n = 142)			.48
Mexico	44 (62.0)	49 (69.0)	
United States	8 (11.3)	9 (12.7)	
Other	19 (26.8)	13 (18.3)	
Education (n = 143)			.09
Less than high school education or general equivalency diploma equivalent	32 (45.1)	39 (54.2)	
High school or general equivalency diploma	20 (28.2)	18 (25.0)	
Some college	16 (22.5)	7 (9.7)	
College	3 (4.2)	8 (11.1)	
Employment (n = 143)			.37
Employed year-round	49 (69.0)	44 (61.1)	
Seasonal	9 (12.7)	7 (9.7)	
Unemployed	10 (14.1)	13 (18.1)	
Disabled/not working	3 (4.2)	8 (11.1)	
Monthly income, $ (n = 141)			
None	12 (16.9)	18 (25.7)	.43
< 1000	16 (22.5)	10 (14.3)	
1000–1999	28 (39.4)	29 (41.4)	
≥ 2000	15 (21.1)	13 (18.6)	

Note. ChiCAS = Chicas *Creando Acceso a la Salud* (Girls Creating Access to Health).
[a]Number for each characteristic may not equal 144 because of missing data.
[b]*P* value from *t*-test statistics for means and χ^2 statistics for %.

TABLE 2— Reported Use of Preexposure Prophylaxis (PrEP), Condoms, and Medically Supervised Hormone Therapy Among ChiCAS Participants at Baseline and Follow-up by Intervention Group: North and South Carolina, 2019–2022

	Intervention			Delayed Intervention			Intervention Effect Unadjusted	Intervention Effect Adjusted[a]
Variable	Baseline, No. (%)	Follow-Up, No. (%)	Unadjusted P[b]	Baseline, No. (%)	Follow-Up, No. (%)	Unadjusted P value[b]	OR (95% CI)	AOR (95% CI)
Current PrEP use[c]	7 (10.6)	21 (31.8)	.002	5 (7.5)	9 (13.4)	.23	3.29 (1.24, 8.75)	4.64 (1.57, 13.7)
Past 30-d consistent condom use among those reporting sex[d]	20 (40.8)	24 (48.9)	.13	17 (38.6)	23 (52.3)	.1	0.81 (0.32, 2.04)	0.76 (0.28, 2.09)
Current use of medically supervised gender-affirming hormone therapy[e]	25 (36.8)	28 (41.2)	.67	25 (39.1)	27 (42.2)	.48	1.04 (0.40, 2.74)	1.29 (0.46, 3.61)

Note. AOR = adjusted odds ratio; ChiCAS = Chicas *Creando Acceso a la Salud* (Girls Creating Access to Health); CI = confidence interval; OR = odds ratio; PrEP = preexposure prophylaxis. Study sample size was n = 144.
[a]Adjusted for baseline, age, education, employment, country of birth, and mode of delivery (in person vs virtual).
[b]Test of within-group differences between baseline and follow-up.
[c]Intervention n = 66; delayed-intervention n = 67 (owing to missing data).
[d]Participants reporting sex in past 30 d, intervention (n = 49) and delayed-intervention(n = 44).
[e]Intervention n = 68; delayed-intervention n = 64 (owing to missing data).

likely as delayed-intervention wait list control participants to report PrEP use ($P = .006$). Adjusting for age, education, employment, country of origin, and mode of intervention delivery, ChiCAS participants' reports of past 30-day condom use and current use of medically supervised gender-affirming hormone therapy were not significantly different at 6-month follow-up (AOR = 0.76; 95% CI = 0.28, 2.09 and AOR = 1.3; 95% CI = 0.46, 3.61, respectively; Table 2).

We observed marked differences in 8 behavioral determinants that the intervention targeted (Table 3). Compared with delayed-intervention wait list control participants at 6-month follow-up, ChiCAS participants reported increases in knowledge of HIV ($P < .001$), STI ($P < .001$), and medically supervised gender-affirming hormone therapy ($P < .01$); PrEP awareness ($P < .001$), knowledge ($P < .001$), and readiness ($P < .001$); condom use skills ($P < .001$); and community attachment ($P < .001$). There were no statistically significant differences between ChiCAS and delayed-intervention wait list control participants in reported internalized transphobia, ethnic group pride, social support, medical mistrust, patient activation, or barriers to health care.

DISCUSSION

Transgender Latinas in the United States are particularly vulnerable to HIV infection, and their PrEP and condom use remain low. However, there are no efficacious HIV prevention interventions for transgender Latinas currently listed in the CDC *Compendium of Evidence-Based Interventions and Best Practices for HIV Prevention* (https://bit.ly/45SSNqp), and the CDC has called for an increased focus on HIV prevention among transgender women, especially Latinas.

We found that ChiCAS participants were more than 4 times as likely as delayed-intervention wait list control participants to report current PrEP use at 6-month follow-up. We did not identify significant changes in the 2 other study outcomes that the intervention was designed to affect: consistent condom use and medically supervised gender-affirming hormone therapy. There are a number of potential explanations for this. First, the ChiCAS trial was powered on PrEP uptake.[11] Furthermore, the onset of the COVID-19 pandemic about halfway through the trial required us to abbreviate the intervention for virtual implementation to continue the trial safely, as previously described.[9] These abbreviations and the absence of in-person interactions during some activities, such as the sexual partner condom use negotiation activities, may have affected intervention efficacy, and the complexities

TABLE 3— Adjusted Means and SE of Behavioral Determinants Among ChiCAS Participants at 6-Month Follow-Up by Intervention Group: North and South Carolina, 2019–2022

	Adjusted Means and SEs at 6-Mo Follow-Up[a]				
Determinant	Adjusted Mean ±SE	Difference of Adjusted Mean ±SE	Degree of Freedom	*t* value	*P*
HIV knowledge		3.7 ±0.48	114	7.67	<.001
Intervention group	16.7 ±0.46				
Control group	13.0 ±0.46				
STI knowledge		2.3 ±0.41	114	5.61	<.001
Intervention group	12.8 ±0.47				
Control Group	10.5 ±0.47				
Gender-affirming hormone therapy knowledge		0.82 ±0.31	114	2.62	.01
Intervention group	8.3 ±0.31				
Control group	7.4 ±0.31				
PrEP awareness		2.2 ±0.37	113	5.81	<.001
Intervention group	7.8 ±0.42				
Control group	5.6 ±0.42				
PrEP knowledge		3.0 ±0.42	114	6.98	<.001
Intervention group	10.7 ±0.40				
Control group	7.7 ±0.40				
PrEP use readiness		1.0 ±0.27	114	3.71	<.001
Intervention group	4.2 ±0.26				
Control group	3.1 ±0.26				
Condom use skills		0.76 ±0.16	114	4.58	<.001
Intervention group	16.1 ±0.18				
Control group	15.4 ±0.18				
Condom use intentions		0.18 ±0.17	111	1.05	.29
Intervention group	4.2 ±0.18				
Control group	4.0 ±0.18				
Internalized transphobia		1.5 ±2.74	113	0.54	.59
Intervention group	62.2 ±2.56				
Control group	60.7 ±2.52				
Multiethnic identity measure/ethnic group pride		0.88 ±0.92	114	0.95	.34
Intervention group	37.0 ±0.92				
Control group	36.1 ±0.94				
Social support		4.2 ±2.41	114	1.76	.08
Intervention group	34.8 ±3.12				
Control group	30.6 ±3.13				
Community attachment		0.82 ±0.21	110	3.86	<.001
Intervention group	3.8 ±0.20				
Control group	3.0 ±0.20				
Medical mistrust		−0.53 ±0.44	113	−1.21	.23
Intervention group	16.3 ±0.44				
Control group	16.9 ±0.44				
Patient activation		−0.98 ±1.12	113	−0.88	.38
Intervention group	43.1 ±1.05				

Continued

TABLE 3— Continued

	Adjusted Means and SEs at 6-Mo Follow-Up[a]				
Determinant	Adjusted Mean ±SE	Difference of Adjusted Mean ±SE	Degree of Freedom	*t* value	*P*
Control group	44.1 ±1.06				
Barriers to health care		−0.33 ±0.38	113	−0.86	.39
Intervention group	0.7 ±0.55				
Control group	1.1 ±0.6				

Note. ChiCAS = Chicas *Creando Acceso a la Salud* (Girls Creating Access to Health); PrEP = preexposure prophylaxis; STI = sexually transmitted infection.
[a]Adjusted means and SEs were based on multivariable random effect linear mixed models with covariates of age, education attainment, employment, model of delivery, and country of origin with corresponding baseline measure.

associated with condom use negotiation and initiation may require additional skills-building support. Furthermore, not all transgender Latinas want to use gender-affirming hormones.

It is noteworthy that we observed favorable changes in 8 critical behavioral determinants that the ChiCAS intervention was designed to affect; specifically, ChiCAS participants had increased knowledge of HIV, STIs, and medically supervised gender-affirming hormone therapy; PrEP awareness and knowledge; readiness to use PrEP; condom use skills; and community attachment. Furthermore, our study had a very high retention rate: 94.4% of all participants completed 6-month follow-up assessments. This may be attributable to the substantial engagement of transgender Latinas at all stages of developing intervention content. ChiCAS was developed to reflect the real-world experiences and priorities of transgender Latinas. Each intervention module and activity was designed to meet Spanish-speaking transgender Latinas' expressed needs and was presented in a manner that was highly engaging and interactive, during both in-person and virtual implementation delivery. Furthermore, many members of the study team who screened and recruited participants and obtained their consent, implemented the intervention, delivered intervention materials, and contacted participants for follow-up assessments reflected the study population (transgender Latinas) or closely aligned with the population (LGBTQ+ community), native Spanish speakers, and were skilled in trust and rapport building.

Limitations

Although we had planned to verify use of PrEP and medically supervised gender-affirming hormone therapy through review of medical records, the onset of the COVID-19 pandemic made this task untenable given that many clinics were understaffed because of the pandemic. Members of our partnership, some of whom represented health departments and clinics, advised us not to place additional burdens on already stressed facilities by conducting medical record reviews. Therefore, we relied on self-reported use of PrEP and medically supervised gender-affirming hormone therapy; however, self-report has been found to be reliable if conducted carefully.[36] In post hoc analyses, 100% of participants who reported use of PrEP and medically supervised gender-affirming hormone therapy at baseline and follow-up were able to provide authenticating details, including the provider and clinic where they obtained their prescriptions and the pharmacy where they filled their prescription.

The lack of significant between-group differences in some of the determinants that we designed the ChiCAS intervention to affect and that have been associated with HIV prevention behaviors suggests a need to reexamine how the intervention addresses these determinants. Finally, although we did control for mode of delivery in our primary outcome analyses, we were unable to test the intervention by mode of delivery (i.e., in person vs virtual) given the small sample size.

Conclusions

Important gaps exist in the current intervention arsenal for reducing HIV risk among sexual and gender minority populations, and nowhere is there a greater need than among transgender Latinas. Thus, ChiCAS offers an urgently needed resource to prevent HIV among Spanish-speaking transgender Latinas who have sex with men. The intervention was efficacious, significantly increasing PrEP use in this trial. It also may serve as

AJPH January 2024, Vol. 114, No. 1

a foundation for interventions designed to increase PrEP use among other transgender populations. AJPH

ABOUT THE AUTHORS

Scott D. Rhodes, Jorge Alonzo, Lilli Mann-Jackson, and Manuel Garcia are with the Department of Social Sciences and Health Policy, Wake Forest University School of Medicine, Winston-Salem, NC. At trial initiation, Lucero Refugio Aviles was with the Triad Health Project, Greensboro, NC; she completed the study while at the Department of Social Sciences and Health Policy, Wake Forest University School of Medicine. Amanda E. Tanner and Tamar Goldenberg are with the Department of Public Health Education, University of North Carolina, Greensboro. Carla A. Galindo, Patricia A. Bessler, and Cari Courtenay-Quirk are with the US Centers for Disease Control and Prevention, Atlanta, GA. Ana D. Sucaldito is with the Clinical and Translational Science Institute, Wake Forest University School of Medicine. Benjamin D. Smart is with the Karolinska Institutet, Stockholm, Sweden. Beth A. Reboussin is with the Department of Biostatistics and Data Sciences, Wake Forest University School of Medicine.

CORRESPONDENCE

Correspondence should be sent to Scott D. Rhodes, Department of Social Sciences and Health Policy, Wake Forest School of Medicine, Division of Public Health Sciences, Medical Center Blvd, Winston-Salem, NC 27157-1063 (e-mail: srhodes@wakehealth.edu). Reprints can be ordered at http://www.ajph.org by clicking the "Reprints" link.

PUBLICATION INFORMATION

Full Citation: Rhodes SD, Alonzo J, Mann-Jackson L, et al. Preexposure prophylaxis uptake among Spanish-speaking transgender women: a randomized controlled trial in North and South Carolina, 2019–2022. *Am J Public Health*. 2024;114(1):68–78.

Acceptance Date: September 3, 2023.

DOI: https://doi.org/10.2105/AJPH.2023.307444

CONTRIBUTORS

S. D. Rhodes coconceptualized and supervised the trial in partnership with colleagues from Triad Health Project, participated in intervention development and refinement; oversaw implementation; collected, analyzed, and interpreted the data; and led article preparation. S. D. Rhodes, J. Alonzo, L. Refugio Aviles, and B. A. Reboussin participated in intervention implementation. J. Alonzo supervised data collection. J. Alonzo and L. Refugio Aviles refined the intervention. J. Alonzo, L. Mann-Jackson, L. Refugio Aviles, C. A. Galindo, P. A. Bessler, C. Courtenay-Quirk, M. Garcia, A. D. Sucaldito, B. D. Smart, T. Goldenberg, and B. A. Reboussin assisted with data interpretation. L. Mann-Jackson oversaw intervention implementation and participant randomization and tracking. L. Refugio Aviles and M. Garcia assisted in participant recruitment and retention and data collection. A. E. Tanner assisted in study implementation and data analysis. C. A. Galindo, P. A. Bessler, and C. Courtenay-Quirk oversaw the study. B. A. Reboussin participated in study development and oversaw data analyses. All authors participated in article preparation.

ACKNOWLEDGMENTS

Funding for the ChiCAS trial was provided by the US Centers for Disease Control and Prevention (CDC; cooperative agreement U01PS005137).

Note. The findings and conclusions in this article are those of the authors and do not necessarily represent the official position of the CDC.

CONFLICTS OF INTEREST

The authors have no conflicts of interest to declare.

HUMAN PARTICIPANT PROTECTION

Human participant oversight was provided by the institutional review board of Wake Forest University School of Medicine. Written informed consent was obtained from each participant.

REFERENCES

1. Becasen JS, Denard CL, Mullins MM, Higa DH, Sipe TA. Estimating the prevalence of HIV and sexual behaviors among the US transgender population: a systematic review and meta-analysis, 2006–2017. *Am J Public Health*. 2019;109(1):e1–e8. https://doi.org/10.2105/AJPH.2018.304727
2. Habarta N, Wang G, Mulatu MS, Larish N. HIV testing by transgender status at Centers for Disease Control and Prevention–funded sites in the United States, Puerto Rico, and US Virgin Islands, 2009–2011. *Am J Public Health*. 2015;105(9): 1917–1925. https://doi.org/10.2105/AJPH.2015.302659
3. Centers for Disease Control and Prevention. HIV infection, risk, prevention, and testing behaviors among transgender women: National HIV Behavioral Surveillance, 7 US cities, 2019–2020. Available at: https://www.cdc.gov/hiv/pdf/library/reports/surveillance/cdc-hiv-surveillance-special-report-number-27.pdf. Accessed November 1, 2023.
4. Sullivan PS, Mena L, Elopre L, Siegler AJ. Implementation strategies to increase PrEP uptake in the South. *Curr HIV/AIDS Rep*. 2019;16(4): 259–269. https://doi.org/10.1007/s11904-019-00447-4
5. Rhodes SD, Alonzo J, Mann-Jackson L, et al. A peer navigation intervention to prevent HIV among mixed immigrant status Latinx GBMSM and transgender women in the United States: outcomes, perspectives and implications for PrEP uptake. *Health Educ Res*. 2020;35(3): 165–178. https://doi.org/10.1093/her/cyaa010
6. Centers for Disease Control and Prevention. *Preexposure Prophylaxis for the Prevention of HIV Infection in the United States—2021 Update. A Clinical Practice Guideline*. 2021. Available at: https://www.cdc.gov/hiv/pdf/risk/prep/cdc-hiv-prep-guidelines-2021.pdf. Accessed November 1, 2023.
7. Holder CL, Perez-Gilbe HR, Fajardo FJ, Garcia S, Cyrus E. Disparities of HIV risk and PrEP use among transgender women of color in South Florida. *J Natl Med Assoc*. 2019;111(6):625–632. https://doi.org/10.1016/j.jnma.2019.08.001
8. Collier KL, Colarossi LG, Hazel DS, Watson K, Wyatt GE. Healing our women for transgender women: adaptation, acceptability, and pilot testing. *AIDS Educ Prev*. 2015;27(5):418–431. https://doi.org/10.1521/aeap.2015.27.5.418
9. Rhodes SD, Tanner AE, Mann-Jackson L, et al. Adapting a group-level PrEP promotion intervention trial for transgender Latinas during the COVID-19 pandemic. *AIDS Educ Prev*. 2022;34(6): 481–495. https://doi.org/10.1521/aeap.2022.34.6.481
10. Poteat T, Wirtz A, Malik M, et al. A gap between willingness and uptake: findings from mixed methods research on HIV prevention among Black and Latina transgender women. *J Acquir Immune Defic Syndr*. 2019;82(2):131–140. https://doi.org/10.1097/QAI.0000000000002112
11. Rhodes SD, Kuhns LM, Alexander J, et al. Evaluating homegrown interventions to promote PrEP among racially/ethnically diverse transgender women in the United States: a unique CDC initiative. *AIDS Educ Prev*. 2021;33(4):345–360. https://doi.org/10.1521/aeap.2021.33.4.345
12. Rhodes SD, Alonzo J, Mann L, et al. Using photovoice, Latina transgender women identify priorities in a new immigrant-destination state. *Int J Transgend*. 2015;16(2):80–96. https://doi.org/10.1080/15532739.2015.1075928
13. Smart BD, Mann-Jackson L, Alonzo J, et al. Transgender women of color in the US South: a qualitative study of social determinants of health and healthcare perspectives. *Int J Transgend*. 2020;23(1-2):164–177. https://doi.org/10.1080/26895269.2020.1848691
14. Rivera AV, Lopez JM, Braunstein SL. Exploring the association between gender affirmation and PrEP use among transgender women in New York City. *AIDS Behav*. 2023;27(5):1523–1530. https://doi.org/10.1007/s10461-022-03944-7
15. Sevelius JM, Patouhas E, Keatley JG, Johnson MO. Barriers and facilitators to engagement and retention in care among transgender women living with human immunodeficiency virus. *Ann Behav Med*. 2014;47(1):5–16. https://doi.org/10.1007/s12160-013-9565-8
16. Sevelius JM. Gender affirmation: a framework for conceptualizing risk behavior among transgender women of color. *Sex Roles*. 2013;68(11–12): 675–689. https://doi.org/10.1007/s11199-012-0216-5
17. Wallerstein N, Duran B. Community-based participatory research contributions to intervention research: the intersection of science and practice to improve health equity. *Am J Public Health*. 2010;100(suppl 1):S40–S46. https://doi.org/10.2105/AJPH.2009.184036
18. Israel BA, Schulz AJ, Parker EA, Becker AB. Review of community-based research: assessing partnership approaches to improve public health. *Annu Rev Public Health*. 1998;19:173–202. https://doi.org/10.1146/annurev.publhealth.19.1.173
19. Rhodes SD, Mann L, Alonzo J, et al. CBPR to prevent HIV within ethnic, sexual, and gender minority communities: successes with long-term sustainability. In: Rhodes SD, ed. *Innovations in*

HIV Prevention Research and Practice Through Community Engagement. New York, NY: Springer; 2014:135–160. https://doi.org/10.1007/978-1-4939-0900-1_7

20. Bandura A. *Social Foundations of Thought and Action: A Social Cognitive Theory*. Englewood Cliffs, NJ: Prentice-Hall; 1986.
21. Freire P. *Education for Critical Consciousness*. New York, NY: Seabury Press; 1973.
22. Neumann MS, Finlayson TJ, Pitts NL, Keatley J. Comprehensive HIV prevention for transgender persons. *Am J Public Health*. 2017;107(2): 207–212. https://doi.org/10.2105/AJPH.2016.303509
23. Mizuno Y, Koenig LJ, Wilkes AL, et al. Utilization of HIV prevention, care, and treatment services among young men who have sex with men and transgender persons of color in the US South: a qualitative analysis. *AIDS Educ Prev*. 2022;34(6): 512–527. https://doi.org/10.1521/aeap.2022.34.6.512
24. Rhodes SD, McCoy TP, Vissman AT, et al. A randomized controlled trial of a culturally congruent intervention to increase condom use and HIV testing among heterosexually active immigrant Latino men. *AIDS Behav*. 2011;15(8):1764–1775. https://doi.org/10.1007/s10461-011-9903-4
25. Rhodes SD, Alonzo J, Mann L, et al. Small-group randomized controlled trial to increase condom use and HIV testing among Hispanic/Latino gay, bisexual, and other men who have sex with men. *Am J Public Health*. 2017;107(6):969–976. https://doi.org/10.2105/AJPH.2017.303814
26. Villarruel AM, Jemmott JB III, Jemmott LS, Ronis DL. Predictors of sexual intercourse and condom use intentions among Spanish-dominant Latino youth: a test of the planned behavior theory. *Nurs Res*. 2004;53(3):172–181. https://doi.org/10.1097/00006199-200405000-00004
27. Perez-Brumer A, Hatzenbuehler ML, Oldenburg CE, Bockting W. Individual- and structural-level risk factors for suicide attempts among transgender adults. *Behav Med*. 2015;41(3):164–171. https://doi.org/10.1080/08964289.2015.1028322
28. Phinney J. The Multigroup Ethnic Identity Measure: a new scale for use with adolescents and young adults from diverse groups. *J Adolesc Res*. 1992;7(2):156–176. https://doi.org/10.1177/074355489272003
29. Gilbert PA, Rhodes SD. Psychometric performance of a novel measure of social support among Spanish-speaking immigrant Latino gay men. *Hisp J Behav Sci*. 2012;34(3):491–504. https://doi.org/10.1177/0739986312446290
30. O'Donnell L, Agronick G, San Doval A, Duran R, Myint UA, Stueve A. Ethnic and gay community attachments and sexual risk behaviors among urban Latino young men who have sex with men. *AIDS Educ Prev*. 2002;14(6):457–471. https://doi.org/10.1521/aeap.14.8.457.24109
31. Vissman AT, Young AM, Wilkin AM, Rhodes SD. Correlates of HAART adherence among immigrant Latinos in the Southeastern United States. *AIDS Care*. 2013;25(3):356–363. https://doi.org/10.1080/09540121.2012.701722
32. Hibbard JH, Mahoney ER, Stockard J, Tusler M. Development and testing of a short form of the patient activation measure. *Health Serv Res*. 2005;40(6, pt 1):1918–1930. https://doi.org/10.1111/j.1475-6773.2005.00438.x
33. Rhodes SD, Hergenrather KC, Zometa C, Lindstrom K, Montaño J. Characteristics of immigrant Latino men who utilize formal healthcare services in rural North Carolina: baseline findings from the HoMBReS Study. *J Natl Med Assoc*. 2008;100(10):1177–1185.
34. Friedman LM, Furberg CD, DeMets DL. *Fundamentals of Clinical Trials*. 3rd ed. New York, NY: Springer-Verlag; 1998. https://doi.org/10.1007/978-1-4757-2915-3
35. Wolfinger R, O'Connell M. Generalized linear mixed models: a pseudo-likelihood approach. *J Stat Comput Simul*. 1993;48(3-4):233–243. https://doi.org/10.1080/00949659308811554 .
36. Qasmieh S, Nash D, Gandhi M, et al. Self-reported use of HIV preexposure prophylaxis is highly accurate among sexual health clinic patients in New York City. *Sex Transm Dis*. 2022;49(11):790–793. https://doi.org/10.1097/OLQ.0000000000001622

Conducting Health Research with Native American Communities

Edited by Teshia G. Arambula Solomon, PhD and Leslie L. Randall, RN, MPH, BSN

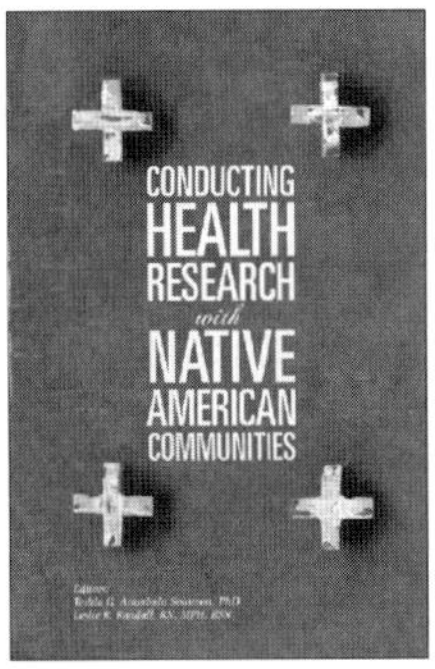

The current research and evaluation of the American Indian and Alaska Native (AIAN) people demonstrates the increased demand for efficiency, accompanied by solid accountability in a time of extremely limited resources. This environment requires proficiency in working with these vulnerable populations in diverse cross-cultural settings. This timely publication is the first of its kind to provide this information to help researchers meet their demands.

This book provides an overview of complex themes as well as a synopsis of essential concepts or techniques in working with Native American tribes and Alaska Native communities. *Conducting Health Research with Native American Communities* will benefit Native people and organizations as well as researchers, students and practitioners.

APHA PRESS
AN IMPRINT OF AMERICAN PUBLIC HEALTH ASSOCIATION

2014, 340 pp., softcover, ISBN 978-0-87553-2028
Available as an eBook and softcover
ORDER ONLINE at www.aphabookstore.org

Untangling Concepts of Financial Circumstances for Public Health Professionals and Scholars: A Glossary and Concept Map

Candace I. J. Nykiforuk, PhD, CE, Ana Paula Belon, PhD, and Lisa K. Allen Scott, PhD, MBT

Public health discipline and practice have prioritized work on poverty and populations at high risk for material deprivation, with less consideration for the full spectrum of financial circumstances relative to well-being. Public health can make a much-needed contribution to this area, which is currently dominated by the financial industry, focused on individual behaviors, and lacking the definitional consensus needed for research and evaluation. A population-level lens can reveal the social determinants and health consequences of real or perceived poor financial circumstances.

This article aims to improve conceptual understanding of financial circumstances among public health scholars and professionals. We identified concepts through a critical literature review of peer-reviewed and practice-based resources on financial well-being and financial strain. We developed a glossary of concepts related to financial circumstances and categorized concepts according to their level of influence using an approach informed by socioecological models. We provide a concept map that illustrates the relationships between concepts in the context of their levels of influence.

This article will help to advance an agenda on financial well-being promotion in public health research and practice. (*Am J Public Health*. 2024;114(1):79–89. https://doi.org/10.2105/AJPH.2023.307449)

AJPH January 2024, Vol. 114, No. 1

The health effects of financial circumstances (the state of one's financial affairs) have not fully garnered the attention of public health researchers and practitioners. Financial circumstances, beyond poverty, dictate individuals' and populations' relative access to the necessities of life and intersect with other factors in shaping experiences of power and privilege that affect health. Yet, the limited public health research on financial circumstances starkly contrasts with the abundance of research on poverty and material deprivation with respect to health outcomes. Missing dialogue between experts in financial circumstance–related fields (e.g., financial inclusion, security) and public health may explain this knowledge gap.[1] In addition, conceptual limitations[1–3] and divergent concept operationalization for data analysis[1,3–5] may have discouraged public health professionals from venturing into this arena, instead retaining a focus on poverty as the chronic financial circumstance in most urgent need of attention.

Contemporary public health policies and programs have mostly targeted populations experiencing or at high risk of poverty and severe material deprivation, which are typically determined through predefined cutoff points for individual or household income. Reducing the burden of poor financial circumstances among the most disadvantaged populations is an unquestionable priority. However, poverty and material deprivation must be understood—and intervened with—relative to impacts on population health over the life course rather than particular cut points for individuals at any moment in time to shift the population distribution of risk.[6] Analysis of different aspects of financial circumstances over time may reveal that nuances matter to health and overall well-being.[7] Thus, in addition to high-risk approaches, population-wide approaches are necessary to address the root causes of poor financial circumstances and shift population risk levels.

Despite the limited focus to date, financial circumstance–related concepts have recently started to be incorporated into public health scholarship and practice. Much of the scarce public health literature has explored the relationship between perceived or objective financial circumstances and perceived stress manifested through physiological or emotional arousal.[8–10] Few studies have focused on how and to what extent concepts related to poor financial circumstances weaken physical,[8,11–13] mental,[8,14,15] and social health.[8,16,17] Recently, Weida et al.[1] innovatively presented financial health as a social determinant of health. This promising work signals the need for clarity on existing financial circumstance–related concepts, especially those relative to public health action on social determinants of health.

When researchers and professionals share a common understanding of terminology to inform research and intervention design, delivery, and evaluation, it can improve coordination of efforts and collective effects on population health. Dismantling the cacophony of current concepts to lay out a solid foundation based on a common language will facilitate communication and intelligibility among multiple public health actors and agencies in research, government, and community settings. Consequently, it will create a fertile space for coproduction of knowledge and advancement of the diverse fields working to improve people's financial circumstances.

This study mobilizes our efforts toward advancing an agenda for promoting financial well-being in public health research and practice. It was a secondary study of a larger project that culminated in an international public health framework[18] and guidebook of strategies and indicators[19] to inform population-level initiatives for financial well-being promotion and financial strain reduction. That larger project employed multiple methods through which we systematically collected concepts and definitions related to financial circumstances.

First, we undertook a critical narrative literature review of theoretical articles and practice-based resources on concepts related to financial strain and financial well-being used in social sciences, economics, consumer research, and public health literatures. The practice-based search targeted institutions such as the Financial Consumer Agency of Canada and the Consumer Financial Protection Bureau. The purpose of that review was to clarify definitions of financial strain and financial well-being as foundations to the larger project. We created a preliminary list of concepts and definitions that informed the search strategies used in the other 2 methods.

Second was a systematic rapid review of peer-reviewed literature and practice-based resources on financial well-being and financial strain initiatives in high-income countries published between 2015 and 2020. This was combined with a critical realist analysis to determine the underlying generative mechanisms of financial strain and financial well-being initiatives.[20,21] It included 39 peer-reviewed resources and 36 practice-based reports. Simultaneously, our third method was a targeted review of frameworks related to financial strain and financial well-being published in the academic and practice-based literature. Fourteen frameworks from areas such as social policy and marketing were fully assessed. A careful analysis of the included resources from the rapid review and the review of frameworks led to revision and expansion of the original list of concepts and definitions.

Building on that foundational work, this article aims to provide conceptual clarity on the current financial circumstance–related literature by specifically introducing the various concepts with definitions. We provide a map that depicts the conceptual relationships between terms and according to different levels of influence. Conceptual clarity will help to advance the public health debate on this area. Although a comprehensive discussion of the health effects and social determinants of financial circumstances is beyond this article's scope, a brief overview is necessary to contextualize the glossary and concept map that follow.

LIFE EVENTS THAT MATTER TO HEALTH AND EQUITY

People's perceived or objective financial circumstances vary across the life course[22] because of expected or unexpected changes in life circumstances. Attending college or university, experiencing the death of the family's primary income earner, having or adopting a child, and obtaining a loan for a home purchase are a few examples of life events that may negatively impact people's financial circumstances.[23] These negative impacts can be temporary or permanent and affect people's lives and health, whether to a lesser or greater extent. Such events may directly or indirectly influence health-related behaviors, health status, morbidity, mortality, and quality of life over the short and the long term.[8,11,12,24]

Although feeling or being under financial pressure and having limited access to financial support are unavoidable life events for many, some populations are at higher risk for such experiences and have lower chances of a quick financial recovery. For example, low-income households, single-parent families, undocumented immigrants, and Indigenous communities are particularly vulnerable to these adverse experiences.[9,22] Population groups with intersecting disadvantaged identities (e.g., older African American women[25] or socially isolated rural residents[15]) are also more vulnerable to negative health consequences of poor financial circumstances. The nefarious relationship between financial circumstances and health may intensify inequalities, entrapping some people in poverty and increasing health gaps. These relationships call for public health attention, particularly from a population-level perspective.

APPLYING A POPULATION-LEVEL LENS

Current work from consumer research, economics, and the financial industry provides a narrow view of individual and household financial circumstances that eclipses analyses of external factors such as housing crises, discriminatory hiring practices, and rising tuition costs.[3,5,26] The use of such a narrow focus to inform policy, program, and service development and delivery is worrisome because it may unintentionally perpetuate systemic discrimination and stigma and entrench poverty and social and health inequities, especially among the most vulnerable.[5] A population-level lens can instead unveil the external, negative forces that may drastically reduce the chances of people enjoying better financial circumstances in the present and future. It helps end the shaming of those who have financial struggles or are unable to build wealth as a result of their so-called lack of financial knowledge and skills or inadequate, unsustainable consumerism. A contextual perspective widens the domain of financial circumstances from the sphere of individual responsibility to collective responsibility.

The need for a population health approach that considers the full spectrum of financial circumstances relative to health and well-being confirms the much-needed contributions that public health can make in this arena. It can position the discussion of financial circumstances within neoliberal systems to uncover fundamental environmental (or population-level) and structural drivers such as economic recessions, financial speculation, predatory and discriminatory lending practices, socialization of economic losses vis-à-vis profit privatization, and debt crises.

A population health lens can thus support theoretical and causal analyses of pathways linking these drivers with financial circumstances and limited or no access to formal or semiformal financial products and services, which may exacerbate financial circumstance–related inequalities and health inequities. Application of a population health approach that considers socioecological and life course frameworks can widen practice-based and scholarly understanding, fostering analysis and inclusion of the myriad belief systems and modus operandi of different population groups relative to their financial resources. Such an understanding is critical for designing effective policies, programs, and services that address unmet basic needs and chronic socioeconomic disadvantage and, over the longer term, shifting risk factors for financial strain and financial well-being at population levels.

CONCEPTUALIZATION OF FINANCIAL CIRCUMSTANCES

Box 1 provides a glossary of single-level and multilevel concepts related to financial circumstances with definitions and by level of influence.[4,10,22,24,26–45] We used a socioecological-informed approach to organize concepts according to their level of influence: individual (personal factors); psychosocial (perceptions and feelings relative to others); family, household, and community (social relationships); and environment (contextual factors). Here individual level concerns money management; psychosocial level refers to control and freedom of choice; family, household, and community level describes concepts of social dynamics and networks; and environment level comprises related infrastructure (e.g., financial services and products). As all multilevel concepts fall under the individual level, the terms are aligned with that concept heading. However, the definitions of the multilevel concepts cross multiple levels. A discussion of the definitions by level follows.

Figures 1 and 2 and Figure A (available as a supplement to the online version of this article at http://www.ajph.org) present and unpack a concept map depicting the conceptual relationships between the various financial

BOX 1— Glossary of Single-Level and Multilevel Concepts Related to Financial Circumstances

Concept	Definitions
	Single-level concepts
Individual level	
Financial empowerment	Acquisition of financial knowledge and skills to make responsible financial decisions,[27,28] become financially stable, and be included in the financial system[29]
Financial fragility	Individuals' or households' abilities to access emergency funds (e.g., savings, alternative credit system) to deal with an unexpected financial shock[30,31]
Financial/economic/ material hardship	Disadvantageous financial circumstances experienced at the individual or household level[10] according to objective measures[32]
Financial literacy	Knowledge and skill development for sound financial decisions[33,34]
Financial knowledge	Understanding of key financial terms and facts[35,36,38] to support choice of financial services and products and financial planning[37]
Financial situation	Objective facts of one's financial circumstances (e.g., income, savings, debt management)[22,38]
Financial skills	Ability to navigate financial systems and identify, process, and act on financial information (e.g., seeking and using financial advice)[34–36,38]
Psychosocial level	
Financial attitudes	Positive or negative assessment of the value of proactive money management[33]
Financial behaviors	Day-to-day money management actions[36–38]
Financial happiness	Short-term feelings about one's financial situation[22]
Financial satisfaction	Long-term feelings about one's financial situation[22]
Financial (in)security	Positive feeling of being able to adapt and cope with adverse financial events (situated at the upper end of the financial resilience spectrum)[39,40]
Financial self-efficacy	Confidence in one's ability to reach financial goals, track money, and choose financial services and products[33,34,41]
Financial strain	Feeling anxious or worried about inabilities to cope with financial hardships and make ends meet[24]
Financial stress/vulnerability (often presented as synonymous with financial strain)	Feeling stressed or vulnerable about not being able to adapt to and cope with adverse financial events (situated at the lower end of the financial resilience spectrum)[24,39,40]
Perceived financial well-being	Perception of current money management combined with sense of future financial security[42]
Family, household, and community level	
Financial abuse	Control over of another person's financial resources to the point that the victim loses access to financial information, disposable income, assets, and power to make financial decisions; becomes financially dependent on the perpetrator[22,34]; or becomes involved in financial fraud[43]
Financial role	Position, responsibilities, and level of agency one may have in making financial decisions[44] (e.g., decision-maker, dependent, contributor)
Financial social capital	One's ability to rely on financial or in-kind support from relatives, neighbors, friends, and governments in times of financial adversity[38,44]
Environment level	
Financial inclusion	Access to appropriate, accessible, and affordable formal, semiformal, or even informal financial services and products[22,26]
	Multilevel concepts: definitions
Individual	Psychosocial
Financial well-being	State of being in which a person can meet current expenses and short- and long-term financial goals, has money left over to absorb financial shocks, has financial freedom (affording "wants"), and feels financially secure for present and future situations[22,36,37,45]
Individual	Psychosocial/environment
Financial capability	Knowledge, skills, behaviors, attitudes, self-efficacy, and financial inclusion (access to appropriate financial services and products) for effective management of financial resources[4,33,36]
Individual	Psychosocial/family, household, and community/environment

Continued

BOX 1— Continued

Concept	Definitions
Financial health	Knowledge, skills, behaviors, financial situation, financial inclusion, and financial support from community allowing one to build resilience from financial setbacks and reach financial goals (e.g., paying off a student loan)[44]
Financial resilience	Financial capability, financial inclusion, financial situation, and financial social capital shaping one's ability to draw on internal capabilities and appropriate, acceptable, and accessible external resources to meet individual needs and preferences[39]

circumstance–related terms that appear in the literature across several disciplines (e.g., consumer research, economics, social sciences). The dashed-line arrows in Figure 1 show what concepts are amalgamated by others. The concepts of financial knowledge and financial skills, for instance, are part of financial literacy.

Some of the concepts presented in Figure 1 embrace more than 1 level (indicated by dashed-line arrows). Thus, different symbols represent the corresponding levels. For example, financial well-being comprises concepts from individual and psychosocial levels. The full-line arrows in Figure 2 indicate that 1 concept may be the goal of another. For example, financial well-being is envisioned as the goal of financial literacy, financial capability, financial resilience, and financial inclusion.[22,41,46] Therefore, full-line arrows connect those latter concepts to the former. Figure A juxtaposes Figures 1 and 2 to illustrate the area's conceptual complexity.

Individual Level: Money Management

Spending, saving, borrowing, and planning are cornerstone behaviors targeted by most financial circumstance–related work led by economists, financial education professionals, the financial services industry, consumer researchers, and government agencies. Their main concern is the (im)balance of income and assets and discretionary and nondiscretionary expenditures. Financial education emerges as a solution to improve one's financial situation, alleviate poverty, and create "good financial citizens."[29] In response, public, private, and not-for-profit organizations offer financial education programs[33,41] (e.g., financial coaching and counseling) predominantly to individuals.[29]

Extant criticisms on the concepts at this level decry their focus on people's knowledge and skills as a mechanism for them to exert greater control over their own financial situation. This emphasis on optimal financial decision-

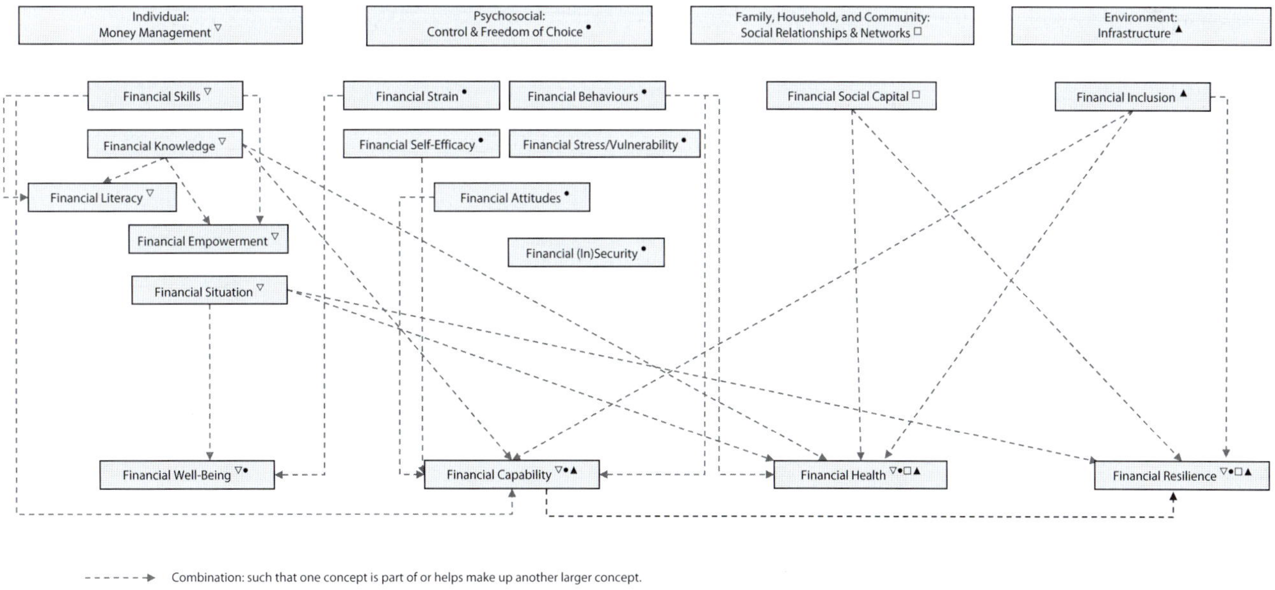

FIGURE 1— Concept Map Showing Combination of Concepts Into Overarching Constructs

Note. ▽ = individual: money management level; ● = psychosocial level; □ = family, household, and community level; ▲ = environment level.

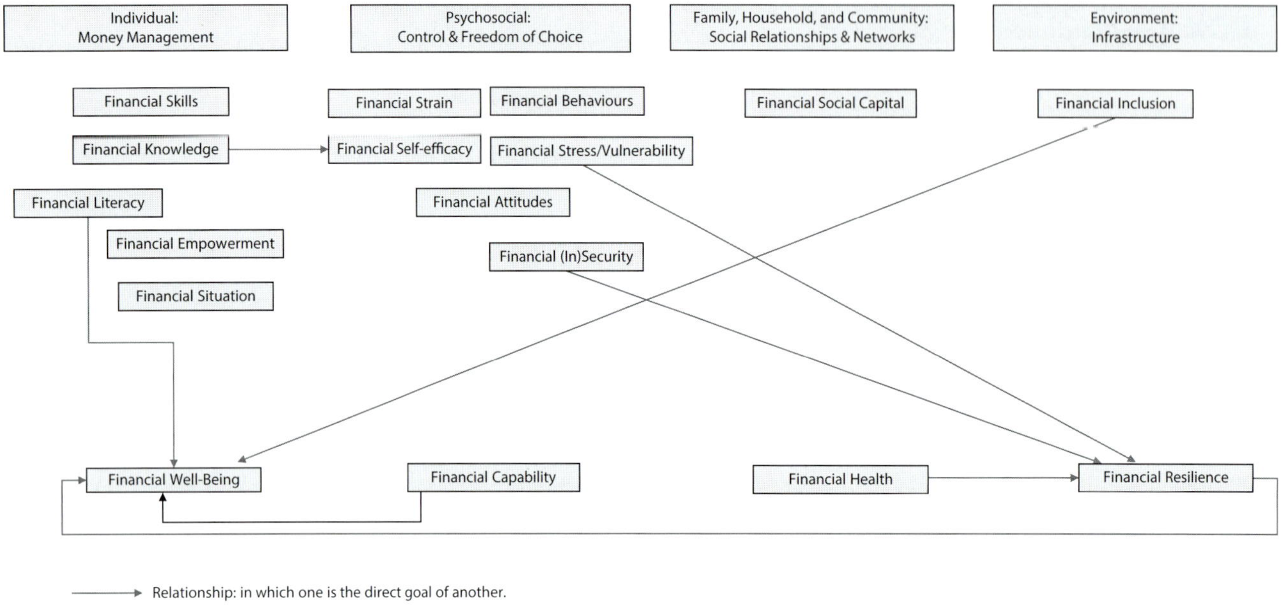

FIGURE 2— Concept Map Showing Concepts That Are Goals of Other Concepts

making disregards both the contexts in which people live (including forces beyond their control, irrespective of their knowledge and skills) and their immediate needs (e.g., prioritizing rising daily costs over contributions to longer-term saving). Such concepts may be less meaningful in application and, worse, result in unintended harmful consequences for the poorest populations who are struggling with day-to-day survival.[4] For instance, despite including the role of agency and adopting a less paternalistic approach, the concept of financial empowerment still places the onus of good financial circumstances primarily on the individual[29] rather than targeting the intersectional structural and societal forces shaping the individual's circumstances.

Psychosocial Level: Control and Freedom of Choice

At the psychosocial level are control and freedom of choice, which implicate the feelings of financial security. These concepts refer to perceptions of one's financial situation and latitude in decision-making, indirectly implicating the role of agency, which is an individual's feeling of control over taking actions that lead to particular effects. Research shows that perceived control and freedom to make financial decisions influence health independently of one's objective financial circumstances.[2] That is, feeling secure, happy, satisfied, confident, and less financially vulnerable or strained alongside financial attitudes and beliefs are distinct dimensions linked to financial circumstances. Exploring these subjective constructs may provide a unique interpretation of their effects on individual and population health and well-being, revealing varied patterns that are independent of objective measures of income and assets.

However, an overemphasis on perceptions of control and freedom of choice may result in oversight of the varied sociocultural, economic, and political factors that limit people's abilities to control and make financial decisions.[4,5] Thus, it is important to contextualize an individual's perceptions and experiences of lack of control or limited freedom of choice relative to these system factors to illuminate potential causes of inequities when using subjective indicators of financial circumstances.

The debate on the importance of an individual's freedom of choice clashes with the ideal of responsible financial choices. Although freedom of choice is important to financial circumstances at the individual level, that freedom seems to be allowed only for those who are not in debt or struggling to make ends meet. Freedom of choice seems to become attainable only when one has accumulated sufficient disposable resources through "optimal" behaviors and skills: only they could meritoriously enjoy latitude in decision-making without putting themselves at financial risk. This is problematic because it relates to a paternalistic view that does not give the opportunity for all people to choose to live the life they value.[4]

Family, Household, and Community Level: Social Relationships and Networks

At this level, concepts refer to the place people hold within a family, household, or community and their horizontal and vertical relationships with peers and institutions. For instance, people's responses to financial well-being are dependent on the financial role they hold within a family (nuclear or extended) or household.[44] The same responses may also shape individuals' reliance on their social or cultural networks or on nonprofit or charitable organizations in their social or community networks that provide (formal or informal) support.

Shaped by power, cultural context, and identity, these social interactions are relevant to financial practices. The reason is that financial resources acquire intrinsic and symbolical values at the family, household, and community levels. Therefore, analysis of the social relationships and networks around financial circumstances can reveal the local cultures and values attributed to financial practices. This may shed light on psychosocial-level concepts by broadening understanding of why people believe, feel, and intend to act in certain ways.

Power dynamics, participation in social networks, and the strength of social connections may buffer the effects of financial hardships at this level; however, they may also restrict people's abilities and freedom to access their own financial resources or make financial decisions. Negative relationships with family members, friends, acquaintances, or strangers may increase restrictions on individual financial freedom and expose disadvantaged individuals and populations to financial abuse through, for example, interception of their financial resources or coercion to be part of financial fraud. A further criticism of concepts at this level is the potential for problematic downloading of responsibility (by the government) for providing support onto nonprofit or charitable community organizations without also providing the resources for those agencies to adequately support people experiencing poor financial well-being.

Environment Level: Infrastructure

This level refers to the availability and quality of the environment to support people's financial actions as currently described in related literature. The concept of financial inclusion refers directly to accessibility of financial services and products (mainly bank accounts, credit cards, and insurance) and indirectly to regulation of the financial industry.[5] Financial inclusion has slowly evolved to include concepts related to inclusiveness, affordability, convenience, flexibility, acceptability, and safety.[4] Although the financial industry often alludes to financial inclusion as a solution to individuals' financial instability,[29] this concept has been criticized for ignoring people's needs, wants, and ways of being and doing.[47] Instead of a user-centric focus, financial inclusion seems to be guided by a top-down approach with the ideal of a universal set of financial products and services that automatically would result in optimal financial behaviors and practices.[4,5] Also missing from the financial inclusion concept is the context of financial industry deregulation, which expands profit-oriented banking strategies.[48] This further excludes people from the formal financial system and aggravates inequalities in financial circumstances.

Multilevel Concepts

Some concepts used in the literature span different levels. For example, the definition of financial well-being encompasses both individual and psychosocial levels because it includes real and perceived aspects of financial circumstances: having the ability to meet regular expenses, having sufficient financial resources to buy "wants," exerting control over finances, and feeling financially secure. These multilevel concepts are built on previous financial circumstance–related concepts and sometimes corresponding measures and indicators.[44] They translate the progress of theoretical and empirical evidence in the field.

Notwithstanding the intrinsic strengths of the multifaced nature of these concepts, some limitations are present. For instance, the strength of the financial resilience concept is the recognition of contextual factors and inequities beyond one's control.[22] However, some criticisms refer to its emphasis on an individual's adaptation even in scenarios of uncertainty and insecurity.[5] As a concept, financial resiliency encompasses the expectation for individuals to learn new ways of consumption (e.g., reducing grocery costs by buying discount products or buying less or in bulk to combat rising grocery prices) rather than a socioeconomic systems approach to addressing costs in the supply chain.

DISCUSSION

We have introduced financial circumstance–related concepts from various disciplines and explained their interrelationships to increase understanding for public health action and research. Many concepts are intimately related and some multidimensional (Figures 1 and 2 and Figure A). The categorization of concepts by their level of influence builds public health's capacity to broadly conceptualize and act on financial circumstances at a population level. Our categorization process maps the concepts to socioecological models (either explanatory or action oriented),[49] which are popularly used for targeting health promotion actions.

Our concept map clearly shows the imbalance of financial circumstance–related concepts across levels, with most belonging to the individual and psychosocial levels. For instance, apart from financial inclusion, there are no other environment-level (or system) concepts accounting for the role of the financial sector or the influence of societal structures. In addition, as this area has begun to evolve, some concepts have been combined to create new terms, blending different definitions. Conceptual clarity is needed for effective measurement of and intervention on financial circumstances: without it, the relative impact of actions will be difficult to ascertain.

Public health can address theoretical gaps concerning environment-level influences to better conceptualize and measure financial circumstances. This will lead to a clearer analysis of intervention gaps and more effective population health interventions within and across the different "levels" implicated in financial well-being. Furthermore, public health scholarship and practice can expand their current horizons by ensuring that intersectional (e.g., power imbalances) and external structural (e.g., racial discrimination) factors are incorporated into emerging concepts and definitions.

Understanding the theoretical and applied relationships between concepts is critical to advancing public health action. This concept map and glossary can help public health professionals and scholars choose the most appropriate concepts for their practice or research questions. Our work offers a stepping stone for the analysis of underlying external drivers of financial circumstance–related constructs and the selection or development of measures and indicators accordingly. It also provides a foundation for a common, interdisciplinary understanding of financial circumstance–related concepts to advance intersectoral collaboration with professionals from other sectors. Interdisciplinary work could better reveal the big-picture system factors (e.g., inflation, income inequality, rising tuition, discriminatory and oppressive practices in banking institutions) that shape financial well-being. This would support the design of evidence-based, equitable interventions to address the drivers of poor financial circumstances.

Building such an evidence base may reveal the need for coordinative, system-level healthy public policies that strategically target proximal and distal determinants of poor financial circumstances. Multilevel concepts, although relatively underarticulated, may offer a more solid foundation for public health intervention and evaluation to explore nuanced associations with health outcomes and health inequities, which together drive decision-making. Recognizing its ethos and praxis, public health can make a substantive and innovative contribution to this field through deeper investigation of these complex, multidimensional concepts.

This article's theoretical and practical contributions should be contextualized within its limitations. Our overview of concepts from various disciplines provides a glossary and relational concept map for those working with these terms; granular nuances of each concept were not captured. Despite the systematic process of gathering concepts and definitions through methods designed to develop public health resources on financial well-being and financial strain, the list of concepts included was not exhaustive. Our glossary may need to be expanded to include missed or emergent terms as the field evolves.

Furthermore, there are no generally acceptable definitions for many financial concepts.[26,50] For example, Storchi and Johnson's[4] definition of financial capability involves wider social and cultural contexts beyond financial contexts. Another example is financial health, which has been used in the financial industry as a proxy equation for savings and spending.[51] The lack of definitional and conceptual consensus may be partly due to efforts of researchers and practitioners to develop culturally grounded and context-specific definitions[52] for particular uses, populations, or settings. Although important for addressing local needs, this can contribute to disagreement on standardized measures. Finally, some measures (e.g., those for financial well-being) are at an earlier stage of development than measures of financial knowledge or financial literacy.[5,50]

MOVING FORWARD

This article has addressed the current fragmented understanding of financial

AJPH January 2024, Vol. 114, No. 1

circumstance–related concepts by untangling a myriad of terms in use across several disciplines. We have presented them as separate constructs and illustrated their interrelationships. This is a much-needed first step toward improving conceptual clarity for using public and population health approaches to address entrenched poverty and other poor financial circumstances. Our article offers a more sophisticated understanding of financial circumstance–related terms, reveals critical conceptual gaps problematic for intervention and measurement, and presents a solid starting point for conceptual debate. It also contributes to an interdisciplinary discussion on the benefits of advancing a population-wide approach over (or alongside) a high-risk population-focused approach, shifting the focus from individuals to populations.

A population-level approach is urgently needed to address the root causes of poor financial circumstances and shift risk levels for the entire population. Grounded in systems thinking, a population-level approach would facilitate the analysis of higher-order structural and environmental factors to better reveal the societal forces and inequities that shape agency, power, and privilege: factors that pose significant barriers for disadvantaged individuals or groups to enjoy better financial circumstances.

As we have discussed elsewhere,[7] individual- and household-level concepts related to financial circumstances require further advancement in public health scholarship and practice. Indeed, public health professionals are well positioned to offer a fresh perspective on the deleterious effects of financial circumstances on people's lives, health, and well-being. Thanks to their training and experience in social determinants of health, health equity, life course approaches, socioecological models, and population health, public health professionals can support the transition from a limited interpretation of people's financial circumstances to a broader contextualization in which people's knowledge, attitudes, behaviors, and decision-making are understood relative to distal social determinants, relative power, and structural inequities.

Future endeavors could integrate these concepts into public health and build a consensus on how to best measure financial circumstance–related concepts at individual, household, or population levels or combined levels. A consolidated list of indicators may further clarify the direction and dimension of the impact of financial circumstance–related concepts on health and support the development of more extensive analyses (see our related work on indicators as a starting point[19]). Moreover, use of a common set of indicators may result in a stronger evidence base indicating where interventions can achieve larger impacts on population health. Well-originated indicators beyond household income will facilitate exploration of causal links and associations between financial circumstances and health outcomes to drive action. Public health research and practice can play a critical role in advancing a global agenda on financial well-being promotion. AJPH

ABOUT THE AUTHORS

Candace I. J. Nykiforuk and Ana Paula Belon are with the Centre for Healthy Communities, School of Public Health, University of Alberta, Edmonton, Alberta, Canada. Lisa K. Allen Scott is with Provincial Population and Public Health, Alberta Health Services, Calgary, Alberta, Canada.

CORRESPONDENCE

Correspondence should be sent to Candace I. J. Nykiforuk, PhD, CE, Centre for Healthy Communities, School of Public Health, University of Alberta, ECHA 3-300, 11405-87 Ave, Edmonton, Alberta, Canada, T6G 1C9 (e-mail: candace.nykiforuk@ualberta.ca). Reprints can be ordered at http://www.ajph.org by clicking the "Reprints" link.

PUBLICATION INFORMATION

Full Citation: Nykiforuk CIJ, Belon AP, Allen Scott LK. Untangling concepts of financial circumstances for public health professionals and scholars: a glossary and concept map. *Am J Public Health*. 2024;114(1):79–89.

Acceptance Date: September 9, 2023

DOI: https://doi.org/10.2105/AJPH.2023.307449

CONTRIBUTORS

C. I. J. Nykiforuk and A. P. Belon contributed equally as co–first authors. C. I. J. Nykiforuk conceptualized the article. A. P. Belon wrote the first draft and was responsible for the revisions. L. K. Allen Scott contributed to initial conceptualization and provided feedback to inform revisions. All of the authors critically reviewed the article.

ACKNOWLEDGMENTS

We are grateful to the research staff members and scientists at the Centre for Healthy Communities (Canada) and Centre for Health Equity Training, Research and Evaluation (Australia) and the team at Alberta Health Services (Canada) who were involved in related projects on financial strain and financial well-being over the past five years, all of which inspired this work. More information about those projects can be found at healthiertogether.ca and https://www.ualberta.ca/public-health/research/centres/centre-for-healthy-communities/what-we-do/financial_wellbeing.html. The subproject described in this article used findings from a literature review that was conducted as part of an overarching project on financial well-being and financial strain funded by the Canadian Institutes of Health Research.

CONFLICTS OF INTEREST

The authors declare no conflicts of interest.

HUMAN PARTICIPANT PROTECTION

No protocol approval was necessary because no human participants were involved in this study.

REFERENCES

1. Weida EB, Phojanakong P, Patel F, Chilton M. Financial health as a measurable social determinant of health. *PLoS One*. 2020;15(5):e0233359. https://doi.org/10.1371/journal.pone.0233359
2. Sehrawat K, Vij M, Talan G. Understanding the path toward financial well-being: evidence from India. *Front Psychol*. 2021;12:638408. https://doi.org/10.3389/fpsyg.2021.638408
3. Brüggen EC, Hogreve J, Holmlund M, Kabadayi S, Löfgren M. Financial well-being: a conceptualization and research agenda. *J Bus Res*. 2017;79:228–237. https://doi.org/10.1016/j.jbusres.2017.03.013

4. Storchi S, Johnson S. Financial capability for well-being: an alternative perspective from the capability approach. Available at: http://hdl.handle.net/10419/179371. Accessed August 20, 2023.
5. Bowman D, Banks M, Fela G, Russell R, de Silva A. Understanding financial well-being in times of insecurity. Available at: http://library.bsl.org.au/jspui/bitstream/1/9423/1/Bowman_etal_Understanding_financial_wellbeing_2017.pdf. Accessed August 20, 2023.
6. Rose G. *Strategy of Preventive Medicine.* New York: Oxford University Press; 1992.
7. Glenn NM, Nykiforuk CIJ. The time is now for public health to lead the way on addressing financial strain in Canada. *Can J Public Health.* 2020;111(6):984–987. https://doi.org/10.17269/s41997-020-00430-2
8. Turunen E, Hiilamo H. Health effects of indebtedness: a systematic review. *BMC Public Health.* 2014;14(1):489. https://doi.org/10.1186/1471-2458-14-489
9. Okechukwu CA, El Ayadi AM, Tamers SL, Sabbath EL, Berkman L. Household food insufficiency, financial strain, work-family spillover, and depressive symptoms in the working class: the Work, Family, and Health Network study. *Am J Public Health.* 2012;102(1):126–133. https://doi.org/10.2105/AJPH.2011.300323
10. Park N, Heo W, Ruiz-Menjivar J, Grable JE. Financial hardship, social support, and perceived stress. *Financ Couns Plan.* 2017;28(2):322–332. https://doi.org/10.1891/1052-3073.28.2.322
11. Kendzor DE, Businelle MS, Costello TJ, et al. Financial strain and smoking cessation among racially/ethnically diverse smokers. *Am J Public Health.* 2010;100(4):702–706. https://doi.org/10.2105/AJPH.2009.172676
12. Davis CG, Mantler J. *The Consequences of Financial Stress for Individuals, Families, and Society.* Ottawa, Ontario, Canada: Centre for Research on Stress, Coping and Well-being, Carleton University; 2004.
13. White ND, Packard K, Kalkowski J. Financial education and coaching: a lifestyle medicine approach to addressing financial stress. *Am J Lifestyle Med.* 2019;13(6):540–543. https://doi.org/10.1177/1559827619865439
14. Szanton SL, Thorpe RJ, Whitfield K. Life-course financial strain and health in African-Americans. *Soc Sci Med.* 2010;71(2):259–265. https://doi.org/10.1016/j.socscimed.2010.04.001
15. Frank C, Davis CG, Elgar FJ. Financial strain, social capital, and perceived health during economic recession: a longitudinal survey in rural Canada. *Anxiety Stress Coping.* 2014;27(4):422–438. https://doi.org/10.1080/10615806.2013.864389
16. Afifi TD, Davis S, Merrill AF, Coveleski S, Denes A, Shahnazi AF. Couples' communication about financial uncertainty following the great recession and its association with stress, mental health and divorce proneness. *J Fam Econ Iss.* 2018;39(2):205–219. https://doi.org/10.1007/s10834-017-9560-5
17. Pinto AD, Da Ponte M, Bondy M, et al. Addressing financial strain through a peer-to-peer intervention in primary care. *Fam Pract.* 2020;37(6):815–820. https://doi.org/10.1093/fampra/cmaa046
18. Centre for Healthy Communities. Action-oriented public health framework on financial well-being and financial strain: executive summary. Available at: https://www.ualberta.ca/public-health/research/centres/centre-for-healthy-communities/what-we-do/framework_eng_2022.pdf. Accessed August 20, 2023.
19. Centre for Healthy Communities. Guidebook of strategies and indicators for action on financial well-being and financial strain: executive summary. Available at: https://www.ualberta.ca/public-health/research/centres/centre-for-healthy-communities/what-we-do/guidebook_eng_2022.pdf. Accessed August 20, 2023.
20. Glenn NM, Yashadhana A, Jaques K, et al. The generative mechanisms of financial strain and financial well-being: a critical realist analysis of ideology and difference. *Int J Health Policy Manag.* 2023;12:6930. https://doi.org/10.34172/ijhpm.2022.6930
21. Yashadhana A, Glenn NM, Jaques K, et al. A rapid review of initiatives to address financial strain and wellbeing in high-income contexts. *Public Health Res Pract.* 2023;33(2):e3322315. https://doi.org/10.17061/phrp3322315
22. Muir K, Hamilton M, Noone JH, Marjolin A, Salignac F, Saunders P. Exploring financial wellbeing in the Australian context. Available at: https://assets.csi.edu.au/assets/research/Exploring-Financial-Wellbeing-in-the-Australian-Context-Report.pdf. Accessed August 20, 2023.
23. Noone J, Muir K, Salignac F, et al. *An Australian Framework for Financial Wellbeing.* Melbourne, Australia: RMIT University; 2016.
24. French D, Vigne S. The causes and consequences of household financial strain: a systematic review. *Int Rev Financ Anal.* 2019;62:150–156. https://doi.org/10.1016/j.irfa.2018.09.008
25. Szanton SL, Allen JK, Thorpe RJ Jr, Seeman T, Bandeen-Roche K, Fried LP. Effect of financial strain on mortality in community-dwelling older women. *J Gerontol B Psychol Sci Soc Sci.* 2008;63(6):S369–S374. https://doi.org/10.1093/geronb/63.6.S369
26. Fu J. Ability or opportunity to act: what shapes financial well-being? *World Dev.* 2020;128:104843. https://doi.org/10.1016/j.worlddev.2019.104843
27. Franz C. Financial empowerment and health related quality of life in Family Scholar House participants. *J Financ Therapy.* 2016;7:1. https://doi.org/10.4148/1944-9771.1099
28. Murray JM, Mulholland E, Slade R. Financial counselling for people living on low incomes: international scan of best practices. Available at: https://prospercanada.org/getattachment/ea318ed1-9eb7-4ec5-85c8-adcc89e9cfda/Financial-Counselling-for-people-Living-on-Low-Inc.aspx. Accessed August 20, 2023.
29. Loomis JM. Rescaling and reframing poverty: financial coaching and the pedagogical spaces of financial inclusion in Boston, Massachusetts. *Geoforum.* 2018;95:143–152. https://doi.org/10.1016/j.geoforum.2018.06.014
30. Financial Consumer Agency of Canada. Canadians and their money: key findings from the 2019 Canadian Financial Capability Survey. Available at: https://www.canada.ca/en/financial-consumer-agency/programs/research/canadian-financial-capability-survey-2019.html. Accessed August 20, 2023.
31. Lusardi A, Schneider DJ, Tufano P. Financially fragile households: Evidence and implications. Available at: https://www.brookings.edu/articles/financially-fragile-households-evidence-and-implications. Accessed August 20, 2023.
32. Friedline T, Chen Z, Morrow S. Families' Financial stress & well-being: the importance of the economy and economic environments. *J Fam Econ Issues.* 2021;42(suppl 1):34–51. https://doi.org/10.1007/s10834-020-09694-9
33. Stuart G. What is financial capability? Available at: https://www.centerforfinancialinclusion.org/what-is-financial-capability. Accessed August 20, 2023.
34. Financial Consumer Agency of Canada. Financial literacy and retirement well-being in Canada: an analysis of the 2014 Canadian Financial Capability Survey. Available at: https://www.canada.ca/content/dam/fcac-acfc/documents/programs/research-surveys-studies-reports/financial-literacy-retirement-well-being.pdf. Accessed August 20, 2023.
35. Bureau of Consumer Financial Protection. Measuring financial skills. Available at: https://files.consumerfinance.gov/f/documents/bcfp_financial-well-being_measuring-financial-skill_guide.pdf. Accessed August 20, 2023.
36. Consumer Financial Protection Bureau. Financial well-being: the goal of financial education. Available at: https://files.consumerfinance.gov/f/201501_cfpb_report_financial-well-being.pdf. Accessed August 20, 2023.
37. Financial Consumer Agency of Canada. Financial well-being in Canada: survey results. Available at: https://www.canada.ca/content/dam/fcac-acfc/documents/programs/research-surveys-studies-reports/financial-well-being-survey-results.pdf. Accessed August 20, 2023.
38. Bureau of Consumer Financial Protection. Pathways to financial well-being: the role of financial capability. Research brief. Available at: https://files.consumerfinance.gov/f/documents/bcfp_financial-well-being_pathways-role-financial-capability_research-brief.pdf. Accessed August 20, 2023.
39. Muir K, Reeve R, Connolly C, Marjolin A, Salignac F, Ho K. Financial resilience in Australia 2015. Available at: https://www.nab.com.au/content/dam/nabrwd/documents/reports/financial/2015-financial-resilience.pdf. Accessed August 20, 2023.
40. Weier M, Dolan K, Powell A, Muir K, Young A. Money stories: financial resilience among Aboriginal and Torres Strait Islander Australians. Available at: https://assets.csi.edu.au/assets/research/Indigenous-Financial-Resilience-Report.PDF. Accessed August 20, 2023.
41. Consumer Financial Protection Bureau. Effective financial education: five principles and how to use them. Available at: https://www.consumerfinance.gov/data-research/research-reports/effective-financial-education-five-principles-and-how-use-them/c. Accessed August 20, 2023.
42. Netemeyer RG, Warmath D, Fernandes D, Lynch JG Jr. How am I doing? Perceived financial well-being, its potential antecedents, and its relation to overall well-being. *J Consum Res.* 2018;45(1):68–89. https://doi.org/10.1093/jcr/ucx109
43. Criminal Justice, Government of Canada. Elder abuse: financial fraud by strangers. Available at: https://www.justice.gc.ca/eng/rp-pr/cj-jp/fv-vf/eldfr-ainfr/eldfr-ainfr.html. Accessed October 24, 2022, 2022.
44. Ladha T, Asrow K, Parker S, Rhyne E, Kelly S. Beyond financial inclusion: financial health as a global framework. Available at: https://www.centerforfinancialinclusion.org/beyond-financial-inclusion-financial-health-as-a-global-framework. Accessed August 20, 2023.

45. Salignac F, Hamilton M, Noone J, Marjolin A, Muir K. Conceptualizing financial wellbeing: an ecological life-course approach. *J Happiness Stud.* 2020;21(5):1581–1602. https://doi.org/10.1007/s10902-019-00145-3

46. Financial Consumer Agency of Canada. Review of financial literacy research in Canada: an environmental scan & gap analysis. Available at: https://www.canada.ca/en/financial-consumer-agency/programs/research/review-financial-literacy-research.html. Accessed August 20, 2023.

47. Harper A, Baker M, Edwards D, Herring Y, Staeheli M. Disabled, poor, and poorly served: access to and use of financial services by people with serious mental illness. *Soc Serv Rev.* 2018;92(2):202–240. https://doi.org/10.1086/697904

48. Caplan MA, Birkenmaier J, Bae J. Financial exclusion in OECD countries: a scoping review. *Int J Soc Welfare.* 2021;30(1):58–71. https://doi.org/10.1111/ijsw.12430

49. Canadian Council on Social Determinants of Health. A review of frameworks on the determinants of health. Available at: https://nccdh.ca/images/uploads/comments/CCSDH_A-review-of-frameworks-on-the-determinants-of-health_EN.pdf. Accessed August 20, 2023.

50. Kempson E, Poppe C. Understanding financial well-being and capability—a revised model and comprehensive analysis. Available at: https://hdl.handle.net/20.500.12199/5357. Accessed August 20, 2023.

51. Innovations for Poverty Action. Nudges for financial health: global evidence for improved product design. Available at: https://www.poverty-action.org/publication/nudges-financial-health-global-evidence-improved-product-design. Accessed August 20, 2023.

52. Abrantes-Braga FDM, Veludo-de-Oliveira T. Development and validation of financial well-being related scales. *Int J Bank Marketing.* 2019;37(4):1025–1040. https://doi.org/10.1108/IJBM-03-2018-0074

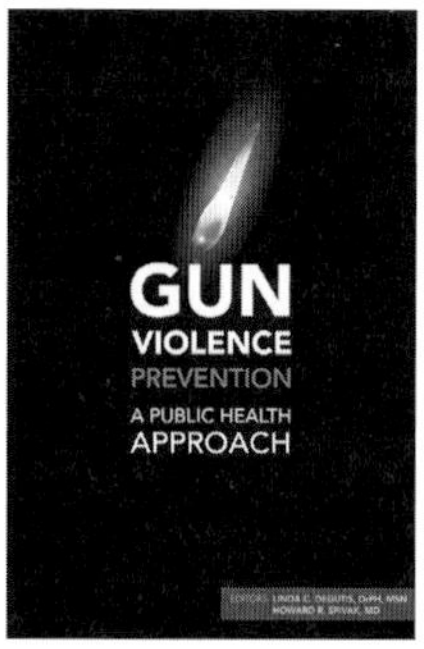

2021, SOFTCOVER
230 PAGES, 9780875533117

Gun Violence Prevention: A Public Health Approach

Edited By: Linda C. Degutis, DrPH, MSN, and Howard R. Spivak, MD

Gun Violence Prevention: A Public Health Approach acknowledges that guns are a part of the environment and culture. This book focuses on how to make society safer, not how to eliminate guns. Using the conceptual model for injury prevention, the book explores the factors contributing to gun violence and considers risk and protective factors in developing strategies to prevent gun violence and decrease its toll. It guides you with science and policy that make communities safer.

APHABOOKSTORE.ORG

APHA PRESS
AN IMPRINT OF AMERICAN PUBLIC HEALTH ASSOCIATION

Tobacco 21 Laws and Youth Tobacco Use: The Role of Policy Attributes

Abigail S Friedman, PhD, Michael F Pesko, PhD

See also Liber, p. 10.

Objectives. To estimate Tobacco-21 policies' relationships to 18- to 20 year-old youth cigarette, cigar, and electronic nicotine delivery system (ENDS) use, and to test for effect modification by policy attributes.

Methods. In fall 2022, we used Tobacco 21 Population Coverage Database data to calculate the percentage of state residents covered by state or local Tobacco 21 (T21) laws monthly through June 2020. Matching T21 coverage to Population Assessment of Tobacco and Health and Behavioral Risk Factor Surveillance System data, we used 2-way fixed effect analyses to assess the relationship between T21 laws and 18- to 20-year-old youth cigarette, cigar, and ENDS use, and tested for differences by policy attributes: possession, use, or purchase (PUP) penalties, retailer noncompliance penalties, and compliance check requirements.

Results. Increased T21 exposure yielded significant reductions in cigarette and cigar use, as well as in ENDS use, when accounting for policy attributes. These effects were dampened in T21 laws with PUP penalties relative to those without.

Conclusions. Tobacco-21 laws yield reductions in 18- to 20-year-old youth cigarette, cigar, and ENDS use, with dampened effects when policies include PUP penalties.

Public Health Implications. State policymakers should consider implementing T21 laws without PUP penalties to reduce underage nicotine and tobacco use. (*Am J Public Health*. 2024;114(1):90–97. https://doi.org/10.2105/AJPH.2023.307447)

AJPH January 2024, Vol. 114, No. 1

Since 2005, when Needham, Massachusetts, became the first US locality to prohibit cigarette sales to people younger than 21 years, US states and localities have increasingly adopted Tobacco 21 (T21) laws, with Hawaii implementing the first state law in 2016. By federal T21's passage in December 2019, 11 states and Washington, DC, had fully implemented their own T21 laws (i.e., without exempting underage youths born before a specific date). At least 27 more states implemented their own T21 laws since then. Indeed, the federal law may have spurred further state adoption, particularly given delays in the US Food and Drug Association's (FDA's) T21 rulemaking, required to make federal T21 fully enforceable.[1]

Quasi-experimental studies of T21 policies across multiple states demonstrate state and local T21 laws' effectiveness at reducing smoking among 18- to 20-year-old youths[2–5] and decreasing sales of cigarette brands favored by young people,[6] with effects on minors typically smaller or nonsignificant depending on the analysis.[4,5] While a longitudinal study of 15 to 21 year-old youths found nonsignificant associations between T21 and cigarette use, and significant positive associations with electronic nicotine delivery system (ENDS) use, that analysis may be biased: it did not adjust for other tobacco policies known to affect behavior (e.g., taxes).[7] More evidence is needed to clarify T21's effects on ENDS and cigar use across the United States.

Furthermore, previous analyses treat T21 laws as homogenous despite differences in key policy attributes, such as whether they penalize youth possession, use, or purchase ("PUP penalties") and legislated penalties for retailer noncompliance. These details matter: research on earlier (T18) sales restrictions link their impact to enforcement and graduated retailer penalties that include retail license suspension, whereas results from PUP penalty analyses are more mixed, with some raising concerns about differential penalization of minoritized youths.[8–12] This research assesses T21 laws' relationships to cigarette, cigar, and ENDS use by those newly subject to age restrictions (i.e., 18- to 20-year-old youths), and tests for effect modification from key policy attributes.

METHODS

Using the University of Michigan's Tobacco 21 Population Coverage Database, we derived each state's percentage of residents living in areas with state or local T21 laws at the start of each month from January 2014–June 2020 (detailed documentation provided here[13]). While later data were not used because the database only verified T21 passage and implementation dates for laws passed before July 2020,[13] we extended the data backward to include the few T21 policies passed before 2014 and adjusted it to reflect states' grandfathering provisions that exempt 18- to 20-year-old adults born before a particular date—in Arkansas, Maine, Massachusetts, Ohio, and Texas—so that state T21 laws only counted as such when they applied to all residents younger than 21 years. State T21 policies attributes were compiled from the Preventing Tobacco Addiction Foundation,[14] CDC STATE,[15] and other publications.[16]

T21 data were matched to restricted-use Population Assessment of Tobacco and Health (PATH) data by respondent state and interview week (PATH's most precise geographic and interview date variables). A longitudinal survey of tobacco and nicotine use behaviors, PATH follows a nationally representative household sample covering 45 971 adults and youths aged 12 years and older at wave 1. Younger minors in sampled households age into the survey across waves, and a 9804-person replenishment sample was added at wave 4. A subset of participants completed wave 4's survey twice. They gave highly concordant responses, suggesting that PATH's tobacco use data are reliable and valid.[17] In this analysis, we used data from waves 1 (fielded September 2013 to December 2014) through 5 (fielded December 2018–November 2019) to assess T21 effects on cigarette, cigar, and ENDS use.

To consider effects on underage tobacco use, the analytic sample was restricted to each respondent's youngest interview between the ages of 18 and 20 years, retaining lagged location and tobacco use (i.e., at their last younger-than-18-years interview) to identify changes in location and behavior. Because state of residence at ages 18 to 20 years may have reflected selection (e.g., if smokers were more likely to move to states with more lenient tobacco control policies), sensitivity tests repeat analyses with the subsample of 18- to 20-year-old respondents who had not moved across state lines since their previous interview.

As a robustness check, we repeated policy attribute analyses with 2011–2020 Behavioral Risk Factor Surveillance System (BRFSS) data, providing nationally and state-representative repeated cross-sections of noninstitutionalized US civilian adults annually. Pre-2011 waves were omitted because of methodological changes that precluded comparisons with earlier years. Merging in T21 policy data by respondent state and interview date limited consideration to pre-July 2020 interviews (because the database's T21 implementation dates were only verified through June of 2020).[13] BRFSS covers a larger sample than PATH ($n \approx 7500$ 18- to 20-year-old youths annually) over more years, and thus provides greater statistical power. However, because BRFSS did not include annual cigar or ENDS use questions, these analyses were limited to cigarette use outcomes.

Outcomes

PATH analyses' outcomes were as indicators for past-30-day use of cigarettes, cigars (including cigarillos), and ENDS. For BRFSS analyses, outcomes were for current established smoking—current cigarette use by those who smoked at least 100 cigarettes in their life—and daily smoking.

Exposures

The main exposure of interest was the percentage of state residents covered by state or local T21 laws 30 days before their interview week (PATH) or interview date (BRFSS), to ensure that exposure preceded the past-30-day outcome period.

With T21 policy attribute data only collected for state-level laws, effect modification analyses split the past-30-day T21 exposure into 2 variables: the percentage of state residents covered by substate T21 laws ("local T21 coverage") versus a binary indicator for state T21 coverage. For BRFSS analyses only (as PATH data predate federal T21 adoption), we used a third T21 variable to capture the percentage of state residents covered by federal T21 alone ("federal T21 coverage").

To assess modifier effects, the state T21 indicator was interacted with policy attribute variables signifying (1) whether state T21 laws included PUP penalties (all but CA, CT, DE, MA, MD, NJ, NY, and KY),[15] (2) whether retailer violation penalties mandate suspending tobacco

AJPH January 2024, Vol. 114, No. 1

product sales for at least a week by the third retailer violation (CA, CT, DC, NY, VT, WA), and (3) legislated compliance check frequency, specifically a categorical measure for requiring at least 1 compliance check per retailer annually (CT, DE, MA, NY) versus compliance checks conducted at random (CA and OR), with unspecified compliance check schedules as the reference group.[14]

Covariates

Covariates included demographics (categorical variables for age, sex, race/ethnicity) and relevant policy variables in the respondent's state 30 days before the interview week for PATH or date for BRFSS (specifically, tax rates for ENDS [standardized as in Cotti et al.[18]], cigarettes, and cigars [separate for per unit vs percentage of cost taxes][15]; indicators for state T19 age restrictions among those younger than 19 years (either explicitly legislated as T19—in AL, AK, NJ, UT, and briefly in NH and NE—or because of expiring grandfather clauses in ME, MA, AR, TX, and OH state T21 laws); the percentage of the state with comprehensive smoke-free worksite laws (i.e., without small business exemptions); and the percentage with comprehensive vape-free worksite laws in that month.[15,19] Covariates also included indicators for state medical and adult recreational cannabis legalization 30 days before the interview week, in case access to cannabis affected tobacco product use.

BRFSS data analyses also included an indicator for surveys conducted by cell phone as opposed to land line (a key sampling variable) and, because BRFSS data extended into 2020, each state's monthly COVID-19 deaths per 100 000 residents to capture the pandemic's potential effects on behavior.[20]

Tobacco 21 Effects on Cigarette, Cigar, and ENDS Use

We used multivariable regressions to estimate how the percentage of state residents covered by T21 laws 30 days before a respondent's interview related to 18- to 20-year-old youths' past-30-day cigarette, cigar, and ENDS use, controlling for quarter-year fixed effects to absorb national time trends in the outcome variable along with age fixed effects and the aforementioned policy covariates. First, a first-difference analysis controlled for a lag of the outcome variable—its previous-wave value, capturing pre–age-18-years behavior but limiting consideration to respondents with a pre–age-18-years observation—as well as the aforementioned covariates and quarter-year fixed effects, so that the T21 coefficient identified the relationship between that policy exposure and changes in the outcome between waves. A second specification estimated 2-way fixed effects regressions to compare outcomes in states with more versus less T21 coverage, before versus after those policies went into effect. Controlling for state and quarter-year fixed effects alongside the aforementioned covariates ensured that resulting policy coefficients were not driven by time-invariant differences between states or nationwide time trends (see Appendix for further detail). All analyses clustered standard errors by state, the level of this study's T21 policy variation and assignment.[21]

While main analyses were run as logistic regressions, specification checks repeated them as linear probability models because of concerns about bias in logistic regressions with large numbers of fixed effects.[22] Sensitivity tests (1) repeated analyses omitting respondents who moved to a different state since the prior interview to address potential selection bias (e.g., if respondents who use tobacco products are less likely to move to states with restrictive tobacco control policies) and (2) repeated ENDS use regressions with the sample limited to pre–August 2019 interviews, to avoid potential effects of the US outbreak of vaping-associated lung injuries.[23]

Tobacco 21 Effect Modification From Policy Attributes

To consider whether specific policy attributes moderated T21 laws' effects, we repeated 2-way fixed effects regressions with 4 interaction terms between binary indicators for the state T21 law and each policy attribute: whether the law included PUP penalties, mandated retailer violation penalties suspending tobacco product sales for at least 1 week by the third retailer violation, required at least 1 compliance check per retailer annually, or required compliance checks conducted at random. Interaction term coefficients therefore indicated whether state T21 laws' relationship to the outcome variable differed with each policy attribute. Absent data on substate T21 policies' attributes, these analyses included the following T21 variables: (1) a state T21 indicator, (2) the proportion of state residents covered by substate T21 laws, and, in BRFSS analyses only, (3) the proportion covered by only federal T21 (because PATH's data predate the federal law), all 30-days before the interview. Absent substate policy attribute data, effect modification analyses omitted states where more than a third of residents were covered by substate T21 laws during the period of analysis, to avoid biasing the policy attribute estimates (see Appendix Section II for further detail).

Causal interpretation of 2-way fixed effect analyses, prior to T1 adoption, is predicated on the assumption that time trends in the outcome variable were parallel in jurisdictions that did versus did not adopt that policy. Because PATH is longitudinal and covers a relatively short window of time, we only ran parallel trends tests for BRFSS analyses, repeating the 2-way fixed effects regressions with the addition of six 1-year leads on the state T21 variable, to confirm whether outcomes differed between states that would versus would not adopt T21 in the future.

All analyses clustered standard errors by state, the level of these data's T21 policy variation and assignment.[21] Regressions were unweighted because neither data set's weights were designed to yield representative estimates for subsamples covering only 3 years of age.

RESULTS

Estimates of T21's relationship to youth cigarette, cigar, and ENDS use are presented first, followed by analyses of effect modification by policy attributes.

Past-30-Day Cigarette, Cigar, and ENDS Use

Figure 1 shows adjusted odds ratios (AORs) from logistic regression analyses of T21's relationship to past-30-day use of cigarettes, cigars, and ENDS, by outcome and regression specification. First-difference specifications linked T21 laws to reductions in 18- to 20-year-old youths' past 30-day cigarette and cigar use, with a nonsignificant relationship to ENDS use. Two-way fixed effects models with state fixed effects generated similar results for cigarettes: full T21 coverage yielded a 40% reduction in the odds of cigarette use (AOR = 0.598; 95% confidence interval [CI] = 0.453, 0.790; *P* < .001), but nonsignificant AORs closer to 1 for cigars and ENDS. However, limiting consideration to nonmovers—62% of our analytic sample—T21 exposure yielded significant reductions in use of cigarettes (AOR = 0.584; 95% CI = 0.407, 0.838; *P* = .003) and cigars (AOR = 0.545; 95% CI = 0.340, 0.874; *P* = .012), and reversed the direction of

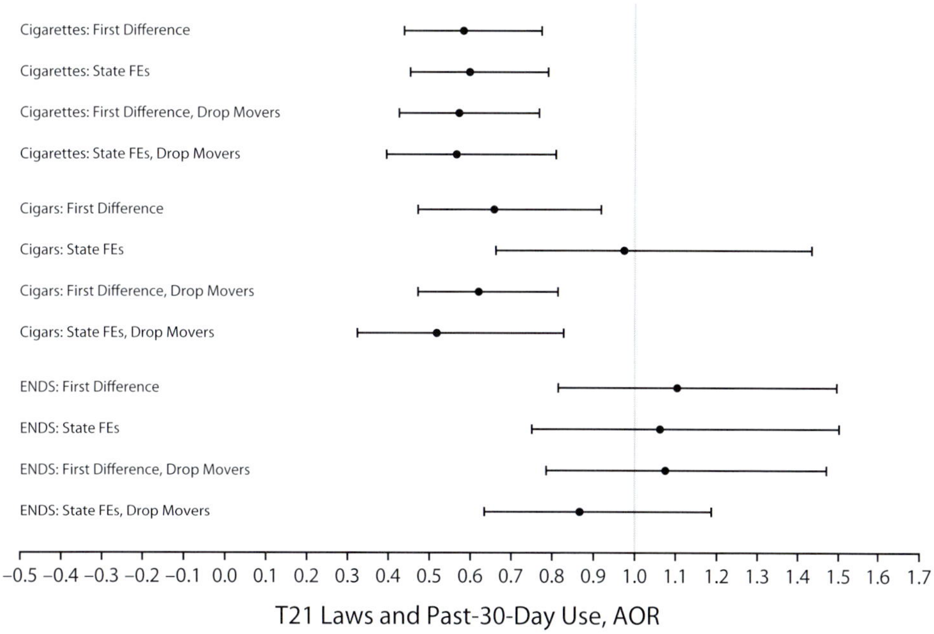

AOR (95% CI)	No.
0.58 (0.44, 0.77)	10 003
0.60 (0.45, 0.79)	15 036
0.57 (0.43, 0.77)	9 324
0.57 (0.40, 0.80)	9 326
0.66 (0.47, 0.92)	9 891
0.97 (0.66, 1.43)	14 969
0.62 (0.47, 0.81)	9 222
0.52 (0.32, 0.83)	9 321
1.10 (0.82, 1.50)	9 949
1.06 (0.75, 1.50)	14 987
1.08 (0.79, 1.47)	9 273
0.87 (0.63, 1.19)	9 293

FIGURE 1— Tobacco-21 Exposure and Past-30-Day Tobacco Product Use Among 18- to 20-Year-Old Youths: United States, Population Assessment of Tobacco and Health Survey, 2013–2019

Note. AOR = adjusted odds ratio; CI = confidence interval; Drop Movers = sample omitted respondents who relocated across state lines since their previous interview; FEs = fixed effects; T21 = Tobacco 21. AORs and 95% confidence intervals (whiskers) reflect estimates for the relationship between the percentage of one's state covered by T21 laws 30 days before the interview and past-30-day use of the tobacco or nicotine product indicated, based on multivariable logistic regression analyses of data from the Population Assessment of Tobacco and Health Survey. All analyses considered 18- to 20-year-old respondents only. Two-way fixed effects analyses use only 1 observation per respondent, while first-difference analyses also control for that respondent's lagged (pre-18-year-old) behavior, restricting consideration to those with a lagged observation. All specifications include demographic and policy covariates described in the Appendix (available as a supplement to the online version of this article at https://www.ajph.org), as well as fixed effects for respondent age and quarter-year. Robust standard errors are clustered by state.

TABLE 1— Two-Way Fixed Effects Estimates of T21 Policy Attributes' Relationships to Tobacco Product Use Among 18- to 20-Year-Old Respondents: United States, PATH 2013–2019 and BRFSS 2011–2020

	PATH Nonmovers, Waves 1–5, AOR (95% CI)			BRFSS, Waves 2011–2020, AOR (95% CI)	
	Past-30-Day Cigarette Use	Past-30-Day Cigar Use	Past-30-Day ENDS Use	Current Cigarette Smoking	Daily Cigarette Smoking
State $T21_{Lag\ 30D}$	0.63 (0.23, 1.75)	0.27 (0.12, 0.61)	0.39 (0.26, 0.57)	0.38 (0.25, 0.57)	0.24 (0.15, 0.40)
State $T21_{Lag\ 30D}$ × PUP provisions	1.50 (0.31, 7.33)	3.61 (1.40, 9.34)	3.15 (1.23, 8.07)	2.53 (1.54, 4.15)	3.86 (1.91, 7.83)
State $T21_{Lag\ 30D}$ × retailer sales banned for ≥ 1 wk at or before third violation	1.92 (0.34, 11.02)	2.93 (0.62, 13.75)	2.40 (0.81, 7.09)	0.79 (0.46, 1.34)	0.87 (0.54, 1.39)
State $T21_{Lag\ 30D}$ × ≥ 1 compliance inspection per retailer annually	. . .[a]	. . .[a]	4.78 (1.51, 15.09)	2.35 (0.53, 10.45)	3.32 (0.56, 19.79)
State $T21_{Lag\ 30D}$ × compliance inspections at random	0.57 (0.15, 2.08)	0.83 (0.39, 1.80)	0.76 (0.30, 1.94)	1.17 (0.84, 1.64)	1.38 (0.91, 2.08)
% substate $T21_{Lag\ 30D}$	0.35 (0.02, 7.26)	0.10 (0.001, 8.55)	0.84 (0.04, 17.36)	0.77 (0.40, 1.47)	0.97 (0.49, 1.92)
% of state covered by federal T21 only $_{Lag\ 30D}$				0.73 (0.53, 0.99)	0.88 (0.55, 1.40)
No.	8275	8264	8245	76 849	76 849
Pseudo-R^2	0.039	0.047	0.069	0.050	0.058
Mean (outcome)	0.152	0.120	0.213	0.123	0.074
Mean (state T21)	0.117	0.117	0.118	0.051	0.051

Note. AOR = adjusted odds ratio; BRFSS = Behavioral Risk Factor Surveillance System; CI = confidence interval; PATH = Population Assessment of Tobacco and Health; PUP = possession, use, or purchase. Multivariable logistic regressions used data on 18- to 20-year-old youths who had not moved to a new state since their previous interview ("nonmovers") from PATH waves 1 (fielded September 2013–December 2014) through 5 (fielded December 2018–November 2019) and 2011–2020 BRFSS data for interviews before July 1, 2020, to assess if and how T21 policy attributes modify these laws' effects on cigarette, cigar, and ENDS use, limiting consideration to states with less than a third of their population covered by local T21 laws throughout the period of analysis. "Lag 30D" subscripts indicate variables coded based on their level 30 days before the respondent's interview. Controls not indicated above include fixed effects for quarter-year, state, and age, as well as demographic and policy variables described in the Appendix. BRFSS analyses include 2 additional covariates: an indicator for cell phone interviews (vs landline, a key BRFSS sampling variable) and, because these include 2020 data, state COVID-19 deaths per capita by month. Robust standard errors are clustered by state.
[a]Multivariable logistic regressions dropped this variable because of collinearity.

the nonsignificant estimate for ENDS. Reestimating specifications as linear probability models yielded similar results (Appendix Figure A). Omitting interviews conducted after July 2019 to avoid potential effects of the 2019 outbreak of vaping-associated lung injuries did not change estimated effects on ENDS use (Appendix Figure B).

Policy Attributes and Tobacco Product Use

To better understand these relationships, we used 2-way fixed effects regressions to test whether T21 associations with cigarette, cigar, and ENDS use varied with state T21 policy details. Because comprehensive policy attribute data were not available for local policies, these analyses omitted states with local T21 laws covering more than one third of residents at any point in the analytic period, to minimize bias from variation in unmeasured local policy attributes. This restriction dropped 3 states with state-T21 laws during our analytic period—Massachusetts, New York, and Illinois.

Of the remaining 12 states and DC with T21 fully in effect before June 1, 2020, 8 had PUP penalties, 5 required retailers to suspend tobacco product sales for at least a week at or before their third violation, 2 mandated at least 1 annual compliance check per retailer, and 2 others mandated randomized compliance checks.[14] Because unmeasured state or policy differences were more likely to drive coefficient estimates where variables were based on only a few states, we interpreted the compliance check interaction terms as controls to ensure that the PUP and retailer violation terms were not driven by differences in compliance check policies, not as indicators of effect modification.

Table 1 shows interaction terms that tested for differential T21 effects by each policy attribute simultaneously, separately controlling for the percentage of a state covered by substate T21 policies and a state-T21 law indicator.

When policy attributes were separately accounted for, state T21 laws were associated with decreases in recent use of ENDS (AOR = 0.387; 95% CI = 0.264,0.569; $P < .001$) and cigars (AOR = 0.267; 95% CI = 0.116, 0.614; $P = .002$). Linear probability models yielded similar results (Appendix Table A).

Considering specific policy attributes, PUP provisions showed significant modifier effects for cigars and ENDS in PATH data and for current and daily smoking in BRFSS, whether using logistic or linear regressions. Relative to T21 laws that did not penalize youth purchase, use, or possession, PUP provisions were associated with increases in past-30-day cigar use (AOR = 3.612; 95% CI = 1.397, 9.337; $P = .008$), past-30-day ENDS use (AOR = 3.146; 95% CI = 1.226, 8.072; $P = .017$), current cigarette smoking (AOR = 2.525; 95% CI = 1.536, 4.151; $P < .001$), and daily cigarette smoking (AOR = 3.862; 95% CI = 1.905, 7.829; $P < .001$). T21 laws with more restrictive retailer violation penalties yielded nonsignificant coefficients in all specifications and outcomes.

Compliance check requirement coefficients were nonsignificant in all but 1 case, where the policy attribute existed in only 2 small states with T21 laws in effect for less than 6 months. This supports interpreting compliance check coefficients as controls, not generalizable estimates of effect modification.

Results were similar when repeating the BRFSS analyses with pre-2020 data only (to avoid COVID-19 effects; Appendix Table B) and when sequentially dropping each T21 state (to confirm that a single state did not drive findings; Appendix Tables C and D).

To test for parallel pretrends—an assumption required for causal interpretation of 2-stage fixed effects estimates—we repeated BRFSS analyses with six 1-year leads on the state T21 variable. Consistent with parallel pretrends, all lead variable coefficients were close to 0 and statistically nonsignificant (Appendix Table E).

DISCUSSION

Contributing to a growing literature assessing T21 laws' effects on youth tobacco and nicotine use, this study's findings link T21 policies to reductions in 18- to 20-year-old youths' use of cigarettes, cigars, and, when policy details were accounted for, ENDS. Moreover, those relationships varied with T21 policy attributes: penalizing youth purchase, use, or possession ("PUP penalties") was associated with significant increases in past-30-day cigar and ENDS use as well as current and daily cigarette smoking, relative to T21 laws without PUP penalties. Further work to determine the most efficacious structure for T21 laws to reduce youth nicotine and tobacco use would be valuable.

The positive association between PUP penalties and use of each product concurs with model T21 policy recommendations.[24] Several mechanisms could explain this result. At the individual level, PUP penalties may deter nicotine dependent youths from seeking help to quit smoking for fear of consequences or promote undesired behavior among marginalized groups.[25] Concurrently, if penalizing underage purchase, use, or possession is seen as placing the responsibility for that behavior on youths, such policies may allow adults to abdicate their responsibility to prevent underage access, reducing barriers to informal sources. The relationship could also stem from differences in resource allocation if penalizing youth behavior pulls concrete resources away from ensuring retailer compliance. In that case, effects may depend on whether funding is allocated to implement the policy, PUP provision enforcement rates, and consequences for violations (e.g., requiring parental involvement, tobacco diversion programs vs fines vs loss of driver's license).[26,27] Indeed, a randomized controlled trial of 24 towns in northern Illinois linked PUP laws to reductions in youth smoking—the opposite of our findings—in a context where PUP enforcement was monitored and both treated and control groups experienced supply side tobacco control activities to reduce youth access.[28] Thus, data on PUP provisions' enforcement and funding might help clarify their effects. Such analyses could be conducted with more recent data, as the federal T21 law does not impose PUP penalties.

This study's findings might also be explained by "crowd out," not only in terms of concrete resources like funding but, less tangibly, in terms of attention and efforts toward policy change. In the former case, if enforcing PUP penalties draws on limited funding or time that would be more impactful if spent elsewhere, their net effect would be increased youth tobacco use. In the latter, PUP laws may divert policymaker, stakeholder, or even enforcing authorities' attention away from more effective regulatory approaches. Critically, evidence on PUP enforcement also raises ethical questions related to divesting industry from their responsibility for youth use, criminalizing youths,[25] and potential inequities in enforcement.

While this analysis assessed T21's relationship to cigarette, cigar, and ENDS use, and applied novel approaches to multiple data sets to evaluate how policy attributes shape T21 laws' effects, it still has several limitations. First, reliance on self-reported data may introduce social desirability bias. However, that should only bias this study's results if T21 adoption per se changes misreporting of tobacco product use and, in the effect modification analyses, if that change in misreporting varies by policy attributes. A second set of concerns relates to generalizability: absent annual BRFSS data on ENDS and cigar use, we cannot test whether PATH results for those outcomes generalize to a larger, more representative sample. The COVID-19 pandemic presents further generalizability questions, because PATH analyses use pre-2020 data and BRFSS analyses overlap only the start of the US outbreak. As pandemic-related restrictions on in-person schooling, masking requirements, and perceived health risks may have affected youth access to and interest in using tobacco and nicotine products, the degree to which this study's results generalize to more recent periods is unclear. A third limitation concerns policy attribute analyses: without data on resources allocated to T21 implementation and enforcement, these analyses cannot pin down the exact mechanisms behind differential smoking-responses to PUP policies. Ongoing assessment of T21 policies' effects accounting for policy attributes and resource allocation is needed to guide policymaking. Fourth, causal interpretation of 2-way fixed effect estimates rests on several assumptions, particularly parallel pretrends. While a variety of studies show parallel pretrends in T21 analyses and we confirm this assumption in the BRFSS data, PATH's longitudinal structure and short period preclude such tests. Thus, findings from PATH analyses that we cannot confirm using BRFSS may be more appropriately interpreted as associations than causal effects.

Finally, whereas the Tobacco 21 Population Coverage Database stopped compiling and validating new data on local T21 laws about 6 months after the federal T21 law was passed, ongoing state T21 adoption suggests added value from these policies, beyond that of the federal law. Thus, to best promote public health, continued analyses are needed to guide T21 policy details at the local, state, and federal level. Future work should assess effects on minors as well as 18- to 20-year-old youths, and test for differential effects on minoritized groups to clarify implications for health equity.

PUBLIC HEALTH IMPLICATIONS

While a federal T21 law was passed in December of 2019, the literature on T21 policies' effects on use of tobacco and nicotine products other than cigarettes remains thin. This study's findings add insight by demonstrating reductions in cigarette, cigar or cigarillo, and ENDS use associated with these policies, and identifying a specific policy attribute that may impede T21's intended effects. State regulators whose T21 laws include PUP penalties should consider removing those provisions as a potential means to amplify reductions in youth cigarette, cigar, and ENDS use. AJPH

ABOUT THE AUTHORS

Abigail S. Friedman is with the Department of Health Policy and Management, Yale School of Public Health, Yale University, New Haven CT. Michael F. Pesko is with the Department of Economics, University of Missouri, Columbia.

CORRESPONDENCE

Correspondence should be sent to Abigail S. Friedman, Associate Professor, Department of Health Policy and Management, Yale School of Public Health, 60 College Street, Rm. 303, New Haven, CT 06520-8034 (e-mail: abigail.friedman@yale.edu). Reprints can be ordered at http://www.ajph.org by clicking the "Reprints" link.

PUBLICATION INFORMATION

Full Citation: Friedman Abigail S, Pesko Michael F. Tobacco 21 laws and youth tobacco use: the role of policy attributes. *Am J Public Health*. 2024; 114(1):90–97.

Acceptance date: September 3, 2023.

DOI: https://doi.org/10.2105/AJPH.2023.307447

CONTRIBUTORS

A. S. Friedman conceptualized the study, carried out empirical analyses, and wrote the first draft. Both authors contributed to the study design, revised the article, and approved the final manuscript as submitted. Both authors agree to be accountable for all aspects of the work.

ACKNOWLEDGMENTS

Research reported in this publication was supported by grant numbers U54DA036151 and R01DA045016 from the National Institute on Drug Abuse (NIDA) and Food and Drug Administration Center for Tobacco Products (CTP), as well as grant number R37CA214787 from the National Cancer Institute of the National Institutes of Health.

Note. The content is solely the authors' responsibility and does not necessarily represent the official views of the National Institutes of Health or the Food and Drug Administration.

CONFLICTS OF INTEREST

The authors have never accepted funding from the tobacco or nicotine industries. Both authors have provided unpaid expert testimony on tobacco and nicotine-related policies. Additionally, A. S. Pesko reports current funding from the National Institutes of Health, American Cancer Society, the US Food and Drug Administration, and Health Canada.

HUMAN PARTICIPANT PROTECTION

Yale University's Human Research Protection Program deemed this research exempt (Protocol ID #2000030989), under 45CFR46.104 (4).

REFERENCES

1. Kaine, McConnell push FDA to Implement new legal tobacco age set by their bill. Available at: https://www.kaine.senate.gov/press-releases/kaine-mcconnell-push-fda-to-implement-new-legal-tobacco-age-set-by-their-bill. Accessed 27 March 2023.
2. Friedman AS, Buckell J, Sindelar JL. Tobacco-21 laws and young adult smoking: quasi-experimental

evidence. *Addiction*. 2019;114(10):1816–1823. https://doi.org/10.1111/add.14653

3. Friedman AS, Wu RJ. Do local tobacco-21 laws reduce smoking among 18 to 20 year-olds? *Nicotine Tob Res*. 2020;22(7):1195–1201. https://doi.org/10.1093/ntr/ntz123
4. Bryan C, Hansen B, McNichols D, Sabia JJ. Do state Tobacco 21 laws work? *NBER Working Paper No. 28173*. https://doi.org/10.3386/w28173
5. Abouk R, De P, Pesko M. Estimating the effects of Tobacco-21 on youth tobacco use and sales. Available at: https://doi.org/10.2139/ssrn.4019077. Accessed January 1, 2023.
6. Liber AC, Xue Z, Cahn Z, Drope J, Stoklosa M. Tobacco 21 adoption decreased sales of cigarette brands purchased by young people: a translation of population health survey data to gain insight into market data for policy analysis. *Tob Control*. 2022;31(3):452–457. https://doi.org/10.1136/tobaccocontrol-2020-055932
7. Patel M, Simard BJ, Benson AF, Donovan EM, Pitzer L. Measuring the impact of state and local Tobacco 21 policies in the United States: a longitudinal study of youth and young adults ages 15–21. *Nicotine Tob Res*. 2023;25(4):631–638. https://doi.org/10.1093/ntr/ntac248
8. Jason LA, Berk M, Schnopp-Wyatt DL, Talbot B. Effects of enforcement of youth access laws on smoking prevalence. *Am J Community Psychol*. 1999;27(2):143–160. https://doi.org/10.1023/A:1022831617055
9. DiFranza JR. Which interventions against the sale of tobacco to minors can be expected to reduce smoking? *Tob Control*. 2012;21(4):436–442. https://doi.org/10.1136/tobaccocontrol-2011-050145
10. Committee on the Public Health Implications of Raising the Minimum Age for Purchasing Tobacco Products; Board on Population Health and Public Health Practice. Evidence on the effects of youth access restrictions. In: Bonnie RJ, Stratton K, Kwan LY, editors. Public Health Implications of Raising the Minimum Age of Legal Access to Tobacco Products. Washington, DC: National Academies Press; 2015, chapter 6.
11. Astor RL, Urman R, Barrington-Trimis JL, et al. Tobacco retail licensing and youth product use. *Pediatrics*. 2019;143(2):e20173536. https://doi.org/10.1542/peds.2017-3536
12. Gottlieb NH, Loukas A, Corrao M, McAlister A, Snell C, Huang PP. Minors' tobacco possession law violations and intentions to smoke: implications for tobacco control. *Tob Control*. 2004;13(3):237–243. https://doi.org/10.1136/tc.2003.003988
13. University of Michigan School of Public Health. Tobacco 21 population coverage database. Available at: https://helper-team.shinyapps.io/t21-data. Accessed 2 November 2022.
14. Preventing Tobacco Addiction Foundation. Tobacco 21 grade cards. Available at: https://tobacco21.org/state-grades. Accessed April 23, 2021.
15. Centers for Disease Control and Prevention. State Tobacco Activities Tracking and Evaluation (STATE) System. Available at: https://www.cdc.gov/statesystem. Accessed October 18, 2022.
16. Marynak K, Mahoney M, Williams KS, Tynan MA, Reimels E, King BA. State and territorial laws prohibiting sales of tobacco products to persons aged <21 years—United States, December 20, 2019. *MMWR Morb Mortal Wkly Rep*. 2020;69(7):189–192. https://doi.org/10.15585/mmwr.mm6907a3
17. Tourangeau R, Yan T, Sun H, Hyland A, Stanton CA. Population Assessment of Tobacco and Health (PATH) reliability and validity study: selected reliability and validity estimates. *Tob Control*. 2019;28(6):663–668. https://doi.org/10.1136/tobaccocontrol-2018-054561
18. Cotti C, Nesson E, Pesko MF, Phillips S, Tefft N. Standardising the measurement of e-cigarette taxes in the USA, 2010–2020. *Tob Control*. 2023;32(e2):e251-e254. https://doi.org/10.1136/tobaccocontrol-2021-056865.
19. American Nonsmokers' Rights Foundation. Percent of US state populations covered by 100% smokefree air laws. Available at: https://no-smoke.org/wp-content/uploads/pdf/percentstatepops.pdf. Accessed November 1, 2022.
20. Centers for Disease Control and Prevention. COVID-19 Response. COVID-19 case surveillance public data access, summary, and limitations. Available at: https://data.cdc.gov/Case-Surveillance/United-States-COVID-19-Cases-and-Deaths-by-State-o/9mfq-cb36. Accessed April 25, 2022.
21. Abadie A, Athey S, Imbens GW, Woolridge J. When should you adjust standard errors for clustering? NBER Working Paper: w24003, November 2017. https://doi.org/10.3386/w24003
22. Greene W. The behaviour of the maximum likelihood estimator of limited dependent variable models in the presence of fixed effects. *Econom J*. 2004;7(1):98–119. https://doi.org/10.1111/j.1368-423X.2004.00123.x
23. Centers for Disease Control and Prevention. CDC clinician outreach and communication activity. Available at: https://web.archive.org/web/20190817233029/ https://emergency.cdc.gov/newsletters/coca/081619.htm. Accessed 28 July 2021.
24. Dobbs PD, Chadwick G. W Ungar K, Dunlap CM, White KA, Kelly MCT, Cheney MK, Development of a Tobacco 21 policy assessment tool and state-level analysis in the USA, 2015–2019. *Tob Control*. 2020;29:487–495.
25. Etter JF. Laws prohibiting the sale of tobacco to minors: impact and adverse consequences. *Am J Prev Med*. 2006;31(1):47–51. https://doi.org/10.1016/j.amepre.2006.03.014
26. Lazovich D, Forster J, Widome R, VanCoevering P. Tobacco possession, use, and purchase laws and penalties in Minnesota: Enforcement, tobacco diversion programs, and youth awareness. *Nicotine Tob Res*. 2007;9(1):S57–S64. https://doi.org/10.1080/14622200601083475
27. Wakefield M, Giovino G. Teen penalties for tobacco possession, use, and purchase: evidence and issues. *Tob Control*. 2003;12(1):i6–i13. https://doi.org/10.1136/tc.12.suppl_1.i6
28. Jason LA, Pokorny SB, Adams M. A randomized trial evaluating tobacco possession-use-purchase laws in the USA. *Soc Sci Med*. 2008;67(11):1700–1707. https://doi.org/10.1016/j.socscimed.2008.09.028

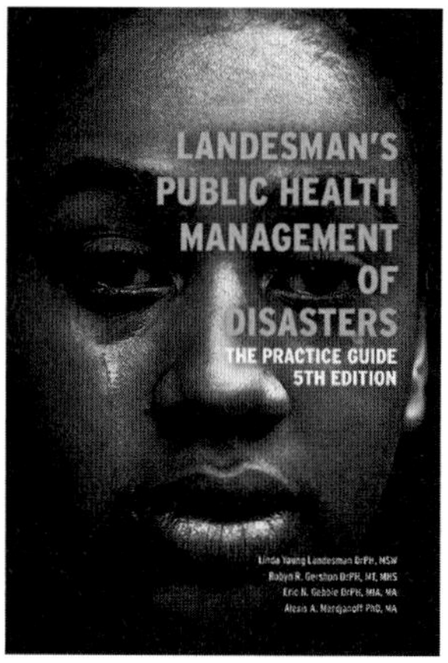

SOFTCOVER, 100 PAGES, 2021
ISBN 978-0-87553-312-6

Landesman's Public Health Management of Disasters: The Practice Guide, 5th Edition

By: Linda Young Landesman, DrPH, MSW; Robyn R. Gershon, DrPH, MT, MHS; Eric N. Gebbie, DrPH, MIA, MA; Alexis A. Merdjanoff, PhD, MA

This new edition is both a comprehensive textbook and an essential tool for those who have a role in disaster management. Every chapter now includes extensive sections on Covid-19 covering all of public health's responsibility as it relates to a pandemic.

APHABOOKSTORE.ORG

APHA PRESS
AN IMPRINT OF AMERICAN PUBLIC HEALTH ASSOCIATION

Cannabis Use Among Adults in Cigarette Smoking Cessation Treatment in Ontario, Canada: Prevalence and Association With Tobacco Cessation Outcome, 2015–2021

Sabrina Voci, PhD, Scott Veldhuizen, PhD, Anna Ivanova, MPH, Osnat C. Melamed, MD, MSc, Peter Selby, MBBS, MHSc, and Laurie Zawertailo, PhD

AJPH January 2024, Vol. 114, No. 1

Objectives. To examine cannabis use prevalence and its association with tobacco cessation among adults enrolled in cigarette smoking cessation treatment before and after Canada legalized recreational cannabis in October 2018.

Methods. The sample comprised 83 206 adults enrolled in primary care–based cigarette smoking cessation treatment between 2015 and 2021 in Ontario, Canada. Past-30-day cannabis use was self-reported at enrollment and cigarette smoking abstinence at 6-month follow-up.

Results. Past-30-day prevalence of cannabis use increased from 20.2% in 2015 to 37.7% in 2021. The prevalence increased linearly both before and after legalization. Cannabis and tobacco co-use was associated with lower odds of self-reported cigarette smoking abstinence at 6-month follow-up than tobacco use only (24.4% vs 29.3%; odds ratio [OR] = 0.78; 95% confidence interval [CI] = 0.75, 0.81). This association was attenuated after adjustment for covariates (OR = 0.93; 95% CI = 0.89, 0.97) and weakened slightly over time.

Conclusions. Cannabis use prevalence almost doubled from 2015 to 2021 among primary care patients in Ontario seeking treatment to quit cigarettes and was associated with poorer quit outcomes. Further research into the impact of cannabis policy on cannabis and tobacco co-use is warranted to mitigate harm. (*Am J Public Health*. 2024;114(1):98–107. https://doi.org/10.2105/AJPH.2023.307445)

Tobacco smoking has declined globally in recent decades but remains a leading preventable cause of death and disability.[1] In contrast, cannabis use has risen,[2] with a growing number of jurisdictions legalizing it for medical and recreational use. Cannabis and tobacco use commonly co-occur.[3,4] In Canada, past-year cannabis use is more than twice as prevalent among people who smoke cigarettes (41%) as among those who do not (17%).[5] Co-use of tobacco and cannabis is associated with increased exposure to toxicants[6,7] and worse respiratory health,[4,8,9] as well as increased risk of dependence and difficulties quitting either substance.[10–15] Cannabis users are also more likely to initiate tobacco smoking than nonusers.[10,16,17] Thus, understanding and monitoring co-use of cannabis and tobacco are important to identify possible harms related to cannabis legalization.

Evidence is beginning to emerge on the effect of cannabis legalization on rates of tobacco and cannabis co-use.

In 2020, regular (at least weekly) cannabis use was higher among adults who smoked cigarettes daily in Canada (27%) and the United States (24%), which have more permissive cannabis laws, than in England (13%) or Australia (12%).[18] Within the United States, the prevalence of cigarette and cannabis co-use is higher in states where recreational or medical cannabis use is legal than in states where it is not.[19]

Canada legalized the use and sale of recreational cannabis to adults on October 17, 2018; before that, cannabis use had been legal for medical purposes since 2001. Sales were initially limited to dried or fresh cannabis and cannabis oil but expanded in January 2020 to include edibles, extracts, and topicals. In Ontario, cannabis was initially available only from a government-run Web site. Retail stores opened beginning in April 2019, with an initial limit on their number that was lifted in March 2020. Thereafter, retail cannabis operations expanded rapidly, from 53 stores in March 2020 to 572 in March 2021[20] and 1460 in March 2022.[21]

In a previous study, we found reduced odds of tobacco cessation among people co-using tobacco and cannabis who enrolled in smoking cessation treatment between 2014 and 2016, before legalization.[22] Legalization of cannabis in various jurisdictions has been accompanied by increased availability, potency, and diversity of cannabis products[23–25]; changes in methods of consumption[26,27]; and increased prevalence of daily use.[26,28] Such changes may occur with expansion of the legal cannabis market, highlighting the importance of examining longer-term trends.[24,29] Examination of trends across sociodemographic groups is also needed to identify and monitor disparities.[19] Thus, further study was warranted to examine whether both cannabis use prevalence and its association with treatment outcome changed after legalization among those seeking treatment to quit smoking tobacco.

In the current study, we examined trends over time and variability across patient characteristics in the prevalence of cannabis use and its association with tobacco cessation among primary care patients who sought treatment to quit cigarette smoking between 2015 and 2021 (approximately 3 years before and 3 years after legalization) in Ontario, Canada. Ontario is Canada's most populous province, with a population of 14.2 million in 2021,[30] and its experience may inform expectations for other jurisdictions beginning or contemplating cannabis legalization.

METHODS

We drew our sample from the Smoking Treatment for Ontario Patients (STOP) study, which provides personalized smoking cessation treatment to residents of Ontario. Participants are seen by health care practitioners throughout the province who are trained in the delivery of tobacco cessation interventions. Treatment consists of nicotine replacement therapy (up to 26 weeks over 12 months) and counseling. We included participants who enrolled at a primary care site between January 1, 2015, and October 31, 2021. Primary care sites comprised 236 family health teams (FHTs), 106 community health centers (CHCs), and 23 nurse practitioner–led clinics (NPLCs). FHTs, CHCs, and NPLCs are interprofessional groups providing primary care services to Ontarians through the province's publicly funded health care system. CHCs also undertake health promotion and community development efforts, prioritizing populations that have traditionally faced barriers to accessing services.[31] The STOP study is publicly funded and is described in more detail elsewhere.[32]

Our initial data set included 117 474 enrollments. We excluded 2037 individuals (1.7%) without a record of consent for research purposes, 486 (0.4%) with incomplete enrollment records, 1052 (0.9%) with no recorded treatment visits, 8190 (7.0%) who were not smoking daily at baseline, and 589 (0.5%) who either were younger than 19 years (the minimum legal age for tobacco and cannabis use in Ontario) or did not provide a date of birth. STOP permits reenrollments 1 year after previous entry. We used probabilistic deduplication[33,34] to identify individuals with multiple enrollments and randomly selected a single enrollment per person. This meant removing 21 914 (18.7%) additional records, leaving an analysis sample of 83 206.

Measures and Data Collection

Data collection. At enrollment, participants self-reported data on sociodemographic characteristics, substance use, and medical history in a baseline questionnaire. At 3, 6, and 12 months after enrollment, participants were invited to self-report information on treatment outcomes. Treatment outcomes could be reported (1) via an online survey, (2) in person with a health care practitioner, or (3) over the telephone with STOP study staff (6 and 12 months only).

Cannabis use. Participants were asked about past-30-day cannabis use at enrollment. Participants enrolling before April 11, 2016, were asked separately about recreational and medical use, whereas later enrollees were asked a

AJPH January 2024, Vol. 114, No. 1

single question about use for any purpose. Participants who reported that they had used cannabis in the past 30 days were classified as cannabis and tobacco co-users, and those who reported that they had not were classified as tobacco-only users.

Cigarette smoking cessation. Smoking status was assessed at each treatment visit and at 3-, 6-, and 12-month follow-ups. Cessation was defined as a response of "no" to the question "Have you smoked a cigarette, even a puff, in the last 7 days?" Cessation at 6-month follow-up was the primary treatment outcome, and data on cessation were available for 50 611 (60.8%) participants. Response rates were slightly lower (51.4%–55.6%) among those who were 25 to 44 years old, those with a lifetime diagnosis of substance use disorder or schizophrenia, those with incomes of $20 000 or less, those from CHCs or NPLCs, those without previous quit attempts, and those who identified their gender as other than male or female; the response rate was lowest (42.3%) among the small subgroup of participants who were younger than 25 years. Smoking cessation rates at 3 and 12 months are not reported because of low response rates.

Baseline covariates. The following baseline variables, known from previous research to be associated with cannabis use or tobacco quit outcome,[22,35,36] were used as covariates: age, gender (self-reported as male, female, or other), employment status, household income, number of previous lifetime quit attempts, cigarettes smoked per day, time to first cigarette after waking, willingness to set a quit date, importance of quitting and confidence in ability to quit (self-rated from 1 to 10), hazardous alcohol use according to the Alcohol Use Disorders Identification Test–Consumption,[37] past-30-day opioid use, rural residence (based on postal code and Rurality Index of Ontario score[38]), treatment setting (FHT, CHC, or NPLC), and presence or absence of a lifetime diagnosis of depression, anxiety, schizophrenia, bipolar disorder, substance use disorder (other than tobacco or caffeine), alcohol use disorder, stroke, diabetes, chronic obstructive pulmonary disease, rheumatoid arthritis, chronic pain, cancer, and heart disease or heart problems.

Analysis

Descriptive statistics, the χ^2 test and *t*-test were used to characterize and compare cannabis and tobacco co-users and tobacco-only users. To test for changes in prevalence of cannabis use at the time of legalization, we used piecewise logistic regression with a prespecified knot at October 17, 2018. To allow for changes in both level and slope, we included an indicator and a spline term. To assess the importance of seasonality, we evaluated indicator-coded quarter of year indicators. Because these indicators changed time coefficients by less than 1%, we omitted them from our final results. We examined time terms and other continuous variables for nonlinearity using descriptive statistics and fractional polynomial models. On the basis of these results, we included all time effects as linear terms but applied a cubic transformation to patient age. We adjusted this model for the baseline covariates just listed. To obtain adjusted prevalence over time, we calculated and plotted predictive margins from our full model.

We also conducted 2 sensitivity analyses. First, to test for important clinic-level differences, we fit a mixed-effects model with a random intercept for clinical site. Second, we fit further models to assess whether prevalence changed at the time our survey items were revised (April 11, 2016) or at the time Ontario declared a state of emergency with the onset of the COVID-19 pandemic (March 17, 2020).

To test whether the prevalence of cannabis use changed at different rates for different patient groups, we fit an additional adjusted model for each covariate including an interaction between that covariate and time. As this was a secondary, exploratory analysis involving a large number of tests, we used the Holm step-down method to adjust significance thresholds for multiplicity.[39] In the case of variables that showed significant differences over time, we calculated unadjusted prevalence for the first and last years of study data along with absolute prevalence differences and prevalence ratios.

To measure the association between cannabis use and quit outcome and to determine whether this association changed over time, we fit logistic models with quit status at 6-month follow-up as the dependent variable. Given the results of our models of change in cannabis use over time, we included time as a single linear term. We fit an initial model including main effects only and then a model including a time by cannabis use interaction. We adjusted both models for our baseline covariates.

To address missing data, we used the Python package miceforest[40] to perform random forest multiple imputation. Random forest imputation is capable of preserving interactions and other complex patterns in imputed data.[40] The imputation model included all variables from our substantive models as well as the following auxiliary variables: number of treatment visits during the 12-month enrollment period, type of nicotine replacement therapy provided at first treatment visit (no nicotine replacement therapy, short acting only, patch only, patch and short acting), and self-reported 7-day point prevalence of abstinence at the 3- and 12-month follow-ups (where available). This approach imputes missing values for all model variables. We produced 20 imputed data sets and used these data for all analyses other than those involving descriptive statistics. We used Stata 16 for all analyses.

RESULTS

Sample characteristics are shown in Table 1 (abbreviated table) and Table A (complete table with all baseline covariates; available as a supplement to the online version of this article at http://www.ajph.org). On average, cannabis and tobacco co-users were younger than tobacco-only users and had lower household incomes; also, a higher proportion were male, smoked cigarettes within 5 minutes of waking, reported hazardous alcohol use or a lifetime history of alcohol use disorder, used opioids, and had lifetime diagnoses of mental health or substance-related disorders. Chronic pain was more common among cannabis co-users, whereas other medical conditions, such as diabetes and heart disease, were more common among tobacco-only users.

Cannabis Use Prevalence

After multiple imputation, the estimated overall prevalence of past-30-day cannabis use was 27.8% (95% confidence interval [CI] = 27.5%, 28.1%). When calculated by year, this percentage rose monotonically from 20.2% (95% CI = 19.5%, 20.9%) in 2015 to 37.7% (95% CI = 36.5%, 38.8%) in 2021. In our piecewise regression model, cannabis use increased until the date of legalization (per-year odds ratio [OR] = 1.21; 95% CI = 1.19, 1.24; $P < .001$). At this time, the level of use increased slightly (OR = 1.07; 95% CI = 1.01, 1.15; $P = .03$) but the rate of increase slowed (per-year OR = 1.13; 95% CI = 1.09, 1.16; $P < .001$; P for change in slope < .001). Results of the full model are presented in Table B (available as a supplement to the online version of this article at http://www.ajph.org). Adjusted predicted probabilities are plotted in Figure 1, along with the unadjusted prevalence for each month. These 2 series diverge slightly toward the end of the study period owing to case-mix changes associated with the COVID-19 pandemic[41] that produced a small difference between adjusted and unadjusted estimates.

Adding interaction terms to this model revealed that changes over time (per year) in the odds of cannabis use varied by gender (with male as the reference group; female OR = 1.04; 95% CI = 1.02, 1.06; $P < .001$; other gender OR = 1.11; 95% CI = 0.92, 1.34; $P = .27$; overall P for interactions < .001), income (OR = 1.02 per level of the 8-level income variable [see Table 2 footnote]; 95% CI = 1.01, 1.02; $P < .001$), and treatment setting (with FHT as the reference group; CHC OR = 0.95; 95% CI = 0.93, 0.97; $P < .001$; NPLC OR = 0.97; 95% CI = 0.92, 1.01; $P = .16$; overall P for interactions < .001). Results of interaction tests for all variables are presented in Table C (available as a supplement to the online version of this article at http://www.ajph.org). Table 2 presents the prevalence of cannabis use in 2015 and 2021 for these 3 variables, along with the absolute and relative changes over time; Table D (available as a supplement to the online version of this article at http://www.ajph.org) shows the prevalence in each year from 2015 to 2021.

Association of Cannabis Use With Cigarette Smoking Cessation

At the bivariate level, co-use of cannabis was associated with a lower probability of quitting cigarettes at 6 months (24.4% for co-users vs 29.3% for tobacco-only users; OR = 0.78; 95% CI = 0.75, 0.81; $P < .001$). This association was attenuated by adjustment for covariates (OR = 0.93; 95% CI = 0.89, 0.97; $P = .001$). In our adjusted model including a cannabis use by time interaction, the interaction term was marginally significant (per-year OR = 1.03; 95% CI = 1.00, 1.05; $P = .03$), suggesting that the association between cannabis use and treatment outcome weakened slightly over the study period. However, incorporating age and gender interactions into our adjusted model showed that there was no significant difference in the association by age ($P = .79$) or gender ($P = .60$).

Sensitivity Analyses

We did not observe significant changes in time slopes or intercepts at the time of the COVID-19 state of emergency (joint $P = .33$) or with the change in survey items (joint $P = .13$). Including a random intercept for site showed that site-level variances were small (0.06 for cannabis use, 0.04 for tobacco cessation) and that all coefficients for time variables changed by 1% or less; we therefore have reported single-level regression results.

TABLE 1— Sample Characteristics at Enrollment in Primary Care–Based Smoking Cessation Treatment by Self-Reported Past-30-Day Cannabis Use: Ontario, Canada, 2015–2021

Characteristic	Total	Past-30-Day Cannabis Use, No. (%) or Mean ± SD	
		No	Yes
Overall	83 206	58 284 (72.2)	22 401 (27.8)
Age, y			
<25	2473 (3.1)	1260 (2.2)	1213 (5.4)
25–44	22 091 (27.4)	13 691 (23.5)	8400 (37.5)
45–64	42 750 (53.0)	31 388 (53.9)	11 362 (50.7)
≥65	13 371 (16.6)	11 945 (20.5)	1426 (6.4)
Gender			
Male	38 396 (47.6)	26 004 (44.7)	12 392 (55.4)
Female	42 047 (52.2)	32 140 (55.2)	9907 (44.3)
Other	152 (0.2)	75 (0.1)	77 (0.3)
Treatment setting			
Family health team	62 043 (76.9)	45 757 (78.5)	16 286 (72.7)
Community health center	16 301 (20.2)	11 039 (18.9)	5262 (23.5)
Nurse practitioner–led clinic	2341 (2.9)	1488 (2.6)	853 (3.8)
Household income, $[a]			
≤20 000	18 278 (35.5)	11 950 (32.9)	6328 (41.7)
20 001–60 000	19 865 (38.6)	14 402 (39.6)	5463 (36.0)
>60 000	13 370 (26.0)	9995 (27.5)	3375 (22.3)
Cigarettes per day	19.8 ± 11.4	19.5 ± 11.4	20.4 ± 11.5
First cigarette within 5 min of waking	31 338 (39.1)	21 751 (37.6)	9587 (43.0)
Confidence in ability to quit (1–10 scale)	7.3 ± 2.1	7.4 ± 2.1	7.2 ± 2.1
Importance of quitting (1–10 scale)	9.1 ± 1.3	9.1 ± 1.3	9.1 ± 1.3
Hazardous alcohol use (AUDIT-C)[b,c]	21 205 (34.0)	13 187 (30.1)	8018 (43.2)
Past-30-day opioid use	12 926 (16.2)	8350 (14.4)	4576 (20.6)
Psychiatric disorders (lifetime)			
Depression	30 953 (39.6)	20 246 (35.8)	10 707 (49.2)
Anxiety	30 241 (38.6)	19 653 (34.8)	10 588 (48.6)
Schizophrenia	2216 (2.8)	1572 (2.8)	644 (3.0)
Bipolar disorder	4651 (6.0)	2841 (5.0)	1810 (8.4)
Substance use disorder[c,d]	5535 (9.0)	2569 (5.9)	2966 (16.2)
Alcohol use disorder[c]	5274 (8.6)	3263 (7.5)	2011 (11.0)

Note. AUDIT-C = Alcohol Use Disorders Identification Test–Consumption. Statistics were calculated with observed data without imputation. Sample sizes vary owing to missing data.

[a]The original variable had 8 levels: no reported income, <$10 000, $10 000–$20 000, $20 000–$40 000, $40 000–$60 000, $60 000–$80 000, $80 000–$100 000, and >$100 000.
[b]AUDIT-C score > 4 for male gender or > 3 for female or other gender.
[c]Not asked before April 11, 2016.
[d]Excluding caffeine and tobacco.

DISCUSSION

The prevalence of past-30-day cannabis use among Ontario primary care patients in cigarette smoking cessation treatment almost doubled between 2015 and 2021. The prevalence of cannabis use in 2021 (38%) was similar to population-level estimates of past-year cannabis use among Canadians smoking tobacco in 2020 (42%[18]; past-month use was not assessed), suggesting that cannabis use may be similarly prevalent among individuals smoking cigarettes whether they have sought treatment to

AJPH January 2024, Vol. 114, No. 1

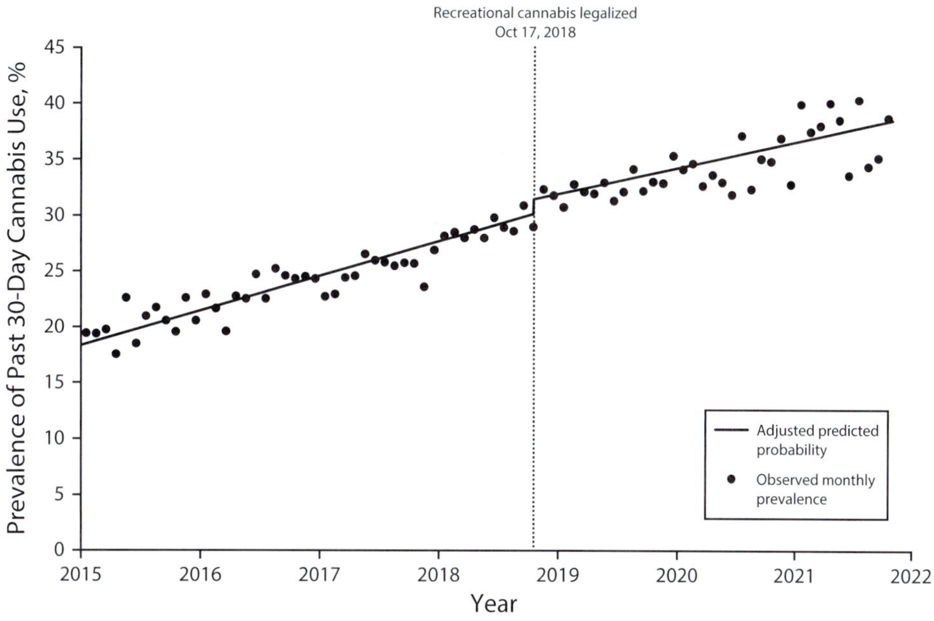

FIGURE 1— Unadjusted Prevalence and Adjusted Predicted Probability of Past-30-Day Cannabis Use Among Adults in Primary Care–Based Smoking Cessation Treatment: Ontario, Canada, 2015–2021.

Note. Adjusted predicted probabilities were estimated with predictive margins from the fully adjusted model.

TABLE 2— Changes in the Prevalence of Past-30-Day Cannabis Use Among Adults in Primary Care–Based Smoking Cessation Treatment From 2015 to 2021 by Gender, Income, and Treatment Setting: Ontario, Canada

	Prevalence, % (95% CI)		Change From 2015 to 2021	
Characteristic	2015	2021	Absolute Prevalence Difference, % (95% CI)	Prevalence Ratio (95% CI)
Gender				
Female	15.9 (15.0, 16.7)	33.8 (32.2, 35.3)	17.9 (16.2, 19.7)	2.13 (1.98, 2.28)
Male	25.1 (24.0, 26.2)	41.9 (40.1, 43.6)	16.8 (14.7, 18.8)	1.67 (1.57, 1.77)
Other[a]	33.3 (16.3, 50.3)	62.5 (38.6, 86.4)	29.2 (0.1, 58.3)	1.88 (0.69, 3.06)
Income, $[b]				
<20 000	25.4 (23.9, 26.9)	41.4 (39.0, 43.9)	16.0 (13.3, 18.7)	1.63 (1.50, 1.76)
20 001–60 000	18.2 (17.0, 19.4)	36.0 (33.8, 38.3)	17.8 (15.3, 20.3)	1.97 (1.80, 2.15)
>60 000	15.0 (13.6, 16.4)	35.4 (32.7, 38.2)	20.5 (17.5, 23.4)	2.36 (2.09, 2.63)
Treatment setting				
Family health team	18.1 (17.4, 18.9)	35.7 (34.4, 37.0)	17.6 (16.1, 19.1)	1.97 (1.86, 2.08)
Community health center	27.3 (25.5, 29.1)	42.4 (40.0, 44.9)	15.1 (12.0, 18.2)	1.55 (1.41, 1.69)
Nurse practitioner–led clinic[a]	31.9 (27.3, 36.4)	50.2 (43.6, 57.0)	18.4 (10.3, 26.5)	1.58 (1.27, 1.88)

Note. CI = confidence interval. CIs are based on logistic approximation.

[a]High sampling variability (relative standard error ≥ 0.30); data should be interpreted with caution.
[b]The original variable had 8 levels: no reported income, <$10 000, $10 000–$20 000, $20 000–$40 000, $40 000–$60 000, $60 000–$80 000, $80 000–$100 000, and >$100 000.

quit or not. Prevalence increased before legalization and continued to increase subsequently, albeit at a somewhat slower rate. Furthermore, cannabis use was associated with decreased odds of 7-day point prevalence smoking abstinence at the 6-month follow-up, with a slight attenuation of this association over time.

The increased prevalence of past-30-day cannabis use in our sample of patients seeking treatment of cigarette smoking is consistent with increases seen in the Canadian population—from 12% in 2015 to 21% in 2019[42]—with a general trend of increasing prevalence beginning before legalization and continuing thereafter.[26,27,43] A similar pattern has also been observed in several US states that have passed recreational cannabis laws.[44] However, this does not exclude the possibility that legalization has had an impact on cannabis use given that legalization is not a discrete, short-term event.

Trends in the prevalence of cannabis use over time varied in our sample by patient gender, income level, and treatment setting. Absolute differences in prevalence over time were roughly similar between groups, but this produced larger relative differences for groups with a lower baseline prevalence. Sex and gender differences in cannabis use trends after legalization in Canada have been inconsistent, with greater increases initially reported among women[26] but more recently among men.[45] The number of individuals who identified their gender as other in our sample was small, resulting in unreliable estimates. Targeted recruitment efforts are needed to obtain sufficient sample sizes to adequately investigate tobacco and cannabis co-use among transgender and gender-diverse individuals, who may be more likely to use both substances.[46,47]

There was some evidence of convergence for income and treatment setting, with absolute differences across categories narrowing somewhat. The prevalence of cannabis use increased more among those with higher levels of income but remained highest in the lowest income group. Thus, individuals with lower incomes do not appear to have been disproportionately impacted by cannabis legalization relative to those with higher incomes, but they remain at greater risk of cannabis-related harms.[48] The greater prevalence increase in FHTs than CHCs may reflect differences in the populations served in these different primary care models.[49] Other surveys have reported greater increases in cannabis prevalence among those with higher educational levels[50] and those with depression.[51] We found a similar interaction with education level that met the traditional definition of statistical significance ($P < .05$; Table C) but failed to meet our more stringent P value cutoff adjusted for multiple comparisons. However, we did not detect an interaction with depression and thus failed to replicate earlier findings.[51]

The negative association between cannabis use and tobacco quit outcome at 6 months was consistent with our earlier findings.[22] Even though there was a slight attenuation of this association over time, the considerable increase in cannabis use means that the net public health impact may have worsened. The attenuation of the association could be due to changes in who is using cannabis as well as why and how they use it. Although smoking is still the most common method of consuming cannabis in Canada (74% in 2021), there has been an increase in vaping and other methods.[45] The common route of administration (inhaling smoke) may play a role in high rates of tobacco and cannabis co-use[4,52,53] whereby the use of one substance acts as a cue and triggers cravings for the other substance. If a shift toward noncombustible methods of consuming cannabis occurred in our sample over time, it may have weakened the association between cannabis use and cigarette smoking cessation outcome.

The association between cannabis use and tobacco cessation outcome may also plausibly be affected by the types and potency of cannabis products used, frequency and duration of use, and whether co-use is simultaneous (e.g., mixing or "chasing"). For example, one study revealed significantly lower rates of tobacco smoking abstinence among frequent cannabis co-users, but not intermittent co-users, relative to nonusers.[54] We have reported an overall effect of general co-use, but co-users are a heterogeneous group. More detailed information about co-use of cannabis among tobacco users is needed in future studies[55] to identify whether there are particular patterns of co-use that should be prioritized for monitoring and clinical interventions, especially in the context of expanding legalization, to mitigate harms.

Patients attempting to quit smoking cigarettes should be asked about their cannabis use and be advised that co-use may adversely affect their quit attempt, and they should be asked whether they might want to stop using cannabis to maximize their chances of quitting. It is especially important that patients smoking cannabis mixed with tobacco are advised to stop this practice, and switching to noncombustible methods of consuming cannabis is also advised to reduce harm.[56] Several studies have shown that interventions addressing co-use are feasible and acceptable; however, most have been pilot studies, and more rigorous research is needed to support wide-scale implementation in clinical and public health settings.[14]

Strengths and Limitations

Strengths of this study include the large real-world sample of primary care patients seeking to quit smoking and adjustment for a wide range of potential confounding variables. However, there were also several limitations. The study was observational, and thus causality cannot be inferred. Given geographical variation in cannabis use and legislation, our findings may not generalize to other jurisdictions, including other Canadian provinces. In addition, treatment was limited to nicotine replacement therapy with counseling, and our results may not generalize to other smoking cessation treatments such as varenicline, which preliminary evidence suggests may be effective for tobacco and cannabis co-use.[57]

Also, cannabis use and smoking abstinence were self-reported and may have been misclassified as a result of social desirability or recall bias; however, biochemical confirmation was not feasible because of the large scale of the study and the fact that follow-up was often conducted remotely. The illegal status of cannabis before October 2018 may have influenced individuals' willingness to report use to a health care provider; however, the small change in prevalence at the time of legalization suggested that this was not a major concern. Finally, tobacco cessation outcome at follow-up was not available for 39% of our sample (a percentage similar to those in other large observational studies[58,59]), with nonresponse slightly higher among some groups. Although our use of multiple imputation will have mitigated any resulting biases, residual confounding by unmeasured variables remains possible.

Conclusion

The prevalence of cannabis use increased among individuals seeking cigarette smoking cessation treatment in Ontario, Canada, in the period leading up to and following recreational cannabis legalization. Of particular concern in the context of rapidly increasing prevalence is the enduring association between cannabis use and decreased odds of tobacco smoking abstinence at follow-up, although this association was slightly attenuated over time. Given the harms of continued smoking and the additive harms to health associated with co-use of the 2 substances, tobacco and cannabis co-users are an important population to monitor. Further research is needed to better understand varying types and patterns of co-use and associated harms to inform interventions tailored for individuals concurrently using tobacco and cannabis. AJPH

ABOUT THE AUTHORS

Sabrina Voci, Scott Veldhuizen, and Anna Ivanova are with the INTREPID Lab, Centre for Addiction and Mental Health, Toronto, Ontario, Canada. Osnat C. Melamed is with the INTREPID Lab, Centre for Addiction and Mental Health, and the Department of Family and Community Medicine, University of Toronto. Peter Selby is with the INTREPID Lab, Centre for Addiction and Mental Health, and the Department of Family and Community Medicine, Department of Psychiatry, and Dalla Lana School of Public Health, University of Toronto. Laurie Zawertailo is with the INTREPID Lab, Centre for Addiction and Mental Health, and the Department of Pharmacology and Toxicology, University of Toronto.

CORRESPONDENCE

Correspondence should be sent to Laurie Zawertailo, PhD, INTREPID Lab, Centre for Addiction and Mental Health, 1025 Queen St W, Toronto, ON M6J 1H4, Canada (e-mail: laurie.zawertailo@camh.ca). Reprints can be ordered at http://www.ajph.org by clicking the "Reprints" link.

PUBLICATION INFORMATION

Full Citation: Voci S, Veldhuizen S, Ivanova A, Melamed OC, Selby P, Zawertailo L. Cannabis use among adults in cigarette smoking cessation treatment in Ontario, Canada: prevalence and association with tobacco cessation outcome, 2015–2021. *Am J Public Health*. 2024;114(1): 98–107.

Acceptance Date: September 3, 2023.

DOI: https://doi.org/10.2105/AJPH.2023.307445

CONTRIBUTORS

S. Voci conceived of this secondary analysis and led the design and writing of the article. S. Veldhuizen conducted the analysis and contributed to the study design and writing. A. Ivanova contributed to the study design and writing. O. C. Melamed contributed to the study design. P. Selby and L. Zawertailo supervised the study. All of the authors reviewed and contributed to the final version.

ACKNOWLEDGMENTS

This work was supported by the Ontario Ministry of Health (grant HLTC5047FL). The funder had no role in the study design, data collection and analysis, interpretation of findings, the writing of the article, or the decision to submit for publication. Peter Selby is the Giblon Professor in Family Medicine Research at the University of Toronto.

Data from this article were presented orally at the European Chapter of the Society for Research on Nicotine and Tobacco's annual conference on September 12, 2023, in London.

Note. The views expressed are those of the authors and not necessarily those of the Ontario Ministry of Health.

CONFLICTS OF INTEREST

Sabrina Voci, Scott Veldhuizen, and Anna Ivanova have no conflicts of interest to declare. Osnat C. Melamed has received peer-reviewed funding and/or salary support from AMS Healthcare and Centre for Addiction and Mental Health (CAMH) Womenmind. Peter Selby reports receiving grants, salary, and/or research support from CAMH, Health Canada, the Ontario Ministry of Health and Long-Term Care, the Canadian Institutes of Health Research (CIHR), the Canadian Centre on Substance Abuse, the Public Health Agency of Canada, Pfizer Inc./Canada, the Ontario Lung Association, the Medical Psychiatry Alliance, ECHO, the Canadian Cancer Society Research Institute, Cancer Care Ontario, Ontario Institute Cancer Research, the Ontario Brain Institute, the McLaughlin Centre, Alternate Funding Plans for Academic Health Science Centres, the Workplace Safety Insurance Board, the National Institutes of Health, the Association of Faculties of Medicine of Canada, Shoppers Drug Mart, Bhasin Consulting Fund Inc., and the Patient-Centered Outcomes Research Institute. He also reports receiving honoraria from Pfizer Canada Inc., ABBVie, and Bristol-Myers Squibb and consulting fees from Pfizer Canada Inc., Evidera Inc., Johnson & Johnson

Group of Companies, Medcan Clinic, Inflexxion Inc., V-CC Systems Inc., MedPlan Communications, Kataka Medical Communications, Miller Medical Communications, the NVision Insight Group, Sun Life Financial, and Myelin & Associates. Through an open tender process, Johnson & Johnson, Novartis, and Pfizer Inc. are vendors of record for providing smoking cessation pharmacotherapy, free or discounted, for research studies in which Selby is the principal investigator or co-investigator. Laurie Zawertailo has received peer-reviewed funding from CIHR, the Canadian Cancer Society, CAMH Womenmind, and Global Research Awards for Nicotine Dependence.

HUMAN PARTICIPANT PROTECTION

This study was approved by the Centre for Addiction and Mental Health research ethics board. Participants provided informed consent before treatment took place.

REFERENCES

1. Murray CJ, Aravkin AY, Zheng P, et al. Global burden of 87 risk factors in 204 countries and territories, 1990–2019: a systematic analysis for the Global Burden of Disease Study 2019. *Lancet*. 2020;396(10258):1223–1249. https://doi.org/10.1016/S0140-6736(20)30752-2
2. United Nations Office on Drugs and Crime. World drug report 2022. Available at: https://www.unodc.org/res/wdr2022/MS/WDR22_Booklet_1.pdf. Accessed August 26, 2022.
3. Agrawal A, Budney AJ, Lynskey MT. The co-occurring use and misuse of cannabis and tobacco: a review. *Addiction*. 2012;107(7):1221–1233. https://doi.org/10.1111/j.1360-0443.2012.03837.x
4. Strong DR, Myers MG, Pulvers K, Noble M, Brikmanis K, Doran N. Marijuana use among US tobacco users: findings from wave 1 of the Population Assessment of Tobacco Health (PATH) study. *Drug Alcohol Depend*. 2018;186:16–22. https://doi.org/10.1016/j.drugalcdep.2017.12.044
5. Statistics Canada. Alcohol and drug use in Canada, 2019. Available at: https://www150.statcan.gc.ca/n1/daily-quotidien/211220/dq211220c-eng.htm. Accessed August 26, 2022.
6. Smith DM, O'connor RJ, Wei B, Travers M, Hyland A, Goniewicz ML. Nicotine and toxicant exposure among concurrent users (co-users) of tobacco and cannabis. *Nicotine Tob Res*. 2020;22(8):1354–1363. https://doi.org/10.1093/ntr/ntz122
7. Meier E, Vandrey R, Rubin N, et al. Cigarette smokers versus co-users of cannabis and cigarettes: exposure to toxicants. *Nicotine Tob Res*. 2020;22(8):1383–1389. https://doi.org/10.1093/ntr/ntz199
8. Taylor DR, Fergusson DM, Milne BJ, et al. A longitudinal study of the effects of tobacco and cannabis exposure on lung function in young adults. *Addiction*. 2002;97(8):1055–1061. https://doi.org/10.1046/j.1360-0443.2002.00169.x
9. Correa JB, Myers MG, Tully LK, Doran N. Co-occurring use of cannabis and tobacco and the presence of acute respiratory symptoms among young adult light and intermittent smokers. *Subst Use Misuse*. 2020;55(13):2129–2137. https://doi.org/10.1080/10826084.2020.1793366
10. Weinberger AH, Delnevo CD, Wyka K, et al. Cannabis use is associated with increased risk of cigarette smoking initiation, persistence, and relapse among adults in the United States. *Nicotine Tob Res*. 2020;22(8):1404–1408. https://doi.org/10.1093/ntr/ntz085
11. Gourlay SG, Forbes A, Marriner T, Pethica D, McNeil JJ. Prospective study of factors predicting outcome of transdermal nicotine treatment in smoking cessation. *BMJ*. 1994;309(6958):842–846. https://doi.org/10.1136/bmj.309.6958.842
12. Agrawal A, Madden PA, Bucholz KK, Heath AC, Lynskey MT. Transitions to regular smoking and to nicotine dependence in women using cannabis. *Drug Alcohol Depend*. 2008;95(1–2):107–114. https://doi.org/10.1016/j.drugalcdep.2007.12.017
13. Weinberger AH, Pacek LR, Wall MM, Gbedemah M, Lee J, Goodwin RD. Cigarette smoking quit ratios among adults in the USA with cannabis use and cannabis use disorders, 2002–2016. *Tob Control*. 2020;29(1):74–80. https://doi.org/10.1136/tobaccocontrol-2018-054590
14. McClure EA, Rabin RA, Lee DC, Hindocha C. Treatment implications associated with cannabis and tobacco co-use. *Curr Addict Rep*. 2020;7(4):533–544. https://doi.org/10.1007/s40429-020-00334-8
15. Weinberger AH, Pacek LR, Wall MM, et al. Trends in cannabis use disorder by cigarette smoking status in the United States, 2002–2016. *Drug Alcohol Depend*. 2018;191:45–51. https://doi.org/10.1016/j.drugalcdep.2018.06.016
16. Patton GC, Coffey C, Carlin JB, Sawyer SM, Lynskey M. Reverse gateways? Frequent cannabis use as a predictor of tobacco initiation and nicotine dependence. *Addiction*. 2005;100(10):1518–1525. https://doi.org/10.1111/j.1360-0443.2005.01220.x
17. Mayer ME, Kong G, Barrington-Trimis JL, McConnell R, Leventhal AM, Krishnan-Sarin S. Blunt and non-blunt cannabis use and risk of subsequent combustible tobacco product use among adolescents. *Nicotine Tob Res*. 2020;22(8):1409–1413. https://doi.org/10.1093/ntr/ntz225
18. Gravely S, Driezen P, McClure EA, et al. Differences between adults who smoke cigarettes daily and do and do not co-use cannabis: findings from the 2020 ITC four country smoking and vaping survey. *Addict Behav*. 2022;135:107434. https://doi.org/10.1016/j.addbeh.2022.107434
19. Weinberger AH, Wyka K, Kim JH, et al. A difference-in-difference approach to examining the impact of cannabis legalization on disparities in the use of cigarettes and cannabis in the United States, 2004–17. *Addiction*. 2022;117(6):1768–1777. https://doi.org/10.1111/add.15795
20. Ontario Cannabis Retail Corporation. Ontario Cannabis Store 2020–2021 annual report. Available at: https://www.doingbusinesswithocs.ca/wp-content/uploads/2022/12/OCS-2021-22-Annual-Report_F.pdf. Accessed August 26, 2022.
21. Ontario Cannabis Retail Corporation. Ontario Cannabis Store 2021–2022 annual report. Available at: https://www.doingbusinesswithocs.ca/wp-content/uploads/2022/12/OCS-2021-22-Annual-Report_F.pdf. Accessed August 26, 2022.
22. Voci S, Zawertailo L, Baliunas D, Masood Z, Selby P. Is cannabis use associated with tobacco cessation outcome? An observational cohort study in primary care. *Drug Alcohol Depend*. 2020;206:107756. https://doi.org/10.1016/j.drugalcdep.2019.107756
23. Matheson J, Le Foll B. Cannabis legalization and acute harm from high potency cannabis products: a narrative review and recommendations for public health. *Front Psychiatry*. 2020;11:591979. https://doi.org/10.3389/fpsyt.2020.591979
24. Hall W, Lynskey M. Assessing the public health impacts of legalizing recreational cannabis use: the US experience. *World Psychiatry*. 2020;19(2):179–186. https://doi.org/10.1002/wps.20735
25. Myran DT, Staykov E, Cantor N, et al. How has access to legal cannabis changed over time? An analysis of the cannabis retail market in Canada 2 years following the legalisation of recreational cannabis. *Drug Alcohol Rev*. 2022;41(2):377–385. https://doi.org/10.1111/dar.13351
26. Rotermann M. Looking back from 2020, how cannabis use and related behaviours changed in Canada. *Health Rep*. 2021;32(4):3–14. https://doi.org/10.25318/82-003-x202100400001-eng
27. Fischer B, Lee A, Robinson T, Hall W. An overview of select cannabis use and supply indicators pre- and post-legalization in Canada. *Subst Abuse Treat Prev Policy*. 2021;16(1):77. https://doi.org/10.1186/s13011-021-00405-7
28. Weinberger AH, Wyka K, Goodwin RD. Impact of cannabis legalization in the United States on trends in cannabis use and daily cannabis use among individuals who smoke cigarettes. *Drug Alcohol Depend*. 2022;238:109563. https://doi.org/10.1016/j.drugalcdep.2022.109563
29. Myran DT, Pugliese M, Tanuseputro P, Cantor N, Rhodes E, Taljaard M. The association between recreational cannabis legalization, commercialization and cannabis-attributable emergency department visits in Ontario, Canada: an interrupted time-series analysis. *Addiction*. 2022;117(7):1952–1960. https://doi.org/10.1111/add.15834
30. Statistics Canada. Census profile, 2021. Available at: https://www12.statcan.gc.ca/census-recensement/2021/dp-pd/prof/details/page.cfm?Lang=E&SearchText=Ontario&DGUIDlist=2021A000235&GENDERlist=1,2,3&STATISTIClist=1&HEADERlist=0. Accessed July 31, 2023.
31. Collins PA, Resendes SJ, Dunn JR. The untold story: examining Ontario's community health centres' initiatives to address upstream determinants of health. *Healthc Policy*. 2014;10(1):14–29. https://doi.org/10.12927/hcpol.2014.23977
32. Veldhuizen S, Zawertailo L, Noormohamed A, Hussain S, Selby P. Treatment use patterns in a large extended-treatment tobacco cessation program: predictors and cost implications. *Tob Control*. 2022;31(4):549–555. https://doi.org/10.1136/tobaccocontrol-2020-056203
33. Asher J, Resnick D, Brite J, Brackbill R, Cone J. An introduction to probabilistic record linkage with a focus on linkage processing for WTC registries. *Int J Environ Res Public Health*. 2020;17(18):6937. https://doi.org/10.3390/ijerph17186937
34. Kranker K. dtalink: Faster probabilistic record linking and deduplication methods in Stata for large data files. Available at: http://fmwww.bc.edu/repec/scon2018/columbus18_Kranker.pdf. Accessed July 31, 2023.
35. Veldhuizen S, Zawertailo L, Selby P. Variability in outcomes and quality-of-care indicators across clinics participating in a large smoking-cessation program. *J Subst Abuse Treat*. 2021;130:108409. https://doi.org/10.1016/j.jsat.2021.108409
36. Parker MA, Weinberger AH, Eggers EM, Parker ES, Villanti AC. Trends in rural and urban cigarette smoking quit ratios in the US from 2010 to 2020. *JAMA Netw Open*. 2022;5(8):e2225326.

https://doi.org/10.1001/jamanetworkopen.2022.25326

37. Bush K, Kivlahan DR, McDonell MB, Fihn SD, Bradley KA, Project ACQI. The AUDIT alcohol consumption questions (AUDIT-C): an effective brief screening test for problem drinking. *Arch Intern Med.* 1998;158(16):1789–1795. https://doi.org/10.1001/archinte.158.16.1789
38. Kralj B. Measuring "rurality" for purposes of health-care planning: an empirical measure for Ontario. *Ont Med Rev.* 2000;67(9):33–52.
39. Holm S. A simple sequentially rejective multiple test procedure. *Scand J Stat.* 1979;6(2):65–70.
40. Shah AD, Bartlett JW, Carpenter J, Nicholas O, Hemingway H. Comparison of random forest and parametric imputation models for imputing missing data using MICE: a CALIBER study. *Am J Epidemiol.* 2014;179(6):764–774. https://doi.org/10.1093/aje/kwt312
41. Minian N, Veldhuizen S, Tanzini E, et al. Changes in the reach of a smoking cessation program in Ontario, Canada, during the COVID-19 pandemic: a cross-sectional study. *CMAJ Open.* 2021;9(4):E957–E965. https://doi.org/10.9778/cmajo.20210053
42. Government of Canada. Canadian Alcohol and Drugs Survey (CADS): summary of results for 2019. Available at: https://www.canada.ca/en/health-canada/services/canadian-alcohol-drugs-survey/2019-summary.html. Accessed July 31, 2023.
43. Rotermann M, Macdonald R. Analysis of trends in the prevalence of cannabis use in Canada, 1985 to 2015. *Health Rep.* 2018;29(2):10–20.
44. Dills AK, Goffard S, Miron J, Partin E. The effect of state marijuana legalizations: 2021 update. Available at: https://www.cato.org/policy-analysis/effect-state-marijuana-legalizations-2021-update. Accessed July 31, 2023.
45. Government of Canada. Canadian Cannabis Survey 2021: summary. Available at: https://www.canada.ca/en/health-canada/services/drugs-medication/cannabis/research-data/canadian-cannabis-survey-2021-summary.html. Accessed September 12, 2022.
46. Sawyer AN, Bono RS, Kaplan B, Breland AB. Nicotine/tobacco use disparities among transgender and gender diverse adults: findings from wave 4 PATH data. *Drug Alcohol Depend.* 2022;232:109268. https://doi.org/10.1016/j.drugalcdep.2022.109268
47. Somé NH, Shokoohi M, Shield KD, et al. Alcohol and cannabis use during the COVID-19 pandemic among transgender, gender-diverse, and cisgender adults in Canada. *BMC Public Health.* 2022;22(1):452. https://doi.org/10.1186/s12889-022-12779-9
48. Windle SB, Wade K, Filion KB, Kimmelman J, Thombs BD, Eisenberg MJ. Potential harms from legalization of recreational cannabis use in Canada. *Can J Public Health.* 2019;110(2):222–226. https://doi.org/10.17269/s41997-018-00173-1
49. Baliunas D, Zawertailo L, Voci S, et al. Variability in patient sociodemographics, clinical characteristics, and healthcare service utilization among 107,302 treatment seeking smokers in Ontario: a cross-sectional comparison. *PLoS One.* 2020;15(7):e0235709. https://doi.org/10.1371/journal.pone.0235709
50. Lowry DE, Corsi DJ. Trends and correlates of cannabis use in Canada: a repeated cross-sectional analysis of national surveys from 2004 to 2017. *CMAJ Open.* 2020;8(3):E487–E495. https://doi.org/10.9778/cmajo.20190229
51. Pacek LR, Weinberger AH, Zhu J, Goodwin RD. Rapid increase in the prevalence of cannabis use among people with depression in the United States, 2005–17: the role of differentially changing risk perceptions. *Addiction.* 2020;115(5):935–943. https://doi.org/10.1111/add.14883
52. Agrawal A, Lynskey MT. Tobacco and cannabis co-occurrence: does route of administration matter? *Drug Alcohol Depend.* 2009;99(1–3):240–247. https://doi.org/10.1016/j.drugalcdep.2008.08.007
53. Rabin RA, George TP. A review of co-morbid tobacco and cannabis use disorders: possible mechanisms to explain high rates of co-use. *Am J Addict.* 2015;24(2):105–116. https://doi.org/10.1111/ajad.12186
54. McClure EA, Baker NL, Hood CO, et al. Cannabis and alcohol co-use in a smoking cessation pharmacotherapy trial for adolescents and emerging adults. *Nicotine Tob Res.* 2020;22(8):1374–1382. https://doi.org/10.1093/ntr/ntz170
55. Hindocha C, McClure EA. Unknown population-level harms of cannabis and tobacco co-use: if you don't measure it, you can't manage it. *Addiction.* 2021;116(7):1622–1630. https://doi.org/10.1111/add.15290
56. Walsh H, Papadakis S, Ross L, McEwen A. Smoking cessation and cannabis use: a guide for stop smoking practitioners. Available at: https://www.ncsct.co.uk/usr/pub/Smoking%20cessation%20and%20cannabis%20use.pdf. Accessed September 12, 2022.
57. Adams TR, Arnsten JH, Ning Y, Nahvi S. Feasibility and preliminary effectiveness of varenicline for treating co-occurring cannabis and tobacco use. *J Psychoactive Drugs.* 2018;50(1):12–18. https://doi.org/10.1080/02791072.2017.1370746
58. Kerkvliet JL, Wey H, Fahrenwald NL. Cessation among state quitline participants with a mental health condition. *Nicotine Tob Res.* 2014;17(6):735–741. https://doi.org/10.1093/ntr/ntu239
59. Brose LS, Hitchman SC, Brown J, West R, McNeill A. Is the use of electronic cigarettes while smoking associated with smoking cessation attempts, cessation and reduced cigarette consumption? A survey with a 1-year follow-up. *Addiction.* 2015;110(7):1160–1168. https://doi.org/10.1111/add.12917

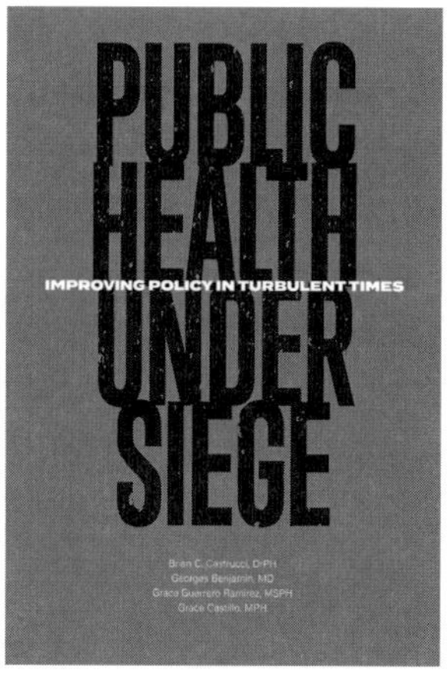

2021, SOFTCOVER, 250 PP
ISBN: 978-0-87553-319-3

Public Health Under Siege: Improving Policy in Turbulent Times

Edited by: Brian C. Castrucci, DrPH, Georges C. Benjamin, MD, Grace Guerrero Ramirez, MSPH, Grace Castillo, MPH

This new book focuses on the importance of health policy through a variety of perspectives, and addresses how policy benefits society, evidently through increased life expectancy and improved health. The book describes how detrimental social determinants can be to the overall population health and emphasizes how the nation is centered on policy change to create equal health care opportunities for all sectors of health.

APHABOOKSTORE.ORG

APHA PRESS
AN IMPRINT OF AMERICAN PUBLIC HEALTH ASSOCIATION

Breastfeeding by Disability Status in the United States: Pregnancy Risk Assessment Monitoring System, 2018–2020

Stephanie Ramer, MPH, Antoinette T. Nguyen, MD, MPH, Jennifer M. Nelson, MD, MPH, Maura K. Whiteman, PhD, Lee Warner, PhD, MPH, JoAnn M. Thierry, PhD, Suzanne Folger, PhD, MPH, Beatriz Salvesen von Essen, MPH, and Katherine Kortsmit, PhD, MPH

See also Brown and Lunsky, p. 7.

Objectives. To describe breastfeeding initiation and breastfeeding at 1, 2, and 3 months, and information sources on breastfeeding among women with a recent live birth by disability status.

Methods. We analyzed October 2018 to December 2020 data from the Pregnancy Risk Assessment Monitoring System for 24 sites in the United States that included the Washington Group Short Set of Questions on Disability (seeing, hearing, walking or climbing stairs, remembering or concentrating, self-care, communicating). We defined disability as reporting "a lot of difficulty" or "cannot do this at all" on any of these questions.

Results. Among 39 673 respondents, 6.0% reported disability. In adjusted analyses, breastfeeding was lower among respondents with disability at 2 (62.6% vs 66.6%; adjusted prevalence ratio [APR] = 0.94; 95% confidence interval [CI] = 0.89, 0.99) and 3 months (54.7% vs 59.6%; APR = 0.92; 95% CI = 0.86, 0.98) than those without disability. Respondents with disability were less likely to receive information from health care providers or support professionals (89.3% vs 92.3%), but as likely from breastfeeding or lactation specialists (78.1% vs 75.3%).

Conclusions. Strategies to ensure women with disability, receive breastfeeding support, including breastfeeding information, could improve breastfeeding outcomes. (*Am J Public Health*. 2024;114(1): 108–117. https://doi.org/10.2105/AJPH.2023.307438)

AJPH January 2024, Vol. 114, No. 1

Approximately 12% to 18% of reproductive-aged women have a disability.[1–3] Disability, as defined by the World Health Organization, encompasses impairments, activity limitations, and participation restrictions a person may experience in their daily lives.[4] Women with disability are as likely as those without disability to desire a future pregnancy, be sexually active, and experience pregnancy.[3,5,6] However, women with disability are less likely to report utilization of reproductive health care and more likely to experience pregnancy complications and adverse birth outcomes.[3,6–9]

The US Dietary Guidelines for Americans, the American Academy of Pediatrics (AAP), the American College of Obstetricians and Gynecologists, and the American Academy of Family Physicians recommend exclusive breastfeeding until about 6 months.[10–14] Many medical organizations recommend physicians and other health care providers offer breastfeeding education and support to patients[11,14–17] and that physicians stay current on best practices and develop skills related to breastfeeding to support patients in overcoming common challenges and continuing to breastfeed as long as desired.[11,14,15] When challenges exceed the expertise of providers, it is recommended that patients be referred to someone with clinical expertise in breastfeeding, such as a lactation consultant.[11,14,16]

National estimates suggest that 83.2%, 78.6%, 73.6%, and 69.1% of infants born in 2019 were ever breastfed, breastfed at 1, 2, and 3 months of age, respectively.[18] Some evidence suggests women with disability breastfeed at lower rates than those without disability[6,19] and are unlikely to receive information concerning how their disability could affect breastfeeding.[20,21] Receipt of some form of breastfeeding education by health care providers is associated with higher breastfeeding rates among the general population.[22] However, data are limited on the breastfeeding experiences among women with disability. Among a large representative sample of women who gave birth during October 1, 2018, to December 31, 2020, we assessed breastfeeding initiation and at 1, 2, and 3 months and sources of breastfeeding information by disability status. We also assessed associations between breastfeeding information sources and breastfeeding outcomes overall and by disability status.

METHODS

We analyzed data from the Pregnancy Risk Assessment Monitoring System (PRAMS), a population-based, site-specific surveillance system, which collects self-reported data on respondent's behaviors and experiences before, during, and shortly after pregnancy. Women with a recent live birth were randomly sampled from site birth certificate files and contacted 2 to 6 months after delivery to participate. PRAMS is conducted by the Centers for Disease Control and Prevention (CDC) in collaboration with site health departments. Data are collected using both mail and telephone survey methods. PRAMS does not collect data on gender identity; therefore, the term "women" was used to align with the birth certificate.

The PRAMS survey includes a core set of questions on all site surveys and, to address emerging topics, sites periodically add supplements to their survey.[23] The PRAMS disability supplement[24] was made available to sites in 2018 to address the gap in availability of population-based data on disability among women. The number of sites that implemented the disability supplement varied during 2018 to 2020. PRAMS methodology[25] and the disability supplement have previously been described.[23]

MEASURES

Disability. To measure disability, respondents were asked the Washington Group Short Set of Questions on Disability (WG-Short Set), a validated instrument with 6 questions on functional ability that measure difficulty with seeing (even when wearing glasses or contact lenses), hearing (even if using hearing aid[s]), walking or climbing stairs, remembering or concentrating, self-care (such as washing all over or dressing), and communicating (for example, understanding or being understood).[26] Respondents selected from the following responses: "no difficulty," "some difficulty," "a lot of difficulty," or "cannot do this at all." As recommended by the Washington Group,[27] we defined disability as reporting "a lot of difficulty" or "cannot do this at all" on any of the 6 questions. We defined no disability as reporting "no difficulty" or "some difficulty" to all questions.

Breastfeeding outcomes: initiation and any breastfeeding at 1, 2, and 3 months. Respondents whose infants were alive and living with them were asked a series of questions on breastfeeding. We considered respondents as having initiated breastfeeding if they answered "yes" to "Did you ever breastfeed or pump breast milk to feed your new baby, even for a short period of time?" To measure any breastfeeding at 1, 2, and 3 months, respondents who had initiated breastfeeding were asked "Are you currently breastfeeding or feeding pumped milk to your new baby?" If respondents were no longer breastfeeding at the time of the survey, they were then asked, "How many weeks or months did you breastfeed or pump milk to feed your baby?" We categorized breastfeeding outcomes into 4 separate dichotomous yes-no variables: (1) breastfeeding initiation; (2) breastfeeding at 1 month (4 weeks); (3) breastfeeding at 2 months (9 weeks); and (4) breastfeeding at 3 months (13 weeks). For all analyses examining breastfeeding at 3 months, we restricted the sample to those who completed the PRAMS survey 3 or more months after delivery (n = 33 704). We conducted analyses on breastfeeding initiation and breastfeeding at 1 and 2 months among this restricted sample, and findings were consistent with results for the full sample. We present results for the full sample for breastfeeding initiation at 1 and 2 months. Respondents who did not initiate breastfeeding were included as "not breastfeeding" for all outcomes.

Sources of breastfeeding information. Respondents were asked, "Before or after your new baby was born, did you receive information about breastfeeding from any of the following sources?" Respondents could select multiple responses. We created 2 categories for sources of information: (1) health care providers and support professionals (hereinafter, health care providers), defined as responding "yes" to any of the following response options: "my doctor," "a nurse/midwife/doula," or "my baby's doctor"; and (2) breastfeeding or lactation specialists, defined as responding "yes" to this response option. We reviewed and recategorized "other" responses if they fit into an existing response option. We also created a composite measure which assessed information from both health care providers and breastfeeding or lactation specialists.

Covariates

We selected covariates a priori that were found to be associated with disability or breastfeeding.[1,2,18] We examined the following respondents' characteristics using birth certificate data available in the PRAMS data set: age (< 20, 20–24, 25–34, ≥ 35 years), race or ethnicity (Hispanic, non-Hispanic American Indian/Alaska Native, non-Hispanic Asian/Pacific Islander, non-Hispanic Black, non-Hispanic other or multiple races [respondents who selected > 1 race or other non-White on the birth certificate], non-Hispanic White), education level (≤ high school, high school diploma or general equivalency diploma [GED], some college or higher), parity (primiparous, multiparous), delivery method (vaginal delivery, cesarean section), participated in the Special Supplemental Nutrition Program for Women, Infants, and Children (WIC) prenatally (yes, no), and gestational age at delivery (preterm, < 37 weeks; term, ≥ 37 weeks). Due to insufficient sample sizes for Native Hawaiian and other Pacific Islander to be presented as disaggregated data, they were combined with Asian to create the category non-Hispanic Asian/Pacific Islander.

Analytical Sample

We analyzed October 1, 2018, to December 31, 2020, data from 24 PRAMS sites (Colorado, District of Columbia, Georgia, Kansas, Louisiana, Massachusetts, Maryland, Maine, Michigan, Mississippi, Missouri, Montana, North Dakota, Nebraska, New Hampshire, New Mexico, New York [excluding New York City], Oregon, Rhode Island, South Dakota, Tennessee, Vermont, Virginia, and West Virginia) that implemented the PRAMS disability supplement and met CDC's 50% response rate threshold for at least 1 study year. Our analytic sample excluded respondents whose infants were not living with them or were deceased (n = 770; 1.1%) at the time of survey completion. After excluding those with missing data on disability (n = 1725; 3.4%), outcomes (range = n = 977; 1.8% to n = 2959; 5.8%), and covariates (n = 812; 2.0%), our final analytic sample included 39 673 respondents (weighted n = 1 767 676).

Statistical Analyses

We performed descriptive statistics (unweighted numbers and weighted percentages and 95% confidence intervals [CIs]) to assess the prevalence of any disability and type of disability overall and by covariates.

We calculated the unadjusted and adjusted prevalence estimates for each breastfeeding outcome using the average marginal predictions approach to logistic regression models and generated prevalence ratios (PRs) with their associated 95% CIs to examine associations between disability status and each breastfeeding outcome. We also calculated unadjusted prevalence estimates and associated 95% CIs for breastfeeding outcomes by type of disability. Because of small sample size for each individual type of disability, we did not conduct further analyses by type of disability. We constructed separate bivariate and multivariable logistic regression models to examine the associations between disability status with each breastfeeding outcome and the source of breastfeeding information. We also examined the adjusted association between each breastfeeding outcome with the breastfeeding information source overall and by disability status. Lastly, we constructed separate multivariable, logistic regression models to examine the adjusted association between each breastfeeding outcome with the breastfeeding information source stratified by disability status. Each multivariable, logistic regression model was adjusted for all aforementioned covariates and PRAMS site.

PRAMS data are weighted for sampling design, noncoverage, and nonresponse to be representative of each site's live birth population. Analyses accounted for PRAMS' complex sampling design by using SAS-callable SUDAAN version 11.0.3 (RTI International, Research Triangle Park, NC).

RESULTS

Among 39 673 respondents, 6.0% reported disability (Table A, available as a supplement to the online version of this article at https://www.ajph.org). Difficulty with remembering (3.7%) was most common, followed by difficulty with seeing (1.6%), walking or climbing stairs (0.6%), hearing (0.6%), communicating (0.5%), and self-care (0.3%). A higher prevalence of respondents with disability than without were non-Hispanic American Indian/Alaska Native (1.3% vs 0.8%), aged 20–24 years (26.8% vs 17.8%), had completed less than high school (15.6% vs 10.1%) or had a high school diploma or GED (36.5% vs 24.7%), were multiparous (65.7% vs 59.6%), participated in WIC prenatally (47.8% vs 31.0%), and had infants who were preterm (11.1% vs 9.0%; Table 1). Prevalence of disability was higher among respondents who were non-Hispanic American Indian/Alaska Native (9.8%) versus those who were non-Hispanic White (5.8%) and non-Hispanic Asian/Pacific Islander (4.0%); were younger than 20 years (8.1%) or aged 20 to 24 years (8.8%) versus aged 25 to 34 years (5.3%) or 35 years or older (5.0%); had completed less than high school (9.0%) or who had a high school diploma or GED (8.7%) versus some college or higher (4.5%); were multiparous (6.6%) versus primiparous (5.2%); had participated in WIC prenatally (9.0%) versus those who had not (4.6%); and whose infants were preterm (7.3%) versus

TABLE 1— Respondent Characteristics by Disability Status: Pregnancy Risk Assessment Monitoring System (PRAMS), 24 US Sites, October 31, 2018–December 31, 2020

Respondent Characteristics	Unweighted No.	Weighted % (95% CI)	
		Disability[a]	No Disability[b]
Total	39 673		
Age at delivery, y			
< 20	1 641	5.4 (4.1, 6.9)	3.9 (3.6, 4.3)
20 – 24	6 782	26.8 (23.8, 29.9)	17.8 (17.1, 18.5)
25 – 34	23 665	52.7 (49.3, 56.0)	59.7 (58.9, 60.6)
≥ 35	7 585	15.2 (12.9, 17.8)	18.6 (17.9, 19.2)
Race/ethnicity			
Hispanic	6 393	14.4 (12.2, 17.0)	14.4 (13.8, 15.1)
Non-Hispanic American Indian or Alaska Native	1 840	1.3 (0.9, 1.9)	0.8 (0.7, 0.8)
Non-Hispanic Asian or Pacific Islander	2 574	2.7 (1.8, 3.9)	4.1 (3.8, 4.5)
Non-Hispanic Black	7 167	21.3 (18.6, 24.2)	18.5 (17.8, 19.1)
Non-Hispanic Other race (not specified or multiple races)	2 029	3.2 (2.3, 4.5)	2.9 (2.6, 3.1)
Non-Hispanic White	19 670	57.1 (53.8, 60.4)	59.4 (58.6, 60.2)
Education level			
< high school	4 231	15.6 (13.3, 18.2)	10.1 (9.6, 10.7)
High school diploma or GED	9 092	36.5 (33.2, 39.9)	24.7 (23.9, 25.4)
≥ some college	26 350	47.9 (44.6, 51.2)	65.2 (64.3, 66.0)
Parity			
Primiparous	15 817	34.3 (31.1, 37.6)	40.4 (39.6, 41.3)
Multiparous	23 856	65.7 (62.4, 68.9)	59.6 (58.7, 60.4)
Delivery method			
Vaginal delivery	26 694	66.5 (63.3, 69.6)	68.7 (67.9, 69.5)
Cesarean section	12 979	33.5 (30.4, 36.7)	31.3 (30.5, 32.1)
Prenatal WIC Participation			
Yes	13 583	47.8 (44.5, 51.2)	31.0 (30.2, 31.8)
No	26 090	52.2 (48.8, 55.5)	69.0 (68.2, 69.8)
Gestational age at delivery, wk			
Preterm, < 37	6 793	11.1 (9.6, 12.8)	9.0 (8.6, 9.4)
Term, ≥ 37	32 880	88.9 (87.2, 90.4)	91.0 (90.6, 91.4)

Note. CI = confidence interval; GED = general equivalency diploma; WIC = Special Supplemental Nutrition Program for Women, Infants, and Children. The 24 PRAMS sites were CO, DC, GA, KS, LA, MA, MD, ME, MI, MS, MO, MT, ND, NE, NH, NM, NY (excluding New York City), OR, RI, SD, TN, VT, VA, and WV.
[a]Disability was defined as having "a lot of difficulty" or "cannot do at all" on 1 or more of the Washington Group Short Set of Questions on Disability (WG-Short Set)[26] that assess difficulty with seeing, hearing, walking/climbing stairs, remembering/concentrating, self-care, and communicating.
[b]No disability was defined as reporting "no difficulty" or "some difficulty" to all of the WG-Short Set.

those whose infants were term (5.9%). The prevalence of disability type by select characteristics generally followed a similar pattern as disability overall (Table A).

In unadjusted analyses, respondents with disability had a lower prevalence of breastfeeding initiation (83.1% vs 87.0%) and breastfeeding at 1 (68.7% vs 76.7%), 2 (56.1% vs 67.0%), and 3 (48.3% vs 60.0%) months than respondents without disability (Table 2). By type of disability: breastfeeding initiation ranged from 72.4% to 84.1% among respondents reporting difficulty communicating and remembering or concentrating, respectively; breastfeeding at 1 month ranged from 57.6% to 71.4% among respondents reporting difficulty communicating and hearing, respectively; breastfeeding at 2 months ranged from 51.5% to 61.6% among respondents reporting difficulty communicating and hearing, respectively; and breastfeeding at 3 months ranged from 45.7% to 54.1% among respondents reporting difficulty remembering or concentrating and hearing, respectively (Table B, available as a supplement to the online version of this article at https://www.ajph.org).

In adjusted analyses, breastfeeding initiation (86.7% vs 86.6%; adjusted PR [APR] = 1.00; 95% CI = 0.97, 1.02) and at 1 month (74.2% vs 76.4%; APR = 0.97; 95% CI = 0.94, 1.01) did not differ by disability status. However, breastfeeding remained lower among respondents with disability at 2 (62.6% vs 66.6%; APR = 0.94; 95% CI = 0.89, 0.99) and 3 months (54.7% vs 59.6%; APR = 0.92; 95% CI = 0.86, 0.98) than among respondents without disability.

Overall, 92.2% of respondents reported receiving breastfeeding information from health care providers, with respondent's doctor being most common (78.3%), followed by nurse, midwife, or doula (75.4%), and baby's doctor (71.0%; data not shown). Precisely 75.5% of respondents received information from breastfeeding or lactation specialists. Overall, 72.3% of respondents received information from both health care providers and breastfeeding or lactation specialists, 19.8% received information from only health care providers, 4.7% did not receive information from either source, and 3.1% received information from only breastfeeding or lactation specialists (Table 3). In adjusted analyses, regardless of disability, respondents who received information from both health care providers and breastfeeding or lactation specialists or received information from only breastfeeding or lactation specialists were more likely to breastfeed across all outcomes than respondents who

TABLE 2— Prevalence and Prevalence Ratios of Breastfeeding Initiation and Any Breastfeeding at 1, 2, and 3 Months by Disability Status: Pregnancy Risk Assessment Monitoring System (PRAMS), 24 US Sites, October 31, 2018–December 31, 2020

	Breastfeeding, Unadjusted			Breastfeeding, Adjusted[a]		
Breastfeeding Outcomes	Disability,[b] Weighted %	No Disability,[c] Weighted %	PR (95% CI)[d]	Disability,[b] Weighted %	No Disability,[c] Weighted %	APR (95% CI)[d]
Breastfeeding Initiation (unweighted n = 39 673)	83.1	87.0	0.96 (0.93, 0.99)	86.7	86.6	1.00 (0.97, 1.02)
Breastfeeding 1 mo (unweighted n = 39 673)	68.7	76.7	0.90 (0.86, 0.94)	74.2	76.4	0.97 (0.94, 1.01)
Breastfeeding 2 mo (unweighted n = 39 673)	56.1	67.0	0.84 (0.79, 0.89)	62.6	66.6	0.94 (0.89, 0.99)
Breastfeeding 3 mo (unweighted n = 33 704)[e]	48.3	60.0	0.80 (0.74, 0.87)	54.7	59.6	0.92 (0.86, 0.98)

Note. APR = adjusted prevalence ratio; CI = confidence interval; PR = prevalence ratio. The 24 PRAMS sites were CO, DC, GA, KS, LA, MA, MD, ME, MI, MS, MO, MT, ND, NE, NH, NM, NY (excluding New York City), OR, RI, SD, TN, VT, VA, and WV.

[a]Adjusted for respondent race or ethnicity; age; education level; parity; type of delivery; participation in Special Supplemental Nutrition Program for Women, Infants, and Children during pregnancy; preterm birth; and PRAMS site. Covariates were obtained from birth certificate data available in the PRAMS data set.

[b]Disability was defined as reporting "a lot of difficulty" or "cannot do at all" on ≥ 1 of the Washington Group Short Set of Questions on Disability (WG-Short Set)[26] that measure difficulty with seeing, hearing, walking/climbing stairs, remembering/concentrating, self-care, and communicating.

[c]No disability was defined as reporting "no difficulty" or "some difficulty" to all of the WG-Short Set.

[d]We constructed separate survey-weighted logistic regression models to examine the association with each breastfeeding outcome by disability status. The reference group for each model was respondents with no disability.

[e]Sample was restricted to those respondents who had completed their PRAMS survey at or after 3 months after giving birth.

TABLE 3— Adjusted Prevalence and Prevalence Ratios of Breastfeeding Outcomes by Sources of Breastfeeding Information and Disability Status: Pregnancy Risk Assessment Monitoring System (PRAMS), 24 US Sites, October 31, 2018–December 31, 2020

Sources of Breastfeeding Information	Weighted %	Breastfeeding Initiation (Unweighted n = 39 673), APR (95% CI)[a,b]	Any Breastfeeding, APR (95% CI)[a,b]		
			1 Month (Unweighted n = 39 673)	2 Months (Unweighted n = 39 673)	3 Months (Unweighted n = 33 704)[c]
Total (n = 39 673)					
Neither source	4.7	1 (Ref)	1 (Ref)	1 (Ref)	1 (Ref)
Health care providers or support professionals only[d]	19.8	1.01 (0.96, 1.07)	1.00 (0.93, 1.07)	0.97 (0.90, 1.05)	0.92 (0.85, 1.01)
Breastfeeding or lactation specialist only	3.1	1.34 (1.26, 1.41)	1.39 (1.29, 1.50)	1.36 (1.24, 1.48)	1.31 (1.17, 1.45)
Both health care providers or support professionals[d] and breastfeeding or lactation specialist	72.3	1.32 (1.26, 1.39)	1.37 (1.29, 1.46)	1.32 (1.23, 1.41)	1.22 (1.13, 1.32)
No disability[e] (n = 37 108)					
Neither source	4.6	1 (Ref)	1 (Ref)	1 (Ref)	1 (Ref)
Health care providers or support professionals only[d]	20.0	1.01 (0.96, 1.07)	1.00 (0.94, 1.07)	0.97 (0.90, 1.05)	0.92 (0.84, 1.00)
Breastfeeding or lactation specialist only	3.1	1.32 (1.25, 1.40)	1.38 (1.28, 1.49)	1.36 (1.24, 1.49)	1.30 (1.16, 1.44)
Both health care providers or support professionals[d] and breastfeeding or lactation specialist	72.4	1.31 (1.25, 1.38)	1.37 (1.28, 1.45)	1.32 (1.23, 1.42)	1.21 (1.11, 1.31)
Disability[f] (n = 2 565)					
Neither source	6.6	1 (Ref)	1 (Ref)	1 (Ref)	1 (Ref)
Health care providers or support professionals only[d]	17.4	0.93 (0.75, 1.16)	0.86 (0.63, 1.16)	0.84 (0.60, 1.19)	0.86 (0.56, 1.34)
Breastfeeding or lactation specialist only	4.4	1.44 (1.20, 1.72)	1.53 (1.15, 2.02)	1.32 (0.89, 1.96)	1.36 (0.81, 2.30)
Both health care providers or support professionals[d] and breastfeeding or lactation specialist	71.6	1.37 (1.15, 1.63)	1.40 (1.09, 1.79)	1.27 (0.95, 1.69)	1.36 (0.94, 1.98)

Note. APR = adjusted prevalence ratio; CI = confidence interval. The 24 PRAMS sites were CO, DC, GA, KS, LA, MA, MD, ME, MI, MS, MO, MT, ND, NE, NH, NM, NY (excluding New York City), OR, RI, SD, TN, VT, VA, and WV.

[a]Adjusted for respondent age; race or ethnicity; education level; parity; type of delivery; participation in Special Supplemental Nutrition Program for Women, Infants, and Children during pregnancy; preterm birth; and PRAMS site. Covariates were obtained from birth certificate data available in the PRAMS data set.

[b]We constructed separate multivariable survey-weighted logistic regression models to examine the association with each breastfeeding outcome by sources of breastfeeding information. The reference group for each model were respondents who reported they had received information on breastfeeding from neither source.

[c]Sample was restricted to those respondents who had completed their PRAMS survey at or after 3 months after giving birth.

[d]Health care provider or support professional included those that reported "my doctor," "my baby's doctor," or "nurse/midwife/doula."

[e]No disability was defined as reporting "no difficulty" or "some difficulty" to all of the Washington Group Short Set of Questions on Disability (WG-Short Set).[26]

[f]Disability was defined as reporting "a lot of difficulty" or "cannot do at all" on 1 or more of the WG-Short Set that measure difficulty with seeing, hearing, walking/climbing stairs, remembering/concentrating, self-care, and communicating.

had not received information from either source.

Respondents with disability were less likely to receive breastfeeding information from health care providers (89.3% vs 92.3%; APR = 0.97; 95% CI = 0.94, 0.99) and as likely to receive information from breastfeeding or lactation specialists (78.1% vs 75.3%; APR = 1.04, 95% CI = 1.00, 1.08) compared with respondents without disability (Table 4). Among respondents without disability only, those who received information from health care providers were more likely to be breastfeeding at 1 and 2 months than respondents who did not receive information from health care providers (Table C, available as a

TABLE 4— Prevalence and Prevalence Ratios of Sources of Breastfeeding Information by Disability Status: Pregnancy Risk Assessment Monitoring System (PRAMS), 24 US Sites, October 31, 2018–December 31, 2020

Source of Breastfeeding Information (Unweighted n = 39 673)	Received Source of Information, Unadjusted			Received Source of Information, Adjusted[a]		
	Disability,[b] Weighted %	No Disability,[c,d] Weighted %	PR (95% CI)	Disability,[b] Weighted %	No Disability,[c] Weighted %	APR (95% CI)[d]
Health care provider or support professional[e]	89.0	92.4	0.96 (0.94, 0.99)	89.3	92.3	0.97 (0.94, 0.99)
Breastfeeding or lactation specialist	76.0	75.4	1.01 (0.97, 1.05)	78.1	75.3	1.04 (1.00, 1.08)

Note. APR = adjusted prevalence ratio; CI = confidence interval; PR = prevalence ratio. The 24 PRAMS sites were CO, DC, GA, KS, LA, MA, MD, ME, MI, MS, MO, MT, ND, NE, NH, NM, NY (excluding New York City), OR, RI, SD, TN, VT, VA, and WV.

[a]Adjusted for respondent race or ethnicity; age; education level; parity; type of delivery; participation in Special Supplemental Nutrition Program for Women, Infants, and Children during pregnancy; preterm birth; and PRAMS site. Covariates were obtained from birth certificate data available in the PRAMS data set.

[b]Disability was defined as reporting "a lot of difficulty" or "cannot do at all" on ≥ 1 of the Washington Group Short Set of Questions on Disability (WG-Short Set)[26] that measure difficulty with seeing, hearing, walking/climbing stairs, remembering/concentrating, self-care, and communicating.

[c]No disability was defined as reporting "no difficulty" or "some difficulty" to all of the WG-Short Set.

[d]We constructed separate multivariable survey-weighted logistic regression models to examine the association with each source of breastfeeding information by disability status. The reference group for each model was respondents with no disability.

[e]Health care provider or support professional included those that reported "my doctor," "my baby's doctor," or "nurse/midwife/doula."

supplement to the online version of this article at https://www.ajph.org). Respondents who received information from breastfeeding or lactation specialists were more likely to be breastfeeding across all outcomes than respondents who did not receive information from breastfeeding or lactation specialists, regardless of disability status.

DISCUSSION

Breastfeeding initiation and breastfeeding at 1, 2, and 3 months were lower among women with disability than without disability in unadjusted analyses by 4 to 12 percentage points. In adjusted analyses, breastfeeding at 2 and 3 months remained lower among women with disability by 4 to 5 percentage points.

Although the absolute differences in prevalence of breastfeeding outcomes were modest, our findings suggest that women with disability might face additional challenges to breastfeeding than those without disability. Regardless of disability, many barriers to breastfeeding exist, including lack of knowledge, poor family and social support, lack of parental leave and lactation support at work, lactation problems, social norms, embarrassment, and health services.[28] In addition, additional challenges accessing breastfeeding support might exist, such as the availability of community support and distance to lactation counselors.[29] Limited evidence exists on breastfeeding experiences of women with disability in the United States. Data on breastfeeding experiences are primarily from qualitative studies with small sample sizes (n ≤ 25) among women who are predominantly White, in their thirties, married, with at least some college education. In these studies, women with a range of disabilities reported challenges, including lack of support, limited information on disability-related health considerations, milk supply and latch problems, and challenges communicating lactation difficulties with lactation consultants.[20,21] Furthermore, women with disability might have difficulty accessing health care,[1] which could impact their ability to seek guidance when they encounter breastfeeding difficulties. Women with disability have also reported breastfeeding facilitators, such as peer support, positive support from health care providers, use of a breast pump, and physical support to breastfeed.[20] In a recent cohort study, conducted in Canada, women with an intellectual or developmental disability or multiple disabilities were less likely to receive in-hospital breastfeeding assistance than women without disability.[30]

Overall, we found respondents who received information from health care providers were more likely to initiate breastfeeding and be breastfeeding at 1 and 2 months than those who did not, suggesting that receiving information from providers may facilitate breastfeeding. However, this association was not found among women with disability at 1 and 2 months, suggesting women with disability may not receive the same benefit from information from providers alone. Regardless of disability status, we found respondents who received information from both health care providers and breastfeeding or lactation specialists and those who received information from only breastfeeding or lactation specialists were more likely to breastfeed than those who received information from only health care providers or neither source. However, respondents with disability were less likely to receive breastfeeding information from health care providers compared with those without disability.

Health care providers might need additional resources to support women who choose to breastfeed, regardless of disability.[11,31] Providing referrals to lactation or breastfeeding specialists for patients, when appropriate, might be another opportunity for health care providers to offer breastfeeding support when they are unable to provide the care directly.[14,16] In a survey of obstetrician-gynecologists, pediatricians, and family physicians, medical education related to breastfeeding was found to be inadequate, and several gaps in training were identified, including the need for breastfeeding education to be prioritized throughout training.[31] Providers might need additional support to follow guidance from professional organizations to support patients in overcoming breastfeeding challenges.[11,14,15] Efforts to improve breastfeeding education among physicians, such as AAPs' Physician Engagement and Training Focused on Breastfeeding Project, a collaborative effort between multiple medical and health organizations, aim to improve physician training to support patients in reaching their breastfeeding goals.[13,32] Provider resources specific to breastfeeding support for women with disability may be needed. Beyond breastfeeding, qualitative studies have demonstrated women with disability face challenges in receiving reproductive health care that is inclusive of their disability.[20,21] Challenges in seeking and receiving health care for women with disability include inaccessible equipment, lack of transportation and lack of provider experience.[7,8,33] In a survey of obstetrician-gynecologists, providers reported that they are not trained to properly care for the needs of women with disability.[34]

Receipt of information on breastfeeding from health care providers that is tailored to the needs of women with disability and referrals to breastfeeding or lactation specialists when warranted might be important strategies to improve breastfeeding outcomes.

LIMITATIONS

This analysis is subject to several limitations. Our findings were limited to PRAMS sites that included the disability supplement on their site-specific survey and met CDC's 50% response rate threshold criteria, limiting the generalizability of our findings. Findings were also subject to recall and social desirability biases. Because we did not disaggregate Asian and Pacific Islander, we may have masked important differences among this population. Due to the small sample size of women with disability, we report the prevalence of each breastfeeding outcome among respondents reporting each type of disability; however, we did not conduct further analyses. Additionally, our definition of disability status is heterogenous and may have masked variability in the associations. While the WG-Short Set is intended to identify persons who report difficulty across 6 functional domains, it might not capture all persons with disability.[35] Our estimates of disability might be an underestimate as the prevalence of disability was lower than what other sources have reported among reproductive-aged women (6% vs 12 − 18%).[1–3] This could be due to differences in how disability was measured or defined, surveys were administered, or differences in disability prevalence in the general versus postpartum population. While PRAMS offers multiple modes to complete the survey,[25] persons with disability might need additional accommodations that are unavailable. We were unable to assess whether there was a difference in survey responses or reasons for nonparticipation by disability status.

The PRAMS core questionnaire does not measure breastfeeding intentions, reasons women breastfed or did not breastfeed (any or exclusivity) and we did not analyze breastfeeding outcomes beyond 3 months. We were therefore unable to assess whether respondents' decision to breastfeed or not was influenced by their disability or other reasons impacted their decision. We were also unable to assess the mode of delivery (in-person, phone, or virtual), content, timing, or frequency of the information received. The category of health care providers included nurse, midwife, and doula; however, the support offered by doulas might differ from other providers. There could be variation in the quality of the information received from breastfeeding or lactation specialists as the training required varies widely.[36] We were also unable to assess respondents' access to breastfeeding information. It is possible that respondents who reported they did not receive information did have access to information, but declined or did not seek or utilize the information for various reasons (e.g., past breastfeeding experiences). There are individual reasons (e.g., stronger desire

AJPH January 2024, Vol. 114, No. 1

to breastfeed) and structural drivers (e.g., socioeconomic inequities) that could affect a person's ability to seek out and access additional support if they were experiencing problems. It's also possible that women with disability might be more likely to be taking medications than women without disability and were advised to pause or stop breastfeeding as a result. However, PRAMS does not have detailed information on medical conditions, including medication use. Few medications are contraindicated while breastfeeding, and in most cases if contraindicated, a safe substitute can be found.[11] However, some evidence suggests women are often advised unnecessarily to stop breastfeeding.[37]

Another limitation of these data is that the latter portion of data were collected during the early part of the COVID-19 pandemic when access to health care was interrupted.[38] While telehealth consultations were more common during the COVID-19 pandemic,[39] we were unable to assess the mode through which women received information on breastfeeding. Lastly, while we were able to adjust for many covariates reported to be associated with breastfeeding[1,2,22] (e.g., race or ethnicity, age), we could not adjust for all factors that could have contributed to differences in breastfeeding outcomes (e.g., breastfeeding intentions).[40] Despite these limitations, this study provides valuable information on breastfeeding outcomes and sources of breastfeeding information by disability status using population-based data.

PUBLIC HEALTH IMPLICATIONS

There is very limited information on how disability affects breastfeeding, and our analyses provide additional insight into how disability might affect breastfeeding. Women with disability generally reported a lower prevalence of breastfeeding at 2 and 3 months than women without disability and were less likely to receive information from health care providers, but as likely to receive information from breastfeeding or lactation specialists. Strategies to ensure women with disability, receive breastfeeding support, including information from health care providers and breastfeeding or lactation specialists can improve breastfeeding outcomes.[21,22] AJPH

ABOUT THE AUTHORS

Stephanie Ramer, Antoinette T. Nguyen, Maura K. Whiteman, Lee Warner, Suzanne Folger, Beatriz Salvesen von Essen, and Katherine Kortsmit are with the Division of Reproductive Health, National Center for Chronic Disease Prevention and Health Promotion, Centers of Disease Control and Prevention (CDC), Atlanta, GA. At the time of the study, Jennifer M. Nelson was is with the Division of Nutrition, Physical Activity and Obesity, National Center for Chronic Disease Prevention and Health Promotion, CDC, Atlanta. JoAnn M. Thierry is with the Division of Human Development and Disability, National Center on Birth Defects and Developmental Disabilities, CDC, Atlanta.

CORRESPONDENCE

Correspondence should be sent to Stephanie Ramer, 4770 Buford Highway, NE, Building 107 Mailstop S107-2, Atlanta, GA 30341 (e-mail: ryi0@cdc.gov).

PUBLICATION INFORMATION

Full Citation: Ramer S, Nguyen AT, Nelson JM, et al. Breastfeeding by disability status in the United States: Pregnancy Risk Assessment Monitoring System, 2018–2020. *Am J Public Health*. 2024; 114(1):108–117.

Acceptance Date: August 30, 2023.

DOI: https://doi.org/10.2105/AJPH.2023.307438

CONTRIBUTORS

S. Ramer conceptualized the study, conducted the analysis, drafted the initial manuscript, and reviewed and revised the manuscript. K. Kortsmit conceptualized the study, supervised and duplicated the analysis, provided significant input on data interpretation and drafting of the manuscript, and reviewed and revised the manuscript. A. T. Nguyen conceptualized the study, assisted with data interpretation, and reviewed and revised the manuscript. J. M. Nelson, M. Whiteman, L. Warner, J. M. Thierry, S. Folger, and B. Salvesen Von Essen contributed to the study design, and reviewed and revised the manuscript. All authors approved the final manuscript as submitted and agree to be accountable for all aspects of the work.

ACKNOWLEDGMENTS

Research reported in this publication was supported by the Eunice Kennedy Shriver National Institute of Child Health and Human Development (NICHD) of the National Institutes of Health under an interagency agreement. S. Ramer was supported by an appointment to the Research Participation Program at the CDC administered by the Oak Ridge Institute for Science and Education through an interagency agreement between the US Department of Energy and the CDC.

We thank the PRAMS Working Group for its role in conducting PRAMS surveillance. PRAMS Working Group Representatives: Tim Feuser, MPH, Alabama; Kathy Perham-Hester, MS, MPH, Alaska; Gina Herrera, MPH, Arizona; Letitia de Graft-Johnson, DrPH, MHSA, Arkansas; Ashley Juhl, MSPH, Colorado; Jennifer Morin, MPH, Connecticut; George Yocher, MS, Delaware; Pamela Oandasan, MPH, District of Columbia; Heather Lake-Burger, MPH, Florida; Jenna Self, MPH, Georgia; Matt Shim, PhD, MPH, Hawaii; Eric Hall, Illinois; Trinity Edinburgh, MPH, Indiana; Jennifer Pham, Iowa; Celina Lopez, Kansas; Tracey D. Jewell, MPH, Kentucky; Dionka Pierce, MPH, Louisiana; Emily Gerety, MSW, Maine; Laurie Kettinger, MS, Maryland; Xiaohui Geng, DrEpi, MSE, Massachusetts; Hannah Sauter, MPH, Michigan; Mira Grice Sheff, PhD, MS, Minnesota; Brenda Hughes, MPPA, Mississippi; Venkata Garikapaty, PhD, Missouri; Miriam Naiman-Sessions, PhD, MPH, Montana; Masoomeh Hajizadeh Oghaz, PhD, Nebraska; Tami M. Conn, MPH, Nevada; Paulette Vallière, MPH, New Hampshire; Sharon Smith Cooley, MPH, New Jersey; Eirian Coronado, MA, New Mexico; Trang Nguyen, MD, DrPH, New York State; Lauren Birnie, MPH, New York City; Heather S. Pangelinan, MS, Northern Mariana Islands; Grace Njau, MPH, North Dakota; Ayesha Lampkins, MPH, Oklahoma; Caitlyn Howell, MA, Oregon; Angelo Santore, MPA, Pennsylvania; Wanda Hernández Virella, MPH, Puerto Rico; Karine Tolentino Monteiro, MPH, Rhode Island; Carlos Avalos, MSPH, South Carolina; Courtney Valencia, South Dakota; Natasha Jahani, MPH, Texas; Angela Miller, PhD, MSPH, Tennessee; Nickee Andjelic, MS, CHES, Utah; Peggy Brozicevic, Vermont; Kay Feagin, MA, Virginia; Linda Lohdefinck, Washington State; Monica Stover, MA, West Virginia; Mireille Perzan, MPH, Wisconsin; Neva Ruso, MPH, Wyoming; CDC PRAMS Team, Women's Health and Fertility Branch, Division of Reproductive Health, National Center for Chronic Disease Prevention and Health Promotion, CDC.

Note. The findings and conclusions in this report are those of the authors and do not necessarily represent the official position of the CDC.

CONFLICTS OF INTEREST

The authors have no conflicts of interest relevant to this article to disclose.

HUMAN PARTICIPANT PROTECTION

The PRAMS protocol was reviewed and approved by CDC's institutional review board (IRB) and each participating site's IRB.

REFERENCES

1. Okoro CA, Hollis ND, Cyrus AC, Griffin-Blake S. Prevalence of disabilities and health care access by disability status and type among adults—United States, 2016. *MMWR Morb Mortal Wkly Rep.* 2018;67(32):882–887. https://doi.org/10.15585/mmwr.mm6732a3
2. Horner-Johnson W, Darney BG, Kulkarni-Rajasekhara S, Quigley B, Caughey AB. Pregnancy among US women: differences by presence, type, and complexity of disability. *Am J Obstet Gynecol.* 2016;214(4):e–e9. https://doi.org/10.1016/j.ajog.2015.10.929
3. Mitra M, Clements KM, Zhang J, Smith LD. Disparities in adverse preconception risk factors between women with and without disabilities. *Matern Child Health J.* 2016;20(3):507–515. https://doi.org/10.1007/s10995-015-1848-1
4. World Health Organization. International Classification of Functioning, Disability and Health (ICF). Available at: https://www.who.int/classifications/international-classification-of-functioning-disability-and-health. Accessed July 18, 2023.
5. Bloom TL, Mosher W, Alhusen J, Lantos H, Hughes RB. Fertility Desires and intentions among US women by disability status: findings from the 2011–2013 National Survey of Family Growth. *Matern Child Health J.* 2017;21(8):1606–1615. https://doi.org/10.1007/s10995-016-2250-3
6. Mitra M, Clements KM, Zhang J, Iezzoni LI, Smeltzer SC, Long-Bellil LM. Maternal characteristics, pregnancy complications, and adverse birth outcomes among women with disabilities. *Med Care.* 2015;53(12):1027–1032. https://doi.org/10.1097/MLR.0000000000000427
7. Sonalkar S, Chavez V, McClusky J, Hunter TA, Mollen CJ. Gynecologic care for women with physical disabilities: a qualitative study of patients and providers. *Womens Health Issues.* 2020;30(2):136–141. https://doi.org/10.1016/j.whi.2019.10.002
8. Holt L, Carney MH, Duncanson L, et al. Perceived barriers to gynecologic care by women who use wheelchairs. *Cureus.* 2021;13(6). https://doi.org/10.7759/cureus.15647
9. Brown HK, Chen S, Guttmann A, et al. Neonatal outcomes of mothers with a disability. *Pediatrics.* 2022;150(3):e2021055318. https://doi.org/10.1542/peds.2021-055318
10. US Department of Agriculture and US Department of Health and Human Services. *Dietary Guidelines for Americans, 2020–2025.* 9th Edition. Available at https://www.DietaryGuidelines.gov. Accessed July 18, 2023.
11. Meek JY, Noble L, Breastfeeding S. Breastfeeding and the use of human milk. *Pediatrics.* 2022;150(1):e2022057988. https://doi.org/10.1542/peds.2022-057988
12. The American College of Obstetricians and Gynecologists. Committee Opinion: Optimizing Postpartum Care. 2018. Available at https://www.acog.org/clinical/clinical-guidance/committee-opinion/articles/2018/05/optimizing-postpartum-care. Accessed July 18, 2023.
13. American Academy of Pediatrics. Physician Education and Training on Breastfeeding. 2021. Available at https://www.aap.org/en/patient-care/breastfeeding/physician-education-and-training-on-breastfeeding. Accessed July 18, 2023.
14. American Academy of Family Physicians. Breastfeeding, Family Physicians Supporting (Position Paper). Available at https://www.aafp.org/about/policies/all/breastfeeding-position-paper.html. Accessed July 18, 2023.
15. The American College of Obstetricians and Gynecologists. Committee Opinion: Optimizing Support for Breastfeeding as Part of Obstetric Practice. Available at: https://www.acog.org/clinical/clinical-guidance/committee-opinion/articles/2018/10/optimizing-support-for-breastfeeding-as-part-of-obstetric-practice. Accessed July 18, 2023.
16. Breastfeeding and the use of human milk. *J Obstet Gynecol Neonatal Nurs.* 2021;50(5):e1–e5. https://doi.org/10.1016/j.jogn.2021.06.006
17. American College of Nurse-Midwives. Position Statement: Breastfeeding. 2016. Available at https://www.midwife.org/acnm/files/ACNMLibraryData/UPLOADFILENAME/000000000248/Breastfeeding-statement-Feb-2016.pdf. Accessed July 18, 2023.
18. Division of Nutrition, Physical Activity, and Obesity, National Center for Chronic Disease Prevention and Health Promotion. Breastfeeding Among US Children Born 2012-2019, CDC National Immunization Survey. Available at https://www.cdc.gov/breastfeeding/data/nis_data/results.html. Accessed July 18, 2023.
19. Mitra M, Parish SL, Clements KM, Cui X, Diop H. Pregnancy outcomes among women with intellectual and developmental disabilities. *Am J Prev Med.* 2015;48(3):300–308. https://doi.org/10.1016/j.amepre.2014.09.032
20. Powell RM, Mitra M, Smeltzer SC, et al. Breastfeeding among women with physical disabilities in the United States. *J Hum Lact.* 2018;34(2):253–261. https://doi.org/10.1177/0890334417739836
21. Andrews EE, Powell RM, Ayers KB. Experiences of breastfeeding among disabled women. *Womens Health Issues.* 2021;31(1):82–89. https://doi.org/10.1016/j.whi.2020.09.001
22. Cohen SS, Alexander DD, Krebs NF, et al. Factors associated with breastfeeding initiation and continuation: a meta-analysis. *J Pediatr.* 2018;203:190–196 e21. https://doi.org/10.1016/j.jpeds.2018.08.008
23. D'Angelo DV, Cernich A, Harrison L, et al. Disability and pregnancy: a cross-federal agency collaboration to collect population-based data about experiences around the time of pregnancy. *J Womens Health (Larchmt).* 2020;29(3):291–296. https://doi.org/10.1089/jwh.2020.8309
24. Division of Reproductive Health, National Center for Chronic Disease Prevention and Health Promotion. PRAMS Disability Supplement 2019–2020. 2019. Available at https://www.cdc.gov/prams/pdf/questionnaire/Disability-Supplement_508.pdf. Accessed July 18, 2023.
25. Shulman HB, D'Angelo DV, Harrison L, Smith RA, Warner L. The Pregnancy Risk Assessment Monitoring System (PRAMS): Overview of Design and Methodology. *Am J Public Health.* 2018;108(10):1305–1313. https://doi.org/10.2105/AJPH.2018.304563
26. Madans JH, Loeb ME, Altman BM. Measuring disability and monitoring the UN Convention on the Rights of Persons With Disabilities: the work of the Washington Group on Disability Statistics. *BMC Public Health.* 2011;11(Suppl 4):1–8. https://doi.org/10.1186/1471-2458-11-S4-S4
27. An Introduction to the Washington Group on Disability Statistics Question Sets. Washington Group on Disability Statistics. Available at: https://www.washingtongroup-disability.com/fileadmin/uploads/wg/The_Washington_Group_Primer_-_English.pdf. Accessed July 18, 2023.
28. Office of Women's Health. The Surgeon General's Call to Action to Support Breastfeeding. Rockville, MD: Office of the Surgeon General; Centers for Disease Control and Prevention; 2011.
29. Grubesic TH, Durbin KM. The complex geographies of telelactation and access to community breastfeeding support in the state of Ohio. *PLoS One.* 2020;15(11):e0242457. https://doi.org/10.1371/journal.pone.0242457
30. Brown HK, Taylor C, Vigod SN, et al. Disability and in-hospital breastfeeding practices and supports in Ontario, Canada: a population-based study. *Lancet Public Health.* 2023;8(1):e47–e56. https://doi.org/10.1016/S2468-2667(22)00310-3
31. Meek JY, Nelson JM, Hanley LE, Onyema-Melton N, Wood JK. Landscape analysis of breastfeeding-related physician education in the United States. *Breastfeed Med.* 2020;15(6):401–411. https://doi.org/10.1089/bfm.2019.0263
32. Division of Nutrition, Physical Activity, and Obesity, National Center for Chronic Disease Prevention and Health Promotion. Physician Education and Training to Support Breastfeeding. 2021. Available at https://www.cdc.gov/breastfeeding/resources/physician-education-and-training.html. Accessed July 18, 2023.
33. Horner-Johnson W, Klein KA, Campbell J, Guise JM. Experiences of women with disabilities in accessing and receiving contraceptive care. *J Obstet Gynecol Neonatal Nurs.* 2021;50(6):732–741. https://doi.org/10.1016/j.jogn.2021.07.005
34. Taouk LH, Fialkow MF, Schulkin JA. Provision of reproductive healthcare to women with disabilities: a survey of obstetrician-gynecologists' training, practices, and perceived barriers. *Health Equity.* 2018;2(1):207–215. https://doi.org/10.1089/heq.2018.0014
35. Rationale for the short set. Washington Group on Disability Statistics. Available at: https://www.cdc.gov/nchs/washington_group/wg_rationale.htm. Accessed July 18, 2023.
36. Lactation support provider (LSP) descriptors. Available at: http://www.usbreastfeeding.org/uploads/1/3/9/7/139788899/2021-08_lsp_descriptor_chart_final.pdf. Accessed November 29, 2023.
37. Sachs HC. Committee On D. The transfer of drugs and therapeutics into human breast milk: an update on selected topics. *Pediatrics.* 2013;132(3):e796–e809. https://doi.org/10.1542/peds.2013-1985
38. Preis H MB, Heiselman C, Lobel M. Vulnerability and resilience to pandemic-related stress among US women pregnant at the start of the COVID-19 pandemic. *Soc Sci Med.* 2020;266:113348. https://doi.org/10.1016/j.socscimed.2020.113348
39. Knierim K, Palmer C, Kramer ES, et al. Lessons learned during COVID-19 that can move telehealth in primary care forward. *J Am Board Fam Med.* 2021;34(Suppl):S196–S202. https://doi.org/10.3122/jabfm.2021.S1.200419
40. Beauregard JL, Nelson JM, Li R, Perrine CG, Hamner HC. Maternity care practices and breastfeeding intentions at one month among low-income women. *Pediatrics.* 2022;149(4):e2021052561. https://doi.org/10.1542/peds.2021-052561

Health Insurance Coverage and Access to Care by Sexual Orientation During the COVID-19 Pandemic: United States, January 2021–February 2022

Kevin H. Nguyen, PhD, Timothy W. Levengood, MPH, Heidi L. Allen, PhD, MSW, and Gilbert Gonzales, PhD, MHA

See also Wootton, p. 12.

Objectives. To compare health insurance coverage and access to care by sex and sexual minority status during the COVID-19 pandemic and assess whether lack of insurance hindered access to care by sexual minority status.

Methods. Using Behavioral Risk Factor Surveillance System data (January 2021–February 2022), we examined differences by sex and sexual orientation among 158 722 adults aged 18 to 64 years living in 34 states. Outcomes were health insurance coverage type and 3 access to care measures.

Results. Sexual minority women were significantly more likely to be uninsured than were heterosexual women, and lack of insurance widened the magnitude of disparity by sexual minority status in all measures of access. Compared with heterosexual men with health insurance, sexual minority men with health insurance were significantly more likely to report being unable to afford necessary care.

Conclusions. During the pandemic, 1 in 8 sexual minority adults living in 34 study states were uninsured. Among sexual minority women, lack of insurance widened inequities in access to care. There were inequities among sexual minority men with health insurance.

Public Health Implications. Sexual minority adults may be disproportionately affected by the unwinding of the COVID-19 public health emergency and may require tailored efforts to mitigate insurance coverage loss. (*Am J Public Health*. 2024;114(1):118–128. https://doi.org/10.2105/AJPH.2023.307446)

AJPH January 2024, Vol. 114, No. 1

Sexual minorities (i.e., people who identify as lesbian, gay, bisexual, or other nonheterosexual identities) have a greater need for, yet fewer opportunities to access, comprehensive health services than do their heterosexual peers.[1] In the United States, well-documented health disparities among sexual minorities (e.g., higher rates of mental health disorders, HIV)[1] are the products of social and structural stigma,[2] but the harms of these conditions may be reduced or rendered manageable with consistent access to appropriate health services.[3] Sexual minority adults have historically faced higher rates of lack of insurance and worse access to care because of structural inequities (e.g., homophobia, barriers to marriage and employer-sponsored insurance).[4,5] Sexual minorities are also more likely to report trouble finding a provider who is informed, affirming, and sensitive to the unique needs of sexual minority patients.[6]

However, previous work suggests that among men, disparities in self-rated health by sexual minority status are narrower in states with more comprehensive legal protections.[7] More broadly, the health equity promotion model—a framework that builds on minority stress theory and the psychological mediation framework—highlights the role of structural and environmental context on mental and physical health for sexual minorities, and there is evidence in the United States and internationally of the association between structural stigma and health inequities among sexual minorities.[1,7–9]

Lack of insurance and access to care among sexual minority adults improved after implementation of the 2010 Affordable Care Act (ACA; e.g., individual mandate, Medicaid expansion, nondiscrimination policies of Section 1557)[10] and the legalization of same-sex marriage via *Obergefell v Hodges* in 2015.[5,10,11] Provisions of the ACA (i.e., Section 2713) also eliminated patient cost sharing for recommended preventive services, such as preexposure prophylaxis to prevent HIV, greatly reducing financial barriers to appropriate care for sexual minority adults at higher risk for HIV. By some estimates, the rate of lack of insurance among sexual and gender minorities (SGM; which includes transgender and gender nonconforming populations) have steadily increased over time from their low of approximately 8% in 2016.[12] Trending increases in lack of insurance parallels that of heterosexual and cisgender populations, likely reflecting the multipronged efforts or the President Donald Trump administration to undermine the ACA.[13]

Meanwhile, the COVID-19 pandemic exacerbated inequities in socioeconomic status, employment, and access to care among marginalized groups in the United States.[14,15] There were concerns that given structural inequities, sexual minority adults would bear disproportionate economic burdens (e.g., employment loss) and pandemic-related barriers to care (e.g., health insurance coverage loss).[16] Survey-based studies found disparities in economic outcomes, with more SGM respondents reporting job loss and food insecurity in the first months of the COVID-19 pandemic in the United States.[17,18] However, no studies to our knowledge have examined health insurance enrollment outcomes for sexual minority adults during the pandemic.[15–18]

We extended previous research by examining detailed health insurance coverage and access to care by sexual minority status using large-scale and population-based data. Specifically, we examined differences in health insurance coverage type (using newly available multistate data) and access to care by self-reported sex and sexual orientation among adults aged 18 to 64 years. We then assessed differences in access to care by self-reported sex, sexual minority status, and lack of insurance status to further explore whether and how health insurance coverage might hinder access to care by sexual minority status. Lastly, in an exploratory analysis, we examined variation in outcomes by state lesbian, gay, bisexual, transgender, or queer (LGBTQ) policy environment.

METHODS

We used data from the 2021 Behavioral Risk Factor Surveillance System (BRFSS), which collected more than 270 000 adult interviews between January 2021 and February 2022. BRFSS is a nationally representative telephone survey administered annually by the US Centers for Disease Control and Prevention and is used to examine health status and access to care for adults in the United States. In addition to the core questionnaire, states can include optional modules each year.[16]

Beginning in 2014, BRFSS included an optional module for states to collect data on a respondent's sexual orientation and gender identity (SOGI). States' inclusion of this module has increased over time, and in 2021 it was used by 34 states (Appendix Table A, available as a supplement to the online version of this article at http://www.ajph.org). Building on previous definitions, we defined an individual as belonging to a sexual minority as one who self-identified as "gay," "lesbian or gay," "bisexual," or "something else" (Appendix Table B, available as a supplement to the online version of this article at http://www.ajph.org).[19] Because most individuals aged 65 years and older have Medicare coverage, we excluded them from the main analysis.

Outcomes

Historically, BRFSS has asked respondents whether they had any health insurance coverage (yes/no), and states had the option of asking respondents their primary health insurance type. However, starting in 2021, the main BRFSS questionnaire asked the specific source of health insurance coverage for all respondents. Building on previous work comparing health insurance coverage type, we created 6 health insurance coverage categories: employer-sponsored insurance, marketplace, Medicare (including Medicare and Medigap), Medicaid and Children's Health Insurance Program, other sources of coverage (e.g., Tricare/CHAMPUS, Indian Health Services, state-sponsored health plan, other government plan), and uninsured with no coverage (Appendix Table B).[20] We then assessed differences in 3 measures in the BRFSS access to care module: having a personal doctor, having a checkup in the past 2 years, and reporting inability to afford needed care in the past 12 months (Appendix Table B). These survey questions have previously been used to assess differences by sexual orientation.[21]

Covariates and Statistical Analysis

We estimated descriptive statistics with the Pearson χ^2 test to compare distributions by sexual minority status. We then used linear probability regression models to examine differences in our outcomes by sexual orientation (sexual minority vs heterosexual). Because of documented differences in health status and access to care by sex and sexual orientation, we ran all analyses separately for men and women.[1,14,22] Specifically, BRFSS asks individuals to self-report their sex ("Are you male or female?"), which we used in our main analyses (Appendix Table B).

For health insurance type outcomes, we adjusted for age, race/ethnicity, educational attainment, household income (measured as a percentage of the federal poverty level according to the US Census),[23] marital status, fair or poor self-reported health status, urban versus rural residence, number of chronic conditions (0, 1, 2, or more), and state policies (e.g., Medicaid expansion and LGBTQ policy environments, as we describe later). For the 3 access to care outcomes, we added indicators for unemployment and lack of insurance to our models. Our main findings included estimates adjusted for the variables specified previously, consistent with our a priori conceptualization (for more detail, we provide stepwise regression estimates in Appendix Tables C and D, available as a supplement to the online version of this article at http://www.ajph.org).

To measure household income as a percentage of federal poverty level, we used a previous method based on the midpoint of household income responses and household sizes.[23] We linked BRFSS data with publicly available state data on Medicaid expansion status and LGBTQ state policy environment, which we measured as a state-level index score of policies related to SGM equality (e.g., related to relationship and parental recognition, nondiscrimination, religious exemptions, SGM youths, health care, criminal justice, and gender identity document changes).[24] The Movement Advancement Project, an independent nonprofit think tank that examines changes in state-level LGBTQ laws and policies, developed the index, which groups states into 1 of 5 categories: negative, low, fair, medium, and high.[24,25] We used data from June 2021, the middle of our study period, to categorize states' LGBTQ policy environments (Appendix Table A).

To assess whether access to care differed by sex, sexual minority status, and health insurance status, we added a 2-way interaction between sexual minority status and lack of insurance (sexual minority × lack of insurance) to our model. The magnitude, direction, and statistical significance of the interaction term indicated whether there were different associations by sexual minority status and lack of insurance to care access. In an exploratory analysis evaluating whether access to care differed by a state's LGBTQ policy environment, we employed similar methods (i.e., adding a 2-way interaction between sexual minority × state LGBTQ policy environment to our model), in which states with negative LGBTQ policy environments were the reference group.

Sensitivity Analyses

We tested the robustness of our main analysis by conducting multiple sensitivity analyses. First, we determined differences for other types of health insurance. Second, we determined sample characteristics, unadjusted differences, and adjusted differences by different sexual orientation categories (e.g., separately for gay or lesbian, bisexual, and individuals reporting something else). Third, we excluded adults for whom we imputed household income from our analysis. Fourth, we used a logistic regression model.

We performed all analyses using Stata version 18 (Statacorp, College Park, TX).

RESULTS

Our study sample included 12 576 sexual minority (7652 women, 4924 men) and 146 146 heterosexual (74 369 women, 71 777 men) adults aged 18 to 64 years living in 34 states (Table 1). Sexual minorities were more likely to be younger, be unmarried, report household income below the federal poverty level, and describe their health as fair or poor (instead of excellent, very good, or good) compared with their heterosexual peers.

Health Insurance Coverage Type

In unadjusted analyses, sexual minority women (42.3%) were nearly 12 percentage points (PPs) less likely to report employer-sponsored coverage than were heterosexual women (54.1%; $P < .001$; Table 2; Appendix Table C, available as a supplement to the online version of this article at http://www.ajph.org). Sexual minority women were significantly more likely to report Medicaid coverage (17.3% vs 11.0%; $P < .001$), other health insurance (9.8% vs 8.3%; $P = .005$), or being uninsured (13.1% vs 8.6%; $P < .001$) than were heterosexual women (Table 2). Sexual minority men (46.0%) were significantly less likely to report employer-sponsored insurance

TABLE 1— Characteristics of Adults Aged 18–64 in 34 States by Sexual Minority Status: United States, 2021

Characteristic	All Women (n = 82 021), %	Sexual Minority Women (n = 7652), %	Heterosexual Women (n = 74 369), %	All Men (n = 76 701), %	Sexual Minority Men (n = 4924), %	Heterosexual Men (n = 71 777), %
Age, y		*	*		*	*
18–34	35.1	67.5	31.0	36.6	58.6	35.1
35–64	64.9	32.5	69.0	63.4	41.4	64.9
Race/ethnicity		*	*			
Non-Hispanic White	62.3	60.3	62.5	62.5	61.1	62.6
Non-Hispanic Black	13.1	10.6	13.4	11.3	10.4	11.4
Hispanic	15.0	17.9	14.7	15.5	16.4	15.4
Non-Hispanic Asian	4.8	4.4	4.8	5.1	5.0	5.1
Non-Hispanic Pacific Islander	0.3	0.1	0.3	0.3	0.3	0.3
Non-Hispanic American Indian or Alaska Native	1.1	1.5	1.0	1.0	1.1	1.0
Non-Hispanic Multiracial	1.5	2.8	1.4	1.5	2.1	1.5
Non-Hispanic other race	0.4	0.6	0.4	0.6	0.7	0.5
Missing race	1.5	1.8	1.5	2.3	2.9	2.2
Married	51.2	25.5*	54.4*	49.6	25.5*	51.3*
Unemployed	7.4	10.4*	7.0*	7.2	11.1*	6.9*
High school diploma or higher	90.5	88.0*	90.9*	88.4	88.7	88.4
Household income, % of FPL		*	*		*	*
< 100	13.8	19.1	13.2	9.5	13.7	9.2
101–138	10.6	13.9	10.2	8.5	10.6	8.3
139–250	21.7	27.3	21.0	21.1	23.9	20.9
251–400	21.0	19.1	21.3	21.3	21.1	21.3
≥ 401	32.9	20.7	34.4	39.6	30.7	40.2
Number of chronic conditions						
0	58.7	58.2	58.7	63.8	63.6	63.8
1	26.5	27.8	26.3	24.7	24.6	24.7
≥ 2	14.9	14.0	15.0	11.5	11.7	11.5
Fair/poor self-reported health	14.9	20.8*	14.1*	13.3	17.3*	13.0*
Reside in a Medicaid expansion state	63.4	66.6*	63.0*	64.1	65.8	63.9
State LGBTQ equality policies		*	*			
Negative	7.2	6.5	7.3	7.0	6.7	7.0
Low	41.8	39.9	42.0	41.0	39.3	41.1
Fair	16.5	16.7	16.5	16.7	16.5	16.8
Medium	4.7	5.6	4.6	4.9	4.6	4.9
High	29.8	31.4	29.6	3.4	33.0	30.2

Note. FPL = federal poverty level (according to the US Census); LGBTQ = lesbian, gay, bisexual, transgender, or queer. The table depicts the authors' analyses of Behavioral Risk Factor Surveillance System, Kaiser Family Foundation, and Movement Advancement Project data (2021). Sample is limited to adults aged 18–64 years residing in 34 US states. We measured state policy environment as an index of laws and policies related to LGBTQ equality. All analyses apply survey weights.

*$P < .05$. P values compare distributions between sexual minority and heterosexual adults for each characteristic using the Pearson χ^2 test.

TABLE 2— Health Insurance Coverage Type and Access to Care for Nonelderly Adults, by Sexual Minority Status: United States, 2021

	Sexual Minority, No. or %	Heterosexual, %	Adjusted Difference (95% CI)
Women			
	7652	74 369	
Health insurance coverage type			
Employer	42.3	54.1	−1.4 (−3.3, 0.4)
Individual/ marketplace	10.4	10.0	0.7 (−0.6, 2.1)
Medicare	6.0	6.6	−1.8 (−3.0, −0.6)**
Medicaid	17.3	11.0	0.2 (−1.4, 1.8)
Other	9.8	8.3	0.4 (−0.8, 1.5)
Uninsured	13.1	8.6	2.4 (0.7, 4.0)**
Access to care			
Has a personal doctor	77.5	86.8	−3.4 (−5.1, −1.7)***
Checkup in the last 2 Years	93.1	96.5	−2.6 (−4.2, −0.9)**
Could not afford care	22.5	11.7	6.8 (5.0, 8.5)***
Men			
	4924	71 777	
Health insurance coverage type			
Employer	46.0	55.9	−2.9 (−5.3, −0.6)*
Individual/ marketplace	11.7	10.2	1.2 (−0.4, 2.8)
Medicare	6.4	5.1	0.3 (−0.9, 1.5)
Medicaid	9.1	5.8	1.1 (−0.2, 2.4)
Other	11.1	9.4	1.2 (−0.4, 2.8)
Uninsured	13.7	11.9	−0.8 (−2.7, 1.2)
Access to care			
Has personal doctor	75.0	76.2	3.6 (1.4, 5.9)**
Checkup in the last 2 years	89.4	90.4	0.3 (−1.5, 2.2)
Could not afford care	17.1	10.2	5.0 (2.9, 7.1)***

Note. CI = confidence interval; LGBTQ = lesbian, gay, bisexual, transgender, or queer. The table depicts the authors' analyses of Behavioral Risk Factor Surveillance System, Kaiser Family Foundation, and Movement Advancement Project data (2021). Sample is limited to adults aged 18–64 years residing in 34 US states. Adjusted differences are measured in percentage points. Adjusted differences for health insurance coverage type measures adjust for sexual orientation, age, educational attainment, marital status, household income measured as a percentage of the federal poverty level (according to the US Census), self-reported health status, number of chronic conditions, urban/rural residence, residence in a Medicaid expansion state, and state policy environment (measured by tally of policies related to LGBTQ equality). Adjusted differences for access to care measures add indicators for unemployment status and lack of insurance. All analyses apply survey weights.
*$P<.05$; **$P<.01$; ***$P<.001$.

compared with heterosexual men (55.9%; $P<.001$; Table 2; Appendix Table D, available as a supplement to the online version of this article at http://www.ajph.org). Sexual minority men were significantly more likely to report Medicaid coverage (9.1% vs 5.8%; $P<.001$) or other health insurance (11.1% vs 9.4%; $P=.03$) than were heterosexual men.

Access to Care

In adjusted analyses, sexual minority women reported worse access to care on all measures relative to heterosexual women: they were less likely to report having a personal doctor (−3.4 PP; 95% confidence interval [CI] = −5.1, −1.7; $P<.001$) or report a checkup in the past 2 years (−2.6 PP; 95% CI = −4.2, −0.9; $P=.002$). Sexual minority women were also significantly more likely to report being unable to afford medical care than were heterosexual women (6.8 PP; 95% CI = 5.0, 8.5; $P<.001$). Although sexual minority men were significantly more likely to report having a personal doctor (3.6 PP; 95% CI = 1.4, 5.9; $P=.002$), they were also significantly more likely to report not being able to afford medical care (5.0 PP; 95% CI = 2.9, 7.1; $P<.001$) in adjusted models.

Access to Care by Lack of Insurance

Barriers to care were significantly larger for uninsured sexual minority women than insured sexual minority women (as indicated by the *P* values in Table 3). The magnitude of disparity between sexual minority and heterosexual women who reported a personal doctor was significantly greater for those who were uninsured (−12.0 PP; 95% CI = −19.0, −5.0; $P<.001$) compared with those with insurance (−2.1 PP; 95% CI = −3.7, −0.5; $P=.007$ for the interaction between sexual orientation and lack of insurance). Similarly, lack of insurance widened the magnitude of disparity for reporting a checkup in the past 2 years between sexual minority and heterosexual women (−15.9 PP; 95% CI = −27.3, −4.5 for uninsured vs −0.9 PP; 95% CI = −1.8, −0.0 for insured individuals; $P=.01$ for interaction).

Sexual minority men were significantly more likely to report a personal doctor than were heterosexual men, irrespective of lack of insurance status. The magnitude of disparity between

TABLE 3— Variation in Access to Care by Sexual Minority Status and Lack of insurance: United States, 2021

	Uninsured			Insured			P
	Sexual Minority, No. or %	Heterosexual, No. or %	Adjusted Difference (95% CI)	Sexual Minority, No. or %	Heterosexual, No. or %	Adjusted Difference (95% CI)	P^a
Women	672	4751		6643	67414		
Access to care							
Has a personal doctor	33.6	48.8	−12.0 (−19.0, −5.0)***	84.6	90.8	−2.1 (−3.7, −0.6)**	.007
Checkup in the last 2 years	67.4	84.2	−15.9 (−27.3, −4.5)**	96.1	97.5	−0.9 (−1.8, −0.0)*	.01
Could not afford care	53.9	42.8	9.4 (0.9, 17.9)*	18.6	8.9	6.4 (4.8, 8.0)***	.49
Men	526	6452		4145	62392		
Access to care							
Has a personal doctor	43.5	32.6	11.6 (3.0, 20.3)**	80.8	82.7	2.3 (0.1, 4.5)*	.04
Checkup in the last 2 years	66.2	69.3	−2.9 (−12.1, 6.4)	92.4	92.8	0.8 (−0.8, 2.4)	.45
Could not afford care	35.8	31.9	2.7 (−5.3, 10.7)	14.7	7.3	5.4 (3.3, 7.4)***	.53

Note. CI = confidence interval; LGBTQ = lesbian, gay, bisexual, transgender, or queer. The table depicts the authors' analyses of Behavioral Risk Factor Surveillance System, Kaiser Family Foundation, and Movement Advancement Project data (2021). Sample is limited to adults aged 18–64 y residing in 34 US states. Adjusted differences are measured in percentage points. Adjusted differences include indicators for sexual minority status, lack of insurance, and their interaction (sexual minority status x lack of insurance). Models also adjust for age, educational attainment, employment status, household income measured as a percentage of the federal poverty level (according to the US Census), marital status, self-reported health status, number of chronic conditions, urban/rural residence, residence in a Medicaid expansion state, and state policy environment (measured by tally of policies related to LGBTQ equality). *P* value represents the interaction between sexual minority status and lack of insurance status. All analyses apply survey weights.
*$P<.05$, **$P<.01$, ***$P<.001$.

sexual minority and heterosexual men was significantly greater among those who were uninsured (11.6 PP; 95% CI = 3.0, 20.3) than those were insured (2.3 PP; 95% CI = 0.1, 4.5; *P* = .04 for interaction). We found significant differences in the ability to afford medical care between sexual minority and heterosexual adults among men with health insurance coverage (5.4 PP; 95% CI = 3.3, 7.4; *P* < .001) and not statistically significant among uninsured men (2.7 PP; 95% CI = −5.3, 10.7; *P* > .05).

Differences by State Policy

For women, disparities in the ability to afford medical care between sexual minority and heterosexual women were significantly narrower in states with high (i.e., more inclusive) policy environments than in states with negative LGBTQ policy environments. For men, disparities in the ability to afford medical care between sexual minority and heterosexual men were significantly narrower in states with more inclusive LGBTQ policy environments (low, fair, medium, or high) when compared with those with negative LGBTQ policy environments (Table 4).

Sensitivity Analyses

Stepwise regression estimates suggest that after accounting for age, race/ethnicity, marital status, and educational attainment, the distinctions between sexual minority and heterosexual adults became less prominent (Appendix Tables C and D). We determined variation across all health insurance coverage types (Appendix Table E, available as a supplement to the online version of this article at http://www.ajph.org) and disaggregated estimates by sexual orientation (Appendix Tables F–I, available as a supplement to the online version of this article at http://www.ajph.org). Our findings were relatively unaffected by other model specifications (Appendix Table J, available as a supplement to the online version of this article at http://www.ajph.org).

DISCUSSION

Using data from 34 states, we found wide variation in health insurance

TABLE 4— Variation in Access to Care by Sexual Minority Status and State LGBTQ Policy Environment: United States, 2021

	Negative (Ref)			Low			Fair			Medium			High		
	Sexual Minority, No. or %	Hetero-sexual, No. or %		Sexual Minority, No. or %	Hetero-sexual, No. or %	P	Sexual Minority, No. or %	Hetero-sexual, No. or %	P	Sexual Minority, No. or %	Hetero-sexual, %	P	Sexual Minority, %	Hetero-sexual, %	P
Women	413	5 308		2 535	27 795		1282	12 516		433	4 046		n = 2989	n = 24 704	
Has a personal doctor	82.4	85.2		82.9	86.4	.81	89.4	88.0	.17	79.1	82.9	.8	81.2	86.9	.32
Checkup in the last 2 years	96.1	95.7		92.1*	96.3*	.04	95.8	96.4	.54	95.3	95.3	.81	94.1	96.8	.07
Could not afford care	25.1	13.6		19.1	12.4	.13	18.8	10.8	.28	21.8	11.3	.79	17.8*	12.8*	.03
Men	261	4 327		1 630	26 465		818	13 087		244	3 616		n = 1971	n = 24 282	
Access to care															
Has a personal doctor	75.7	76.4	Ref	82.7	76.5	.10	82.2	77.8	.23	75.2	72.0	.49	78.0	75.9	.48
Checkup in the last 2 years	89.6	90.0	Ref	91.1	90.1	.68	89.0	88.9	.91	84.0	89.5	.35	92.1	91.5	.76
Could not afford care	25.6	11.0	Ref	15.1*	10.3*	.04	12.8*	8.9*	.02	13.0*	9.7*	.02	15.3*	11.3*	.02

Note. LGBTQ = lesbian, gay, bisexual, transgender, or queer. The table depicts the authors' analyses of Behavioral Risk Factor Surveillance System, Kaiser Family Foundation, and Movement Advancement Project data (2021). Sample is limited to adults aged 18–64 years residing in 34 US states. Estimates provided are predicted values, derived from the Margins command in Stata version 18 (StataCorp LP, College Station, TX). Health insurance coverage outcomes adjust for age, race or ethnicity, educational attainment, employment status, household income measured as a percentage of the federal poverty level (according to the US Census), self-reported health status, number of chronic conditions, urban/rural residence, and residence in a Medicaid expansion state. Access to care models add indicators for unemployment and lack of insurance. All models include indicators for sexual minority status, state LGBTQ policy environment (negative, low, fair, medium, high), and their interaction (sexual minority x state LGBTQ policy environment), where the reference group is states with a negative LGBTQ policy environment. State LGBTQ policy environment is measured as an index of state-level laws and policies related to LGBTQ equality. *P* value represents the interaction between sexual minority status and state LGBTQ policy environment. All analyses apply survey weights.

*$P<.05$; **$P<.01$; ***$P<.001$.

coverage type and access to care by sex and sexual minority status between January 2021 and February 2022. Compared with heterosexual peers, sexual minority women were significantly more likely to be uninsured, and both sexual minority men and women were significantly less likely to report employer-sponsored coverage. Sexual minority women reported less access to care on all metrics than did heterosexual women. Sexual minority men were more likely to report having a personal doctor but more likely to report being unable to afford medical care compared with heterosexual men. Analyses stratified by sex indicated that access to care differed by sexual minority status and lack of insurance for certain outcomes. For both men and women, residence in states with the most inclusive LGBTQ policy environments narrowed disparities in ability to afford necessary medical care by sexual minority status when compared with states with negative LGBTQ policy environments.

Our results are consistent with previous studies that have identified inequities in other access to care measures (e.g., no usual source of care) by sex and sexual minority status, and our results support evidence that sexual minority adults are more likely to delay medical care because of cost than are heterosexual adults.[6,11,19,21,22] A previous study assessed differences by sexual minority and lack of insurance status using 2014–2017 BRFSS data.[21] Compared with these previous estimates—which did not stratify by sex—our findings identified wider inequities in ability to afford medical care by sexual minority status during the pandemic and that there was variation by sex and sexual minority status.[21] These findings suggest that insurance status is an important driver of access to care for sexual minority populations, with substantial disparities in access for those without insurance.

Strategies that promote insurance coverage (e.g., targeted enrollment assistance) may need to be implemented, and policies that threaten insurance coverage (e.g., Medicaid unwinding) should be carefully monitored. Previous work has assessed the association between state LGBTQ policy environment and self-reported health status, and our exploratory analyses extend this work by assessing its association with access to care.[2,7]

Our study has several implications for health equity policy and practice. We identified new disparities in health insurance coverage and potential underinsurance (as measured by financial barriers to care despite having health insurance) by sexual minority status. Recent evidence suggests that, despite substantially fewer people lacking insurance beginning in 2014, lack of insurance rates have gradually increased for adults since their lowest point in 2016.[12] Although lack of insurance rates remain lower than rates before the ACA, about 1 in 8 nonelderly sexual minority adult remained uninsured in 2021 compared with 1 in 10 heterosexual adults.[12]

For sexual minority women, lack of insurance widened existing inequities in having a personal doctor and having a checkup in the previous 2 years, illustrating the unique disparities faced by sexual minority women (e.g., structural-level inequalities related to sexism). However, we found significant differences in ability to afford medical care between sexual minority and heterosexual men among those with health insurance, suggesting that some sexual minority adults may be underinsured. These findings are supported by a recent study suggesting that sexual minority adults are more likely to report money-saving behaviors regarding medications (e.g., skipping medication doses, delaying prescription refills).[26] Future work should examine the role of health insurance benefit design (e.g., high-deductible plans) on inequities in access to care for sexual minorities.

Our study provides new evidence about inequities by sexual minority status during the COVID-19 pandemic. Historically, sexual minority adults have borne the burden of structural inequities, including higher rates of economic hardship, such as poverty and experiencing homelessness.[27] Consequently, there were concerns that sexual minority adults would be disproportionately affected by the pandemic.[15] Some studies have examined health and health care inequities faced by SGM adults in the pandemic: early in the pandemic, more than 13% of SGM adults reported health insurance loss.[28] Apart from a few states (e.g., California and Pennsylvania), there was limited systematic SOGI data collection to understand the impact of the COVID-19 pandemic. In July 2021, the US Census Bureau began ascertaining SOGI information in the Household Pulse Survey and demonstrated that SGM adults experienced substantially higher rates of financial precarity, including food insecurity and loss of employment and income, than did non-SGM adults.[17,18] Additional examination of the long-term impacts of the pandemic on sexual minority adults—including health insurance loss, delays in care, and mental health outcomes—remains critical.[14]

Beginning in March 2020, through COVID-19 emergency declarations and congressional legislation, states were required to provide continuous enrollment for individuals enrolled in Medicaid.

However, Medicaid continuous coverage protections ended on March 31, 2023, and states were permitted to resume Medicaid disenrollments.[29,30] Sexual minority adults—who reported higher rates of Medicaid coverage than heterosexual adults—may be disproportionately affected by the Medicaid continuous enrollment provision ending. Tailored outreach and enrollment assistance to sexual minority adults may be needed to mitigate lapses in health insurance coverage, retain coverage for individuals who remain Medicaid eligible, and transition individuals who are no longer Medicaid eligible to other forms of health insurance coverage.

More broadly, our findings underscore the importance of developing policies that protect and improve the well-being of all vulnerable populations—including SGM populations. Our study used data from 34 states that opted to collect SOGI data. Comprehensive data collection that follows best practices for requiring SOGI data collection is a critical first step for understanding the needs of SGM communities and using reliable SOGI-based information to develop targeted state and federal policies.[31] Inequities in access to care are largely the product of discrimination and other structural barriers to SGM health equity. Nondiscrimination protections for SGM adults may play a crucial role in mitigating inequities in access to care. For example, the August 2022 proposed revision to Section 1557 of the ACA reinstates the prohibition of discrimination based on sexual orientation or gender identity on health insurance benefit design and insurer marketing practices.[32]

Lastly, public policies may play a critical role in reducing health inequities. Should the 10 states that have not yet expanded Medicaid do so, it could reduce insurance coverage inequities for low-income sexual minority adults. Social policies that codify equality by sexual orientation or gender identity may particularly increase financial security and mental well-being.[8] For instance, the December 2022 passage of the Respect for Marriage Act is a positive step forward.[33] Additional policies, such as passage of the federal Equality Act—which would prohibit discrimination based on sexual orientation or gender identity in education, housing, public accommodations, employment, and other federally funded programs—could further advance equity.[34] Efforts to lessen unemployment, in particular, might facilitate the availability of employer-sponsored insurance and decrease income-related delays in care. In the meantime, more evidence is required to understand how structural discrimination creates or ameliorates disparities in health insurance coverage and access to care for SGM population.

Limitations

Our study has several limitations. First, the BRFSS response rate was 44%, which is lower than other federal surveys such as the American Community Survey.[35] Second, because the SOGI module is optional, it includes only 34 states, so the sample may not be nationally representative. However, the SOGI module was used by more states in 2021 than any previous wave of BRFSS and contains the most recent data available. Relatedly, this study is not generalizable to sexual minorities in other countries. Third, it is possible that our approach to measuring household income is imprecise, but we followed previously validated methods.[24] Fourth, health insurance coverage type was self-reported and may have been subject to recall and misreporting biases. Respondents in our sample may have had multiple forms of health insurance coverage, but BRFSS requires respondents to identity their primary source of coverage.

Fifth, although previous work suggests that state policy environments affect health outcomes for sexual minority adults, it is possible that the significant relationship between state LGBTQ policy environments and affordability of care is spurious or possibly attributable to other state-level characteristics.[2,7] Future work should directly test the hypothesis of this potential relationship. Relatedly, state LGBTQ policy environments can change over time. Therefore, our results may differ using different points in time. Sixth, we were unable to further examine mechanisms driving disparities in access to care. For our outcome examining ability to afford care, we were unable to disentangle whether certain types of care (e.g., mental health care, prescription medications) were particularly challenging.

Conclusions

We identified inequities in health insurance coverage and access to care by sex and sexual minority status during the COVID-19 pandemic. To prevent disparities from widening following the decline of the COVID-19 public health emergency, tailored outreach and enrollment assistance to sexual minority adults may be needed. AJPH

ABOUT THE AUTHORS

Kevin H. Nguyen and Timothy W. Levengood are with the Department of Health Law, Policy, and Management, Boston University School of Public Health, Boston, MA. Heidi L. Allen is with the Columbia University School of Social Work, New York, NY. Gilbert Gonzales is with the Department of Medicine, Health, and Society, Vanderbilt University, Nashville, TN.

CORRESPONDENCE

Correspondence should be sent to Kevin H. Nguyen, Boston University School of Public Health, 715 Albany St, Boston, MA 02118 (e-mail: nguyen@bu.edu). Reprints can be ordered at http://www.ajph.org by clicking the "Reprints" link.

PUBLICATION INFORMATION

Full Citation: Nguyen KH, Levengood TW, Allen HL, Gonzales G. Health insurance coverage and access to care by sexual orientation during the COVID-19 pandemic: United States, January 2021–February 2022. *Am J Public Health*. 2024; 114(1):118–128.

Acceptance Date: September 4, 2023.

DOI: https://doi.org/10.2105/AJPH.2023.307446

CONTRIBUTORS

K. H. Nguyen conceptualized and designed the study, conducted the statistical analyses, and wrote the initial draft of the article. T. W. Levengood assisted in writing the initial draft. H. L. Allen and G. Gonzales provided feedback on preliminary findings and each draft of the article and supervised the study.

CONFLICTS OF INTEREST

The authors have no conflicts of interest to declare.

HUMAN PARTICIPANT PROTECTION

The Boston University institutional review board determined that this study did not qualify as human participant research. The study follows the strengthening the reporting of observational studies in epidemiology reporting guidelines for cross-sectional studies.

REFERENCES

1. Fredriksen-Goldsen KI, Simoni JM, Kim HJ, et al. The health equity promotion model: reconceptualization of lesbian, gay, bisexual, and transgender (LGBT) health disparities. *Am J Orthopsychiatry*. 2014;84(6):653–663. https://doi.org/10.1037/ort0000030
2. Hatzenbuehler ML. Structural stigma and the health of lesbian, gay, and bisexual populations. *Curr Dir Psychol Sci*. 2014;23(2):127–132. https://doi.org/10.1177/0963721414523775
3. Hung DY, Rundall TG, Tallia AF, Cohen DJ, Halpin HA, Crabtree BF. Rethinking prevention in primary care: applying the chronic care model to address health risk behaviors. *Milbank Q*. 2007; 85(1):69–91. https://doi.org/10.1111/j.1468-0009.2007.00477.x
4. Gonzales G, Blewett LA. National and state-specific health insurance disparities for adults in same-sex relationships. *Am J Public Health*. 2014; 104(2):e95–e104. https://doi.org/10.2105/AJPH.2013.301577
5. Downing J, Cha P. Same-sex marriage and gains in employer-sponsored insurance for US adults, 2008–2017. *Am J Public Health*. 2020;110(4):537–539. https://doi.org/10.2105/AJPH.2019.305510
6. Dahlhamer JM, Galinsky A, Joestl S, Ward B. Barriers to health care among adults identifying as sexual minorities: a US national study. *Am J Public Health*. 2016;106(6):1116–1122. https://doi.org/10.2105/AJPH.2016.303049
7. Gonzales G, Ehrenfeld JM. The association between state policy environments and self-rated health disparities for sexual minorities in the United States. *Int J Environ Res Public Health*. 2018;15(6):1136. https://doi.org/10.3390/ijerph15061136
8. Raifman J, Moscoe E, Austin SB, McConnell M. Difference-in-differences analysis of the association between state same-sex marriage policies and adolescent suicide attempts. *JAMA Pediatr*. 2017;171(4):350–356. https://doi.org/10.1001/jamapediatrics.2016.4529
9. Bränström R, Fellman D, Pachankis J. Structural stigma and sexual minority victimization across 28 countries: the moderating role of gender, gender nonconformity, and socioeconomic status. *J Interpers Violence*. 2023;38(3-4):3563–3585. https://doi.org/10.1177/08862605221108087
10. Mann S, Carpenter CS, Gonzales G, Harrell B, Deal C. Effects of the Affordable Care Act's Medicaid expansion on health insurance coverage for individuals in same-sex couples. *Health Serv Res*. 2023;58(3):612–621. https://doi.org/10.1111/1475-6773.14128
11. Gonzales G, Henning-Smith C. The Affordable Care Act and health insurance coverage for lesbian, gay, and bisexual adults: analysis of the Behavioral Risk Factor Surveillance System. *LGBT Health*. 2017;4(1):62–67. https://doi.org/10.1089/lgbt.2016.0023
12. Bosworth A, Turrini G, Pyda S, et al. Health insurance coverage and access to care for LGBTQ+ individuals: recent trends and key challenges. June 30, 2021. Available at: https://aspe.hhs.gov/reports/health-insurance-coverage-lgbtq. Accessed November 2, 2023.
13. Thompson FJ. Six ways Trump has sabotaged the Affordable Care Act. October 9, 2020. Available at: https://www.brookings.edu/articles/six-ways-trump-has-sabotaged-the-affordable-care-act. Accessed November 2, 2023.
14. Fish JN, Salerno J, Williams ND, et al. Sexual minority disparities in health and well-being as a consequence of the COVID-19 pandemic differ by sexual identity. *LGBT Health*. 2021;8(4):263–272. https://doi.org/10.1089/lgbt.2020.0489
15. Martino RJ, Krause KD, Griffin M, LoSchiavo C, Comer-Carruthers C, Halkitis PN. Employment loss as a result of COVID-19: a nationwide survey at the onset of COVID-19 in US LGBTQ+ populations. *Sex Res Social Polic*. 2022;19(4):1855–1866. https://doi.org/10.1007/s13178-021-00665-9
16. Gonzales G, Loret de Mola E. Potential COVID-19 vulnerabilities in employment and healthcare access by sexual orientation. *Ann LGBTQ Public Popul Health*. January 2021. Available at: https://connect.springerpub.com/content/sgrlgbtq/early/2021/01/04/lgbtq-2020-0052. Accessed November 2, 2023. https://doi.org/10.1891/LGBTQ-2020-0052
17. Levengood TW, Raifman J. Financial precarity for lesbian, gay, bisexual, and transgender (LGBT) individuals during the US COVID-19 epidemic—a descriptive study. Available at: https://cesr.usc.edu/sites/default/files/A19%20-%20Levengood.pdf. Accessed November 2, 2023.
18. File T, Marshall J. LGBT community harder hit by economic impact of pandemic. August 11, 2021. Available at: https://www.census.gov/library/stories/2021/08/lgbt-community-harder-hit-by-economic-impact-of-pandemic.html. Accessed January 12, 2023.
19. Tran NM, Henkhaus LE, Gonzales G. Adverse childhood experiences and mental distress among US adults by sexual orientation. *JAMA Psychiatry*. 2022;79(4):377–379. https://doi.org/10.1001/jamapsychiatry.2022.0001
20. Gonzales G, Henning-Smith C, Ehrenfeld JM. Changes in health insurance coverage, access to care, and health services utilization by sexual minority status in the United States, 2013–2018. *Health Serv Res*. 2021;56(2):235–246. https://doi.org/10.1111/1475-6773.13567
21. Nguyen KH, Sommers BD. Access and quality of care by insurance type for low-income adults before the Affordable Care Act. *Am J Public Health*. 2016;106(8):1409–1415. https://doi.org/10.2105/AJPH.2016.303156
22. Nguyen KH, Trivedi AN, Shireman TI. Lesbian, gay, and bisexual adults report continued problems affording care despite coverage gains. *Health Aff (Millwood)*. 2018;37(8):1306–1312. https://doi.org/10.1377/hlthaff.2018.0281
23. Tabaac AR, Solazzo AL, Gordon AR, Austin SB, Guss C, Charlton BM. Sexual orientation-related disparities in healthcare access in three cohorts of US adults. *Prev Med*. 2020;132:105999. https://doi.org/10.1016/j.ypmed.2020.105999
24. Sommers BD, Gunja MZ, Finegold K, Musco T. Changes in self-reported insurance coverage, access to care, and health under the Affordable Care Act. *JAMA*. 2015;314(4):366–374. https://doi.org/10.1001/jama.2015.8421
25. Movement Advancement Project. LGBTQ equality by state. Available at: https://www.lgbtmap.org/equality-maps. Accessed January 11, 2023.
26. Greene N, Johnson RM, Rosen J, German D, Cohen JE. Exploring the relationship between the alcohol policy environment and nondiscrimination laws: implications for binge drinking disparities among LGB adults in the United States. *Drug Alcohol Depend*. 2021;225:108749. https://doi.org/10.1016/j.drugalcdep.2021.108749
27. Das RK, Gonzales G. Self-reported behaviors regarding medications to save money among sexual minority adults in the US, 2015–2018. *JAMA*. 2021;326(24):2526–2529. https://doi.org/10.1001/jama.2021.20335
28. Badgett MVL. Left Out? Lesbian, gay, and bisexual poverty in the US. *Popul Res Policy Rev*. 2018; 37(5):667–702. https://doi.org/10.1007/s11113-018-9457-5
29. Movement Advancement Project. Understanding the impact of COVID-19 on the LGBTQI movement. September 2020. Available at: https://www.lgbtmap.org/2020-covid-impact-report. Accessed January 11, 2023.
30. Cubanski J, Kates J, Guth M, Pollitz K, Musumeci MB, Freed M. What happens when COVID-19 emergency declarations end? Implications for coverage, costs, and access. January 31, 2023. Available at: https://www.kff.org/coronavirus-covid-19/issue-brief/what-happens-when-covid-19-emergency-declarations-end-implications-for-

coverage-costs-and-access. Accessed November 2, 2023.

31. National Science and Technology Council. Federal evidence agenda on LGBTQI+ equity. January 2023. Available at: https://www.whitehouse.gov/wp content/uploads/2023/01/Federal Evidence Agenda-on-LGBTQI-Equity.pdf. Accessed February 8, 2023.

32. Notice of proposed rulemaking: nondiscrimination in health programs and activities. *Fed Regist.* 2022; 72:47824–47920. Available at: https://www.federalregister.gov/documents/2022/08/04/2022-16217/nondiscrimination-in-health-programs-and-activities. Accessed November 2, 2023.

33. Respect for Marriage Act. Pub L. No. 117-228. 117th Congress (2022). Available at: https://www.congress.gov/bill/117th-congress/house-bill/8404. Accessed November 2, 2023.

34. Gonzales G, Gavulic KA. The Equality Act is needed to advance health equity for lesbian, gay, bisexual, and transgender populations. *Am J Public Health*. 2020;110(6):801–802. https://doi.org/10.2105/AJPH.2020.305614

35. Czajka JL, Beyler A. Declining response rates in federal surveys: trends and implications. *Math Policy Res.* 2016;1:1–86.

New in the
ESSENTIAL PUBLIC
HEALTH SERIES

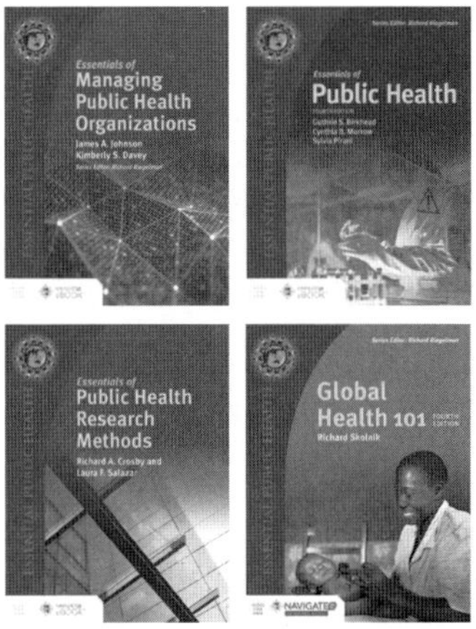

JONES & BARTLETT LEARNING
APHA PRESS
AN IMPRINT OF AMERICAN PUBLIC HEALTH ASSOCIATION

www.essentialpublichealth.com

Read AJPH?

A PUBLICATION OF THE AMERICAN PUBLIC HEALTH ASSOCIATION

Earn Continuing Education credits while you learn

Thanks to APHA's program with the ***American Journal of Public Health***, earning continuing education credits is easy.

By reading select articles from *AJPH*, you can get credits for **CHES®**,**CME**, **CNE**, and **CPH**.

SIGN UP TODAY!

Introductory rate:

APHA members: $10 per credit
Non-members: $20 per credit

ce Online Continuing Education Program

APHA.org/continuing-education

APHA
AMERICAN PUBLIC HEALTH ASSOCIATION
For science. For action. For health.

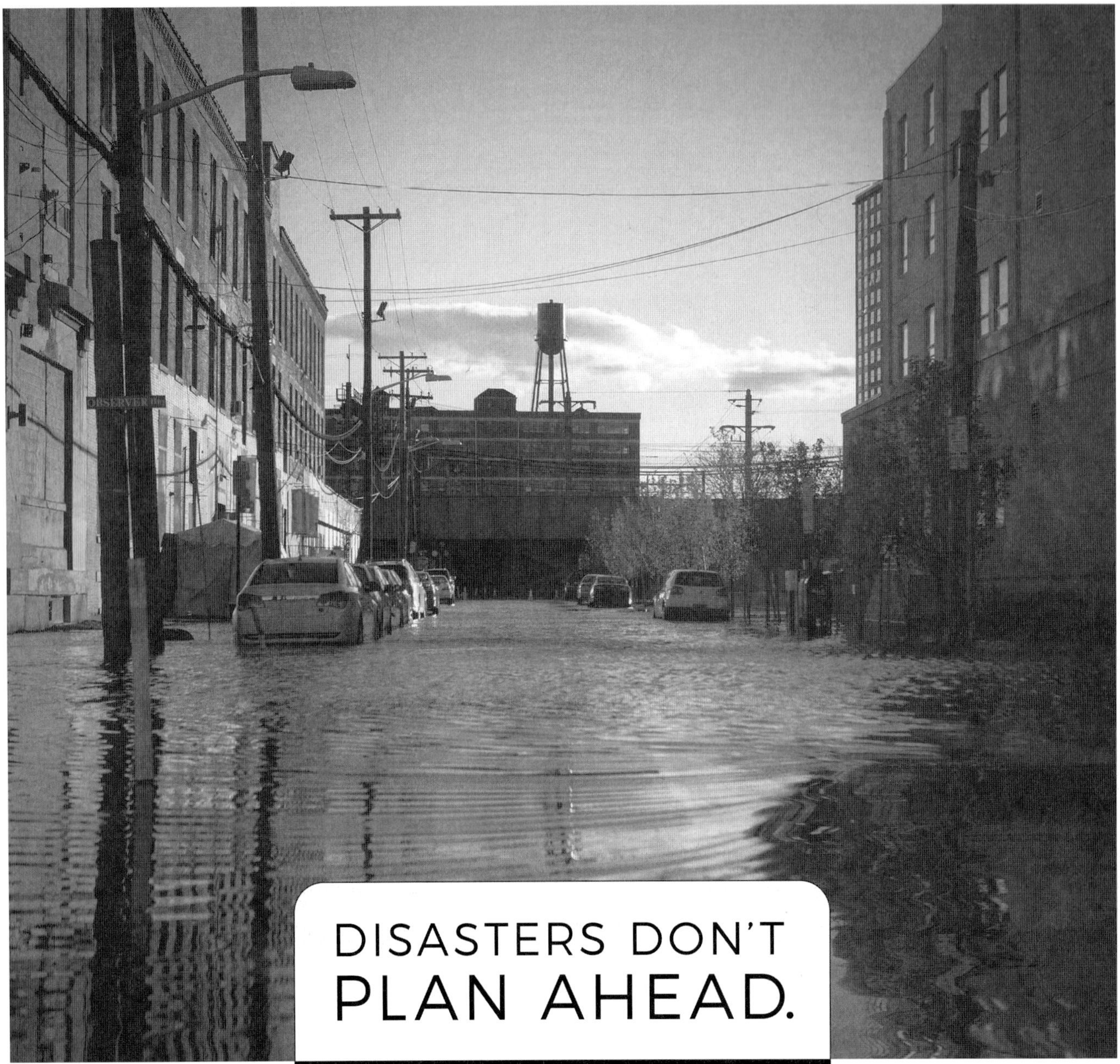

DISASTERS DON'T PLAN AHEAD.

YOU CAN.

DON'T WAIT. COMMUNICATE.

Talk to your loved ones about how you are going to be ready in an emergency.

VISIT READY.GOV/PLAN.

Ad Council Ready® FEMA

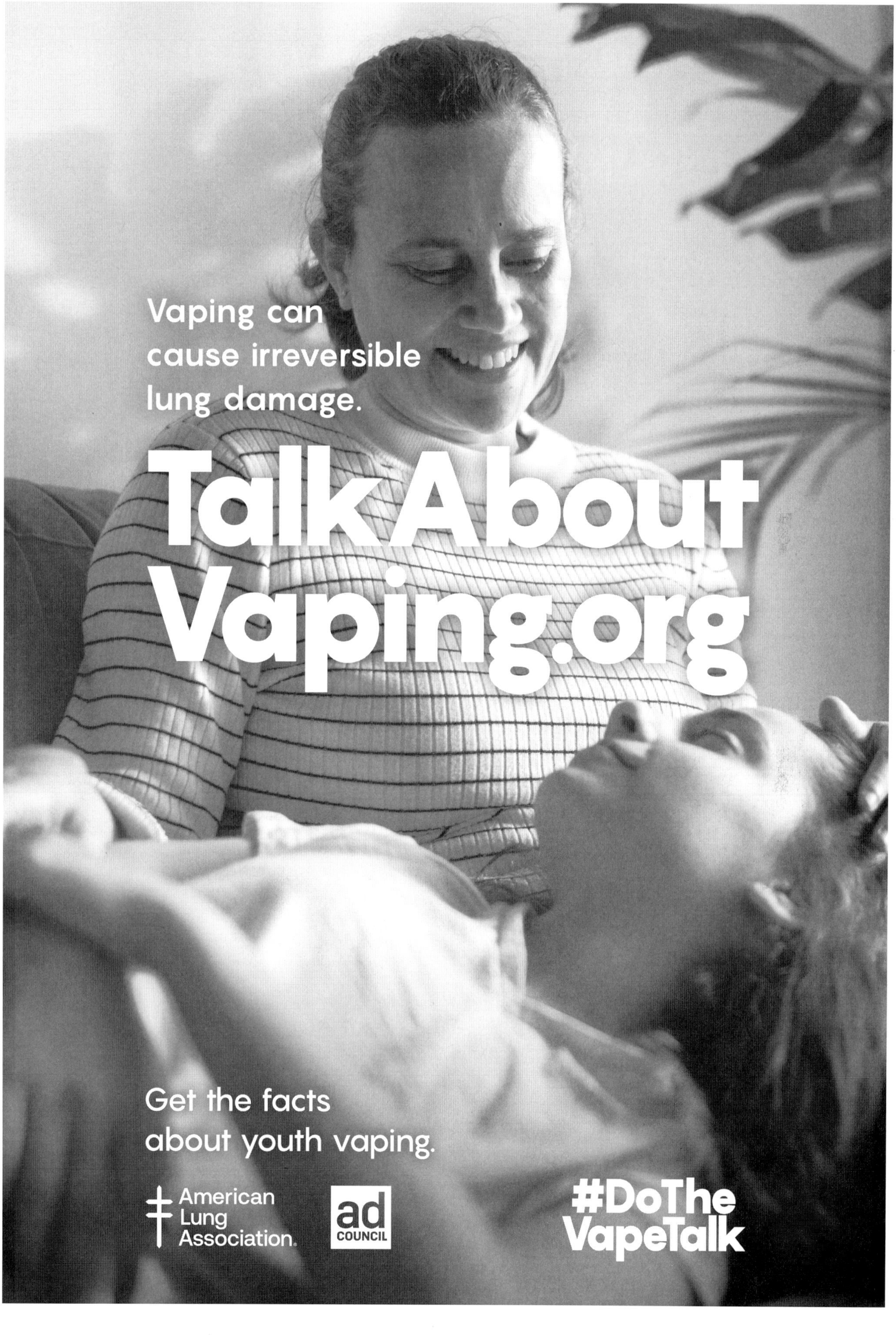
Vaping can
cause irreversible
lung damage.
TalkAbout
Vaping.org
Get the facts
about youth vaping.
American
Lung
Association.
ad
COUNCIL
#DoThe
VapeTalk

GET DOWN WITH YOUR BLOOD PRESSURE™

1 GET IT

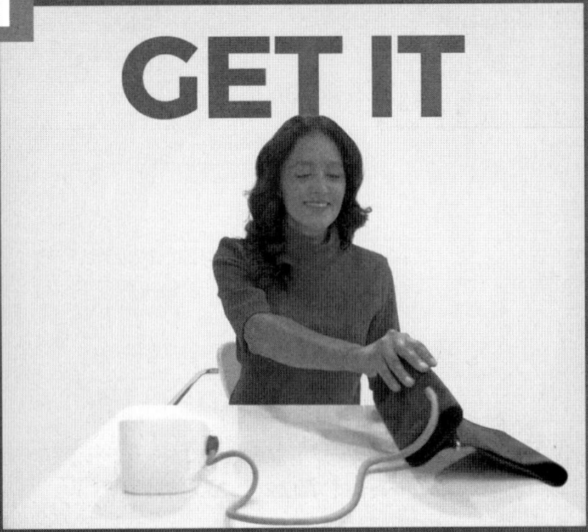

2 SLIP IT

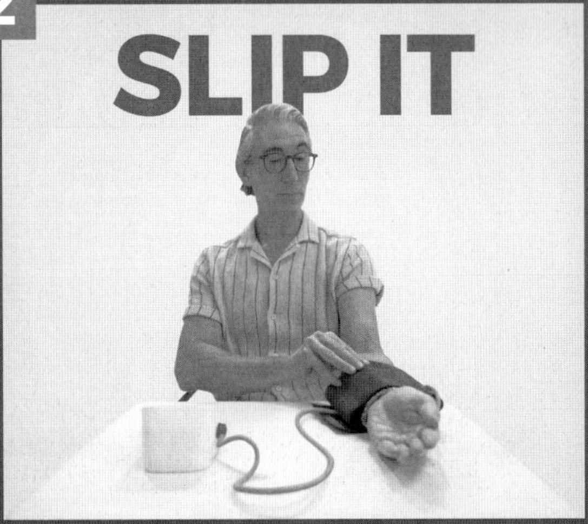

3 CUFF IT

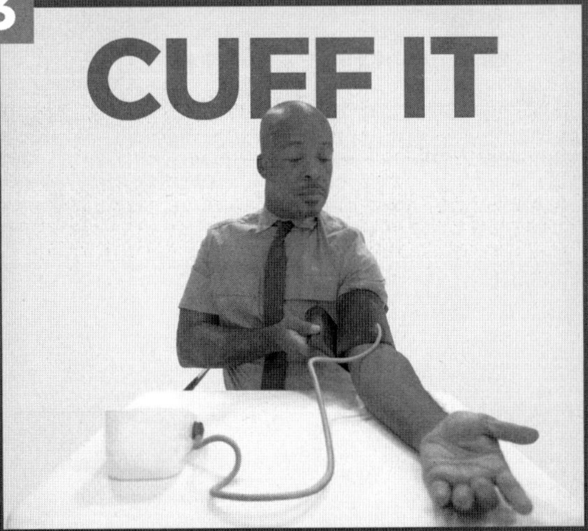

4 CHECK IT

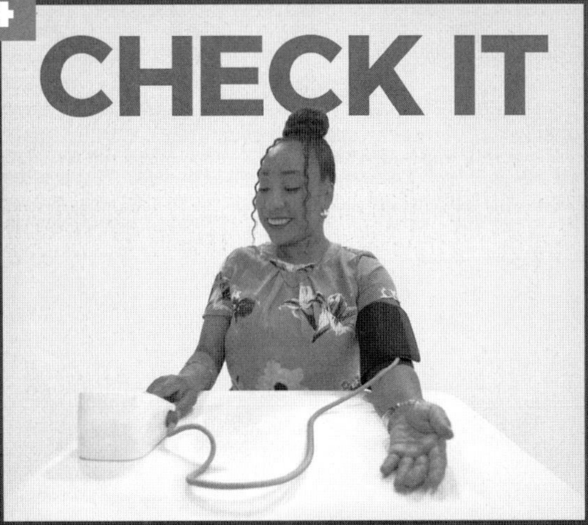

Check it every day. Self-monitoring is power.

ad COUNCIL

American Heart Association

AMA AMERICAN MEDICAL ASSOCIATION

Visit: ManageYourBP.org

Or scan code for more.

In partnership with HHS Office of Minority Health and Health Resources and Services Administration under cooperative agreements CPIMP211227 and CPIMP211228.

AdoptUSKids

ad COUNCIL

His first football season, Isaiah told us, 'Wear a jersey with my name on it. I want everyone to know you're here for me.'

Darnell and Denna, adopted 16-year-old Isaiah

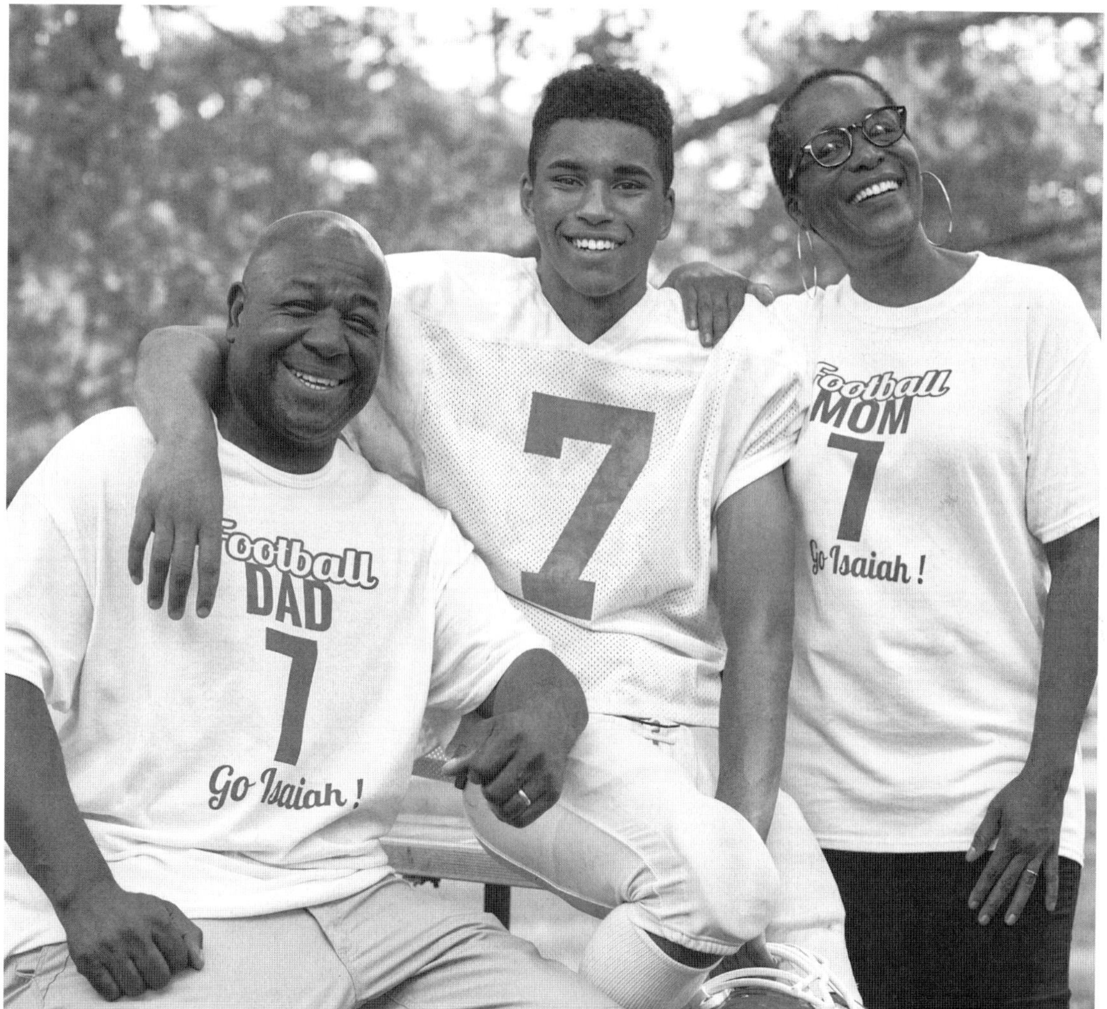

LEARN ABOUT ADOPTING A TEEN
YOU CAN'T IMAGINE THE REWARD

ADOPTUSKIDS.ORG

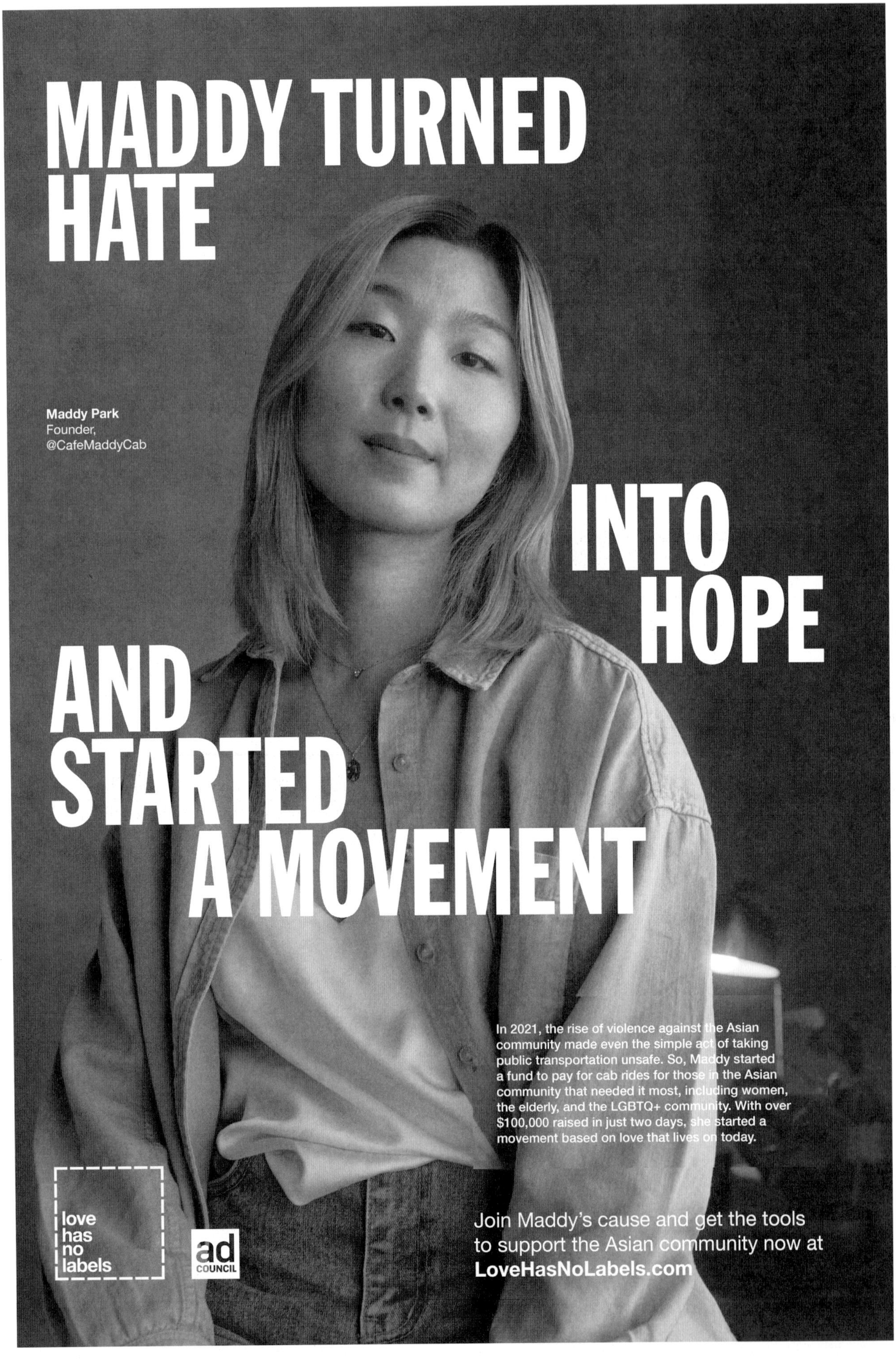
MADDY TURNED HATE
Maddy Park
Founder,
@CafeMaddyCab
INTO HOPE
AND STARTED A MOVEMENT
In 2021, the rise of violence against the Asian community made even the simple act of taking public transportation unsafe. So, Maddy started a fund to pay for cab rides for those in the Asian community that needed it most, including women, the elderly, and the LGBTQ+ community. With over $100,000 raised in just two days, she started a movement based on love that lives on today.
love has no labels
ad COUNCIL
Join Maddy's cause and get the tools to support the Asian community now at LoveHasNoLabels.com

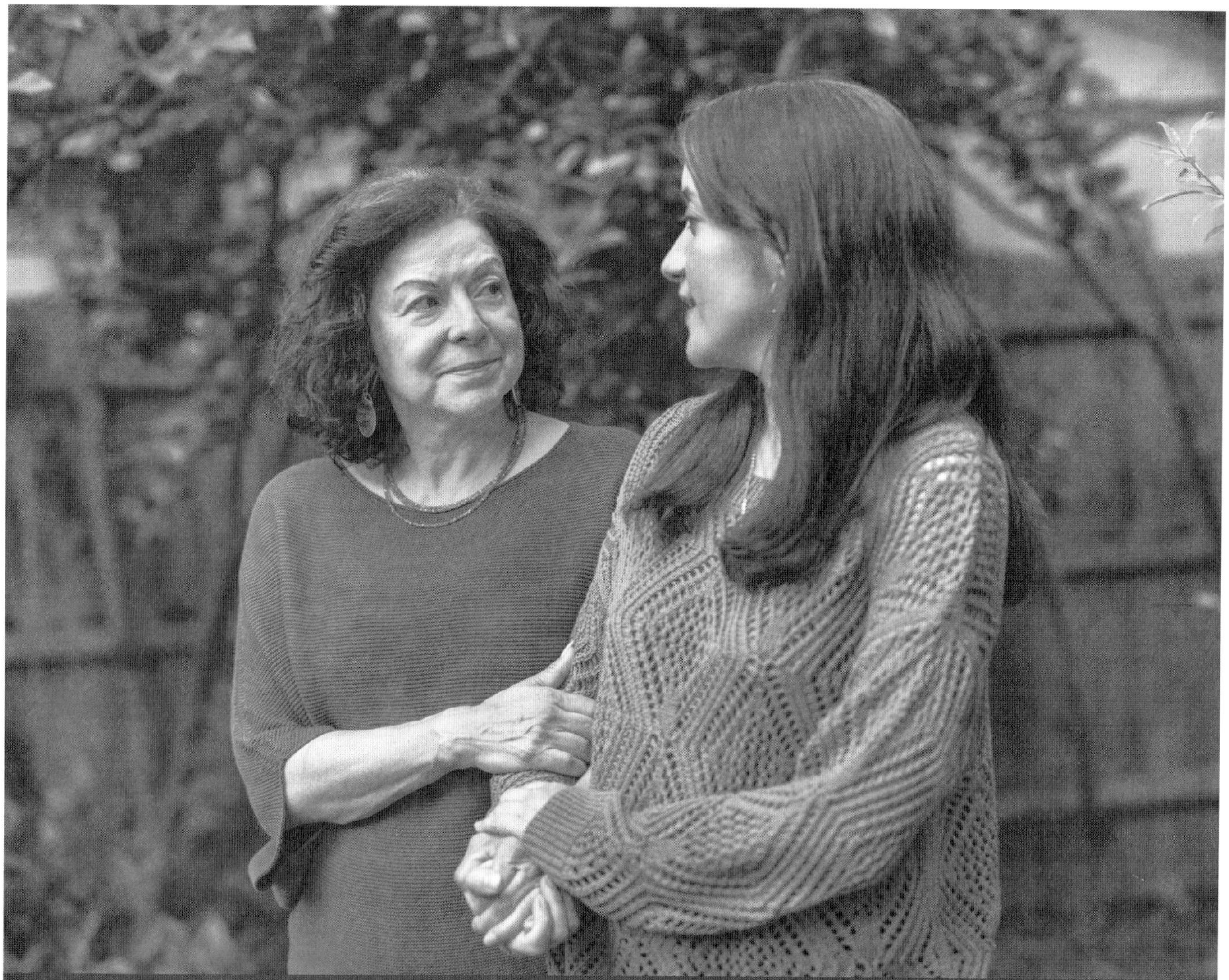

"Early detection allowed us to take control of the situation and make a plan together."

If you're noticing changes, it could be Alzheimer's. Talk about visiting a doctor together.

ALZ.org/TimeToTalk

ad COUNCIL

ALZHEIMER'S® ASSOCIATION

AJPH

A PUBLICATION OF THE
AMERICAN PUBLIC HEALTH ASSOCIATION

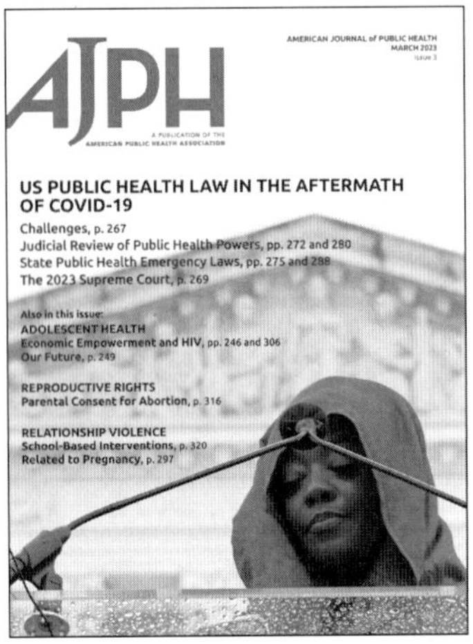

SUBSCRIBE TODAY!

AJPH publishes the highest quality articles in essential areas of research, policy analysis, and program evaluation. Each monthly issue also features critical commentaries, editorials, and letters to the editor.

Mail orders to:

American Public Health Association
800 I St, NW
Washington, DC 20001

E-mail: apha.subscriptions@apha.org

2024 Institutional Pricing:

Online	Tier 2:	☐ $935 (U.S. and International)	
	Tier 3:	☐ $1160 (U.S. and International)	
	Tier 4:	☐ $1390 (U.S. and International)	
Print + Online	Tier 2:	☐ $1150 (U.S.)	☐ $1240 (International)
	Tier 3:	☐ $1415 (U.S.)	☐ $1505 (International)
	Tier 4:	☐ $1670 (U.S.)	☐ $1765 (International)
Print Only		☐ $855 (U.S.)	☐ $955 (International)

The official version of AJPH is our online journal. Please note that print-only subscribers will not have online access to any online-only articles and supplements.

Features of *AJPH* online subscriptions:

- Perpetual access for each year subscribed
- Enhanced search capabilities
- Dynamic PDFs
- Mobile and e-reader options
- Personalization and management tools to view your content
- Access to research online ahead of print
- COUNTER report-availability notification
- Archives dating back to 1911
- Supplement issues

AJPH Highlights

- *AJPH* Global News
- Podcasts in English, Spanish, and Chinese
- E-mail alerts and more
- Special topic collections
- Perspectives from prominent voices in public health
- Book reviews

APHA
AMERICAN PUBLIC HEALTH ASSOCIATION

For more information, visit **www.ajph.org** today!

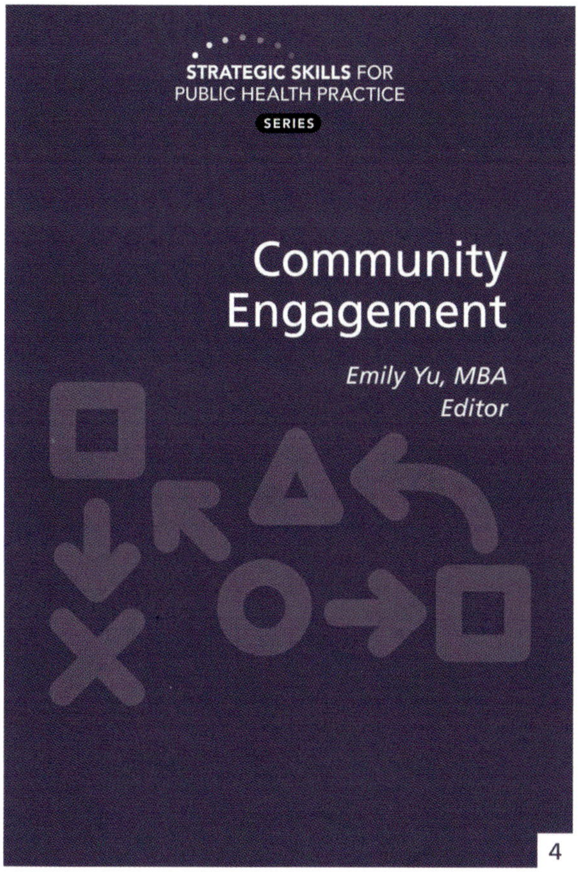

978-087553-3308, 108 PP, DIGITAL & SOFTCOVER

Community Engagement

Edited by Emily Yu, MBA

Community Engagement is the first book to be published from our new *Strategic Skills for Public Health Practice* series. This book brings the concept of community engagement to life through first-person stories, real-world examples and valuable insights from leaders across sectors. Curated specifically for public health practitioners and those interested in supporting community health, the book's chapters, guidance, and perspectives from the field will enhance readers' understanding of community-centered design and provide the tools to support organizational practices that drive better health for all.

APHABOOKSTORE.ORG

APHA PRESS

AN IMPRINT OF AMERICAN PUBLIC HEALTH ASSOCIATION

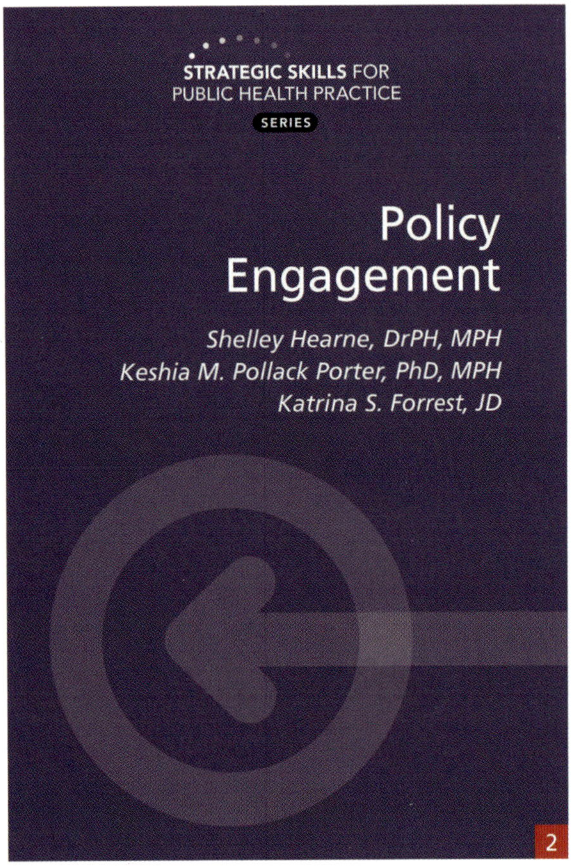

Policy Engagement

By Shelley Hearne, DrPH,
Keshia M. Pollack Porter, PhD,
and Katrina S. Forrest, JD

978-087553-3384, 200 PP., 2023
DIGITAL AND SOFTCOVER

Policy Engagement is a field guide for public health practitioners (from government workers to nonprofit leaders) on engaging with policymakers to create a healthier, more equitable world. This easy-to-read introduction to policy advocacy and decision-making offers a toolkit of concrete, practical, and insightful strategies for informing and influencing policymakers.

Part of the Strategic Skills for Public Health Practice series, *Policy Engagement* demystifies policymaking to help public health professionals become engaged, energized, and effective advocates for policies that drive better health.

APHABOOKSTORE.ORG

APHA PRESS
AN IMPRINT OF AMERICAN PUBLIC HEALTH ASSOCIATION